Key Clinical Topics in

Anaesthesia

D0528992

Key Clinical Topics in
Anaesthesia

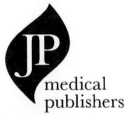

Roger Langford BMBS BMedSci(Hons) FRCA
Consultant in Anaesthesia, Department of Anaesthesia,
Royal Cornwall Hospitals NHS Trust, Truro, Cornwall, UK

David Ashton-Cleary MBChB(Hons) FRCA FHEA DICM
Locum Consultant in Critical Care & Anaesthesia, Department of Anaesthesia,
Royal Cornwall Hospitals NHS Trust, Truro, Cornwall, UK

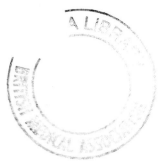

JP
medical
publishers

London • Philadelphia • Panama City • New Delhi

© 2014 JP Medical Ltd.
Published by JP Medical Ltd,
83 Victoria Street, London, SW1H 0HW, UK
Tel: +44 (0)20 3170 8910   Fax: +44 (0)20 3008 6180
Email: info@jpmedpub.com   Web: www.jpmedpub.com

The rights of Roger Langford and David Ashton-Cleary to be identified as editors of this work have been asserted by them in accordance with the Copyright, Designs and Patents Act 1988.

Medical knowledge and practice change constantly. This book is designed to provide accurate, authoritative information about the subject matter in question. However readers are advised to check the most current information available on procedures included and check information from the manufacturer of each product to be administered, to verify the recommended dose, formula, method and duration of administration, adverse effects and contraindications. It is the responsibility of the practitioner to take all appropriate safety precautions. Neither the publisher nor the editors assume any liability for any injury and/or damage to persons or property arising from or related to use of material in this book.

This book is sold on the understanding that the publisher is not engaged in providing professional medical services. If such advice or services are required, the services of a competent medical professional should be sought.

Every effort has been made where necessary to contact holders of copyright to obtain permission to reproduce copyright material. If any have been inadvertently overlooked, the publisher will be pleased to make the necessary arrangements at the first opportunity.

ISBN: 978-1-907816-77-2

British Library Cataloguing in Publication Data
A catalogue record for this book is available from the British Library

Library of Congress Cataloging in Publication Data
A catalog record for this book is available from the Library of Congress

JP Medical Ltd is a subsidiary of Jaypee Brothers Medical Publishers (P) Ltd, New Delhi, India

Commissioning Editor: Steffan Clements
Editorial Assistant: Sophie Woolven
Design: Designers Collective Ltd

Indexed, typeset, printed and bound in India.

Preface

The apparent simplicity of an uneventful surgical intervention with minimal side-effects belies the evolving complexity of the anaesthetic techniques required. New surgical techniques, a shift towards day-case operating and, in particular, an increasingly elderly and co-morbid population make the anaesthetist's task ever more challenging. In the emergency setting, patients are now undergoing procedures where previously there would have been no surgical option. This demands an increasing awareness of peri-operative and intensive care medicine from the anaesthetist. To maintain this knowledge base, a focussed distillation of current literature is required.

Key Topics in Anaesthesia is a succinct reference for the practicing anaesthetist and anaesthetic assistant as well as a structured resource for those preparing for post-graduate examinations in anaesthesia and intensive care medicine. Subject matter has been picked from topical literature, recent examination topics and 'old chestnuts' to cover the breadth of present practice.

A range of authors with specialist interests have been selected to develop the content. This draws on latest standards in clinical best practice, current evidence and guidelines and information on practical considerations. Each alphabetically ordered chapter provides a carefully structured commentary on the topic, suggestions for further reading as well as links to other relevant chapters and, in many cases, online resources.

Roger Langford
David Ashton-Cleary
June 2014

Acknowledgements

Particular thanks must go to Dr Paul Upton and Dr Tim Craft for producing the original concept of this book, 'Key Topics in Anaesthesia', which was an examination 'revision-favourite' for many years. We are grateful for their permission to use and adapt their original structure and content.

The editors would like to thank the following clinicians for their expertise in assisting with the following topics. Dr Pete Stoddart and Ian Jenkins, Bristol Children's Hospital for assistance in the paediatric topics; Dr David Knight, Birmingham Children's Hospital for help with topic 9 (Burns); Dr Cathy Ralph, Royal Cornwall Hospital, for her support with topic 8 (Blood transfusion and salvage) Dr Will Fox, Royal Cornwall Hospital, for his assistance with topics 46 and 47 on obesity.

Finally, we are extremely grateful to our wives, Polly and Gemma, for their patience during the writing and editing of this book.

Roger Langford
David Ashton-Cleary

Contents

Abbreviations

2,3-DPG	2,3-diphosphoglycerate
5HT	5-hydroxytryptamine (serotonin)
AAA	abdominal aortic aneurysm
AAGBI	Association of Anaesthetists of Great Britain and Ireland
ABG	arterial blood gas
ACC/AHA	American College of Cardiology and American Heart Association
ACE	angiotensin converting enzyme
Ach	acetylcholine
ACS	acute coronary syndrome
ACT	activated clotting time
ACTH	adrenocorticotropic hormone
ADH	antidiuretic hormone
ADP	adenosine diphosphate
AF	atrial fibrillation
AHI	apneoa hypopnoea index
AIDS	acquired immunodeficiency syndrome
AKI	acute kidney injury
ALI	acute lung injury
ALS	advanced life support
APLS	advanced paediatric life support
APTT	activated partial thromboplastin time
AR	aortic regurgitation
ARDS	acute respiratory distress syndrome
AS	aortic stenosis
ASA	American Society of Anesthesiologists grading system
ASD	atrial septal defect
ATN	acute tubular necrosis
ATP	adenosine triphosphate
AVR	aortic valve replacement
BiPAP	bilevel positive airway pressure
BLS	basic life support
BMI	body mass index
BP	blood pressure
CABG	coronary artery bypass grafting
CBF	cerebral blood flow
CBW	corrected body weight
CCF	congestive cardiac failure
CICV	'cannot intubate, cannot ventilate' scenario
CKD	chronic kidney disease
CNB	central neuraxial block

CNS	central nervous system
CO	cardiac output (or carbon monoxide)
COPD	chronic obstructive pulmonary disease
CPAP	continuous positive airway pressure
CPB	cardiopulmonary bypass
CPD-A	citrate, phosphate, dextrose, adenine
CPET	cardiopulmonary exercise testing
CPP	cerebral perfusion pressure
CQC	Care Quality Commission
CRBSI	catheter-related bloodstream infections
CSE	combined spinal epidural
CSF	cerebrospinal fluid
CT	computed tomography
CTZ	chemoreceptor trigger zone
CVE	cerebrovascular event
CVP	central venous pressure
CVS	cardiovascular system
CXR	chest X-ray
DAS	Difficult Airway Society
DBD	donation after brain death
DCD	donation after cardiac death
DCI	delayed cerebral ischaemia
DHCA	deep hypothermic circulatory arrest
DIC	disseminated intravascular coagulopathy
DLT	double lumen tube
DMD	Duchenne muscular dystrophy
DNA	deoxyribose nucleic acid
DPP	dipeptidyl peptidase
DVT	deep vein thrombosis
ECMO	extracorporeal membrane oxygenation
ECG	electrocardiogram
ECT	electroconvulsive therapy
ECTAS	electroconvulsive therapy accreditation service
EEG	electroencephalogram
ELISA	enzyme-linked immunosorbent assay
EMG	electromyogram
EMI	electromagnetic interference
EPO	erythropoietin
ENT	ear nose and throat
ERAS	enhanced recovery after surgery
ERPC	evacuation of retained products of conception
ETCO2	end-tidal carbon dioxide
ETT	endotracheal tube

EVAR	endovascular abdominal aortic aneurysm repair
EVD	external ventricular drain
FB	foreign body
FBC	full blood count
FEV	forced expiratory volume
FFP	fresh-frozen plasma
FiO2	fractional inspired oxygen concentration
FRC	functional residual capacity
FVC	forced vital capacity
GA	general anaesthesia
GABA	gamma-aminobutyric acid
GCS	Glasgow Coma Score (Scale)
GFR	glomerular filtration rate
GI	gastrointestinal
GMC	General Medical Council
GP	general practitioner
GTN	glyceryl trinitrate
GUCH	grown-up congenital heart disease
HbA1C	glycosylated haemoglobin
HCAI	healthcare-acquired infection
HDU	high dependency unit
HELLP	haemolysis elevated liver-enzymes low platelets
HEMS	helicopter emergency medical services
HFJV	high-frequency jet ventilation
HFOV	high-frequency oscillatory ventilation
HIV	human immunodeficiency virus
HPA	hypothalamo-pituitary adrenal axis
HPV	human papilloma virus
HTLV	human T-cell lymphotropic virus
IAP	intra-abdominal pressure
IBW	ideal body weight
ICD	implanted cardioverter defibrillator
ICNARC	Intensive Care National Audit and Research Centre
ICP	intracranial pressure
ICS	Intensive Care Society
ICU	intensive care unit (critical care)
IHD	ischaemic heart disease
IHPS	infantile hypertrophic pyloric stenosis
IE	infective endocarditis
IgE	immunoglobulin E
IL-1	interleukin 1
ILMA	intubating laryngeal mask airway
ILS	immediate life support

IMV	intermittent mandatory ventilation
INR	international normalised ratio
IOP	intraocular pressure
IPC	infection prevention and control
IPPV	intermittent positive pressure ventilation
IR	interventional radiology
IRV	inverse ratio ventilation
IUCD	intrauterine contraceptive device
IV	intravenous
IVC	inferior vena cava
LA	local anaesthesis
LDH	lactate dehydrogenase
LASER	Light Amplification by Stimulated Emission of Radiation
LMA	laryngeal mask airway
LMWH	low molecular weight heparin
LSCS	lower segment caesarean section
LVEDP	left ventricular end-diastolic pressure
LVEF	left ventricular ejection fraction
LVH	left ventricular hypertrophy
MAC	minimum alveolar concentration
MAP	mean arterial pressure
MCA	Mental Capacity Act
MCT	mast cell tryptase
MDMA	methylene-dioxy-meth-amphetamine
MET	metabolic equivalent
MG	myaesthenia gravis
MH	malignant hyperpyrexia
MI	myocardial infarction
MILS	manual in-line stabilization
MLT	microlaryngeal tube
MODS	multiple organ dysfunction syndrome
MR	mitral regurgitation
MRI	magnetic resonance imaging
MRSA	methicillin-resistant *Staphylococcus aureus*
MS	mitral stenosis (or muscular sclerosis)
MV	mitral valve
NAP	Royal College of Anaesthetists National Audit Project
NCEPOD	National Confidential Enquiry into Perioperative Deaths
NEC	necrotising enterocolitis
NIBP	noninvasive blood pressure
NICE	National Institute for Health and Care Excellence
NMDA	N-methyl-D-aspartic acid
NMS	neuroleptic malignant syndrome

NNT	number needed to treat
NO	nitric oxide
NPSA	National Patient Safety Agency
NSAID	nonsteroidal anti-inflammatory drug
NSTEMI	non-ST-elevation myocardial infarction
NTS	nucleus tractus solitarius
OCR	oculocardiac reflex
ODP	operating department practitioner
OLV	one lung ventilation
OSA	obstructive sleep apnoea
$PaCO_2$	arterial partial pressure of carbon dioxide
PaO_2	arterial partial pressure of oxygen
PAP	pulmonary artery pressure
PAV	proportional assist ventilation
PCA	patient-controlled analgesia
PCEA	patient-controlled epidural anaesthesia
PCP	Phencyclidine (1-(1-phenylcyclohexyl)-piperidine)
PCV	pressure-controlled ventilation
PDA	patent ductus arteriosus
PE	pulmonary embolism
PEEP	positive end-expiratory pressure
PEFR	peak expiratory flow rate
PEP	post-exposure prophylaxis
PET	positron emission tomography
PFO	patent foramen ovale
PICU	paediatric intensive care unit
PONV	postoperative nausea and vomiting
P-POSSUM	Portsmouth Physiological and Operative Severity Score for the enUmeration of Mortality and morbidity
PPE	personal protective equipment
PRST	blood Pressure, heart Rate, Sweating and Tears
PV	pulmonary valve
PVR	pulmonary vascular resistance
RA	regional anaesthesia
RAE	Ring Adair and Elwyn endotracheal tube
RBC	red blood cell
RCT	randomised-controlled trial
REM	rapid eye movement
RF	radio frequency
RhA	rheumatoid arthritis
RRT	renal replacement therapy
RSI	rapid sequence induction
SACD	sudden adult cardiac death

SAG-M	saline, adenine, glucose, mannitol
SAH	subarachnoid haemorrhage
SAPS	simplified acute physiology score
SBP	systolic blood pressure
SCI	spinal cord injury
SHOT	serious hazards of transfusion
SIMV	synchronised intermittent mandatory ventilation
SIRS	systemic inflammatory response syndrome
SLE	systemic lupus erythematosus
SpO2	pulse-oximetry oxygen saturation
SR	sarcoplasmic reticulum
SSEP	somatosensory evoked potential
SSRI	selected serotonin reuptake inhibitor
STEMI	ST-elevation myocardial infarction
STOP	surgical termination of pregnancy
SV	spontaneous ventilation
SVR	systemic vascular resistance
TACO	transfusion-associated circulatory overload
TARN	Trauma Audit and Research Network
TB	tuberculosis
TBI	traumatic brain injury
TBSA	total body surface area
TBW	total body weight
TCI	target-controlled infusion
TEG	thromboelastography
TIVA	total intravenous anaesthesia
TMJ	temporomandibular joint
TNFα	tumour necrosis factor α
TOE	transoesophageal echocardiography
TRALI	transfusion-related acute lung injury
TURP	transurethral resection of prostate
TV	tricuspid valve
V/Q	ventilation/perfusion
VAP	ventilator-associated pneumonia
VALI	ventilator-associated lung injury
vCJD	variant Creutzfeldt–Jakob disease
VCV	volume-controlled ventilation
VF	ventricular fibrillation
VSD	ventricular septal defect
VT	ventricular tachycardia
VTE	venous thrombo-embolism
WHO	World Health Organization

Contributors

David Adams MBBS BSc MRCP FRCA
Topic 51
Consultant in Anaesthesia, Department of
Anaesthesia, Derriford Hospital, Plymouth
Hospital NHS Trust, Devon, UK

Gilly Ansell MBBS BSc FRCA
Topics 40, 42
Consultant in Anaesthesia, Department of
Anaesthesia, Derriford Hospital, Plymouth
Hospital NHS Trust, Devon, UK

David Ashton-Cleary MBChB FRCA FHEA DICM
Topics 3, 4, 10, 18, 27, 29, 30, 52, 53, 63, 66, 69, 79, 86, 89, 90, 93, 97, 98
Locum Consultant in Critical Care and
Anaesthesia, Department of Anaesthesia, Royal
Cornwall Hospitals NHS Trust, Truro, Cornwall,
UK

Claire Blandford MBBS FRCA
Topic 16
Consultant in Anaesthesia,
Department of Anaesthesia, Torbay Hospital,
South Devon Hospitals NHS Foundation Trust,
Torquay, Devon, UK

Nicholas J Boyd MBChB FRCA
Topic 13, 31
Speciality Registrar in Anaesthesia, Department
of Anaesthesia, Royal Cornwall Hospitals NHS
Trust, Truro, Cornwall, UK

Hentie Cilliers MBChB FRCA
Topic 9
Consultant in Anaesthesia, Department
of Anaesthesia, Queen Elizabeth Hospital,
University Hospitals Birmingham NHS
Foundation Trust, Birmingham, UK

Adrian Clarke BM BSc MRCP FRCA DICM FFICM
Topic 45
Consultant in Anaesthesia and Intensive Care,
Royal Gwent Hospital, Newport, Wales, UK

James Cole MBChB BSc FRCA
Topic 14
Consultant Cardiothoracic Anaesthetist,
Department of Anaesthesia, Derriford Hospital,
Plymouth Hospital NHS Trust, Devon, UK

Dr Nila Cota MBBS FCARCSI FRCA
Topic 8
Locum Consultant Anaesthetist,
Department of Anaesthesia, Royal Cornwall
Hospitals NHS Trust, Truro, Cornwall, UK

Gemma Crossingham MBChB BSc FRCA
Topics 33, 83
Speciality Registrar in Anaesthesia, Department
of Anaesthesia, Derriford Hospital, Plymouth
Hospital NHS Trust, Devon, UK

Susie Davies BMBS BMedSci DCH FRCA
Topics 59, 65
Post CCT Fellow in Anaesthesia,
St Marys Hospital, Central Manchester
University Hospitals NHS Foundation Trust,
Manchester, UK

Sarah Ford MBChB FRCA
Topic 19
Consultant in Anaesthesia, Department of
Anaesthesia, Derriford Hospital, Plymouth
Hospital NHS Trust, Devon, UK

Nicola Freeman MBChB MRCP FRCA
Topics 49, 82
Advanced Trainee in Critical Care, Department
of Anaesthesia, Derriford Hospital, Plymouth
Hospital NHS Trust, Devon, UK

Charles Gibson MBChB BSc MRCP FRCA
Topics 70, 71
Speciality Registrar in Anaesthesia,
Department of Anaesthesia, Derriford
Hospital, Plymouth Hospital NHS Trust,
Devon, UK

Robert Goss MBBS BSc MRCP
Topic 31
Specialty Registrar in Anaesthesia, Department of Anaesthesia, Derriford Hospital, Plymouth Hospital NHS Trust, Plymouth, Devon, UK

Alex Harrison MBBS MRCP
Topics 77, 78
Speciality Registrar in Nephrology and G(I) Medicine, Advanced Trainee in Critical Care, Derriford Hospital, Plymouth Hospital NHS Trust, Devon, UK

Iain Hennessey MBChB BSc MMIS FRCS
Topic 58
Consultant Paediatric Surgeon, Alder Hey Children's Hospital, Alder Hey Children's NHS Foundation Trust, Liverpool, UK

Ben Ivory MBChB MRCP FRCA FFICM
Topics 10, 11
Consultant in Intensive Care and Anaesthesia, Department of Anaesthesia, Torbay Hospital, South Devon Hospitals NHS Foundation Trust, Torquay, Devon, UK

Helen King MBChB FRCA
Topic 75
Speciality Registrar in Anaesthesia, Department of Anaesthesia, Royal Cornwall Hospitals NHS Trust, Truro, Cornwall, UK

Roger Langford BMBS BMedSci FRCA
Topics 2, 5, 7, 12, 15, 17, 20, 22, 23, 25, 28, 35, 37, 38, 39, 43, 44, 54, 55, 68, 73, 74, 80, 81, 84, 85, 91, 95, 96, 99, 100
Consultant in Anaesthesia, Department of Anaesthesia, Royal Cornwall Hospitals NHS Trust, Truro, Cornwall, UK

Tom Lawson BM FRCA
Topics 1, 6, 34, 36, 94
Speciality Registrar in Anaesthesia, Department of Anaesthesia, Royal Cornwall Hospitals NHS Trust, Truro, Cornwall, UK

Paul Margetts MBBS FRCA
Topic 76
Consultant in Anaesthesia and Intensive Care Medicine, Department of Anaesthesia, Derriford Hospital, Plymouth Hospitals NHS Trust, Devon, UK

Cathryn Matthews MBBS BA MRCP FRCA
Topics 48, 50
Speciality Registrar in Anaesthesia, Department of Anaesthesia, Derriford Hospital, Plymouth Hospital NHS Trust, Devon, UK

Alex Mills MBBS BSc FRCA
Topics 46, 47
Speciality Registrar in Anaesthesia, Department of Anaesthesia, Derriford Hospital, Plymouth Hospital NHS Trust, Devon, UK

Gary Minto MBChB FRCA PGCM
Topic 33
Consultant in Anaesthesia, Department of Anaesthesia, Derriford Hospital, Plymouth Hospital NHS Trust, Devon, UK

Ruth Murphy BM BCh BA Phys Sci FRCA
Topics 57, 58, 60
Speciality Registrar in Anaesthesia, Bristol Children's Hospital, University Hospitals Bristol NHS Trust, Bristol, Avon, UK

Amelia Pickard MBChB FRCA
Topics 56, 60
Fellow of Anaesthesia, Department of Anaesthesia, Great Ormond Street Hospital, Great Ormond Street Hospital for Children NHS Foundation Trust, London, UK

David Portch MBChB MRCP FRCA
Topic 32
Consultant in Anaesthesia, Department of Anaesthesia, Torbay Hospital, South Devon Hospitals NHS Foundation Trust, Torquay, Devon, UK

Claire Preedy MBBS MRCS(Ed) FRCA
Topics 41, 67
Locum Consultant Anaesthetist, Department of Anaesthesia, Royal Cornwall Hospitals NHS Trust, Truro, Cornwall, UK

Mark Rockett MBChB PhD FRCA
Topic 62
Consultant in Anaesthesia, Department of Anaesthesia, Derriford Hospital, Plymouth Hospital NHS Trust, Devon, UK

David Sanders MA BM BChD Phil FRCA
Topic 92
Consultant in Anaesthesia, Department of Anaesthesia, Royal Devon and Exeter Hospital, Exeter, Devon, UK

Paul Sice MBBS BSc FRCA
Topic 19
Consultant in Anaesthesia, Department of Anaesthesia, Derriford Hospital, Plymouth Hospital NHS Trust, Devon, UK

Fran Smith MBBCh BSc FRCA
Topic 92
Speciality Registrar in Anaesthesia, Department of Anaesthesia, Royal Devon and Exeter Hospital, Exeter, Devon, UK

Tim Starkie BMedSci BMBS FRCA
Topic 64
Consultant in Anaesthesia, Department of Anaesthesia, Waikato Hospital, Hamilton, New Zealand

Mary Stocker MA MBChB FRCA MA (Healthcare Ethics and Law)
Topic 16
Consultant in Anaesthesia, Department of Anaesthesia, Torbay Hospital, South Devon Healthcare NHS Foundation Trust, Torbay, Devon, UK

Calum Thompson BMBS MCEM MA (Healthcare Ethics and Law)
Topic 24
Specialty Doctor, Department of Emergency, Royal Cornwall Hospital, Royal Cornwall Hospitals Trust, Truro, Cornwall, UK

Andrew Tillyard MBChB B Appl Sc FRCA EDIC
Topic 24
Specialty Doctor, Department of Emergency, Royal Cornwall Hospital, Royal Cornwall Hospitals Trust, Truro, Cornwall, UK

Claire Todd MBChB BSc MRCP FRCA PGDip
Topic 26,
Fellow in Anaesthesia, Department of Anaesthesia, Waikato Hospital, Hamilton, New Zealand

Ruth Treadgold MBBCh FRCA
Topics 87, 88
Locum Consultant in Anaesthesia, Department of Anaesthesia, Derriford Hospital, Plymouth Hospital NHS Trust, Devon, UK

Lauren Weekes BM FRCA
Topics 21, 72
Speciality Registrar in Anaesthesia, Department of Anaesthesia, Derriford Hospital, Plymouth Hospital NHS Trust, Devon, UK

Timothy Wilson MBChB FRCA
Topic 61
Consultant in Anaesthesia and Pain Medicine, Department of Anaesthesia, Derriford Hospital, Plymouth Hospital NHS Trust, Devon, UK

Airway assessment

Key points

- Airway assessment is a dynamic process comprising many different elements
- Bedside tests should not be used in isolation
- The actual assessment is one aspect of a two-part process; equally important is the subsequent airway management plan

A thorough airway assessment is the cornerstone of any anaesthetic assessment, allowing the practitioner to

- Prepare necessary equipment and the environment for airway management
- Summon help if needed

The 4th National Audit Project, conducted by the Royal College of Anaesthetists and the Difficult Airway Society, highlighted that airway assessment (and subsequent planning) in critical incidents was poor and may have contributed towards negative outcomes.

The overall airway assessment is not only aimed at determining ease of intubation, but also that of bag-mask ventilation and laryngoscopy and follows a multimodal approach involving history, examination and investigation.

History

In addition to a previously documented difficult airway, there are various congenital and acquired conditions that may pose problems and should be sought during the preoperative assessment. Some examples include

- Congenital syndromes
  - Down's syndrome
  - Pierre Robin syndrome
  - Treacher Collins syndrome
  - Mucopolysaccharidoses
- Acquired
  - Orthopaedic/rheumatological
    - Rheumatoid arthritis
    - Ankylosing spondylitis
  - Tumour
    - Airway, neck or mediastinal masses, e.g. goitre

- Previous radiotherapy to the neck
  - Traumatic
    - Dental, facial, laryngeal, tracheal trauma
    - Cervical spine injury
    - Acute burns
  - Infection
    - Croup and epiglottitis
    - Oral, pharyngeal, retropharyngeal abscesses
    - Ludwig's angina
  - Endocrine/other
    - Acromegaly
    - Diabetes
    - Obesity and obstructive sleep apnoea
    - Pregnancy

Examination

Examination comprises two parts: a general systemic examination followed by a focused airway examination. General patient features that are associated with difficult airways include

- Presence of stridor
- Short neck
- Small or receding mandible (which may be disguised by a beard)
- Obvious neck swellings, e.g. goitre
- Obesity
- Large breasts
- Evidence of trauma or previous surgery

Specific airway examination

- Teeth
  - Prominent teeth can increase difficulty of laryngoscopy
  - Although the presence of restorative dental work may not directly make the airway difficult, it may be a source of anxiety for the inexperienced laryngoscopist
  - Even though an edentulous mouth can make laryngoscopy easier, it may make bag-mask ventilation more difficult
- Palate
  - High-arched palates are associated with a superiorly displaced tongue, limited

space for laryngoscope insertion and a posterior oropharynx
- Associated conditions include Marfan's syndrome, Pierre Robin syndrome, trisomy 21
- Mouth opening
  - Is a marker of temporomandibular joint (TMJ) mobility and ease of laryngoscope insertion
  - A distance between the upper and lower incisors of <3–4 cm (or three patient finger breadths) is associated with increased difficulty
- Mallampati class
  - Classes are based on the visibility of pharyngeal structures on mouth opening and tongue protrusion without phonation
  - Classes I, II and III were proposed initially with classes 0 (Shashtri) and IV (Samsoon and Young) added later
    - Class 0 = epiglottis seen on mouth opening and tongue protusion
    - Class I = tonsillar pillars, soft palate and uvula visible
    - Class II = tip of uvula masked by base of tongue
    - Class III = soft palate visible only
    - Class IV = hard palate visible only
  - Is a marker of several things
    - Adequacy of mouth opening for laryngoscope insertion
    - Size of tongue relative to oral cavity
    - Potential ease of tongue displacement
  - Mallampati class III or above is associated with increased difficulty
- Prognathism
  - The ability to protrude the mandible
    - Class A = lower incisors protruded anterior to upper incisors
    - Class B = lower incisors in-line with upper incisors
    - Class C = lower incisors cannot reach upper incisors
  - Is a marker of TMJ mobility
  - Limited prognathism is associated with increased difficulty of bag-mask ventilation and laryngoscopy

- Cervical mobility
  - The ability to flex/extend the atlanto-occipital joint
  - Is a marker of the ability to align three axes (oral, pharyngeal and laryngeal) and achieve the 'Sniffing the morning air' position
  - Neck extension <35° is associated with increased difficulty
- Thyromental distance (Patil's test)
  - The distance from the mental process to the thyroid notch when head and neck are extended
  - Is a marker of the submental space and the ease of tongue displacement with the laryngoscope blade
  - A distance of <6 cm is associated with increased difficulty
- Sternomental distance (Savva's test)
  - The distance from mental process to sternal notch when the head and neck are extended
  - Is a marker of head and neck mobility
  - A distance of <12 cm is associated with increased difficulty
- Prayer sign
  - Inability to place both palms flat together
  - Is seen in diabetic patients and is a marker of limited joint mobility
  - It is thought that the same process affects the cervical spine, TMJ and larynx

None of these tests are sensitive or specific in isolation; however, when we amalgamate them into an overall airway assessment their sensitivity and specificity improve. The combination of Mallampati and thyromental distance has been suggested to have the highest discriminative power.

Prediction tools

There are several scoring tools that take these examination findings into account in order to predict likelihood of difficult intubations; however, the most widely cited is the Wilson risk score. A score of 3 or more predicts 75% difficult intubation (12% false positive) (**Table 1**).

Variable	Score
Weight	0 = <90 kg 1 = >90 kg 2 = >110 kg
Head and neck movement	0 = >90° 1 = ~90° 2 = >90°
Jaw movement [interincisor gap (IG) and subluxation (Slux)]	0 = IG >5 cm or SLux >0 1 = IG <5 cm or SLux = 0 2 = IG <5 cm or SLux <0
Receding mandible	0 = Normal 1 = Moderate 2 = Severe
Prominent teeth	0 = Normal 1 = Moderate 2 = Severe

Table 1 Wilson risk score for predicted difficult intubation

Investigations

Other investigations can be used to ascertain underlying anatomy and function, and although they may not predict difficult intubation, they can still provide useful information, e.g. subglottic stenosis. Such techniques include:

- Head, neck and chest X-rays
- CT/MRI of neck and chest
- Fibreoptic techniques, e.g. nasendoscopy or fibreoptic laryngoscopy
- Flow-volume loops

Further reading

Cook TM, Woodall N, Frerk C. Fourth National Audit Project. Major complications of airway management in the UK: results of the Fourth National Audit Project of the Royal College of Anaesthetists and the Difficult Airway Society. Part 1: anaesthesia. Br J Anaesth 2011; 106:617–631.

Mallampati SR, Gatt SP, Gugino LD, et al. A clinical sign to predict difficult tracheal intubation: a prospective study. Can Anaesth Soc J 1985; 32:429–434.

Shiga T, Zen'ichiro W, Inoue T, Sakamoto A. Predicting difficult intubation in apparently normal patients: a meta-analysis of bedside screening test performance. Anaesthesiology 2005; 103:429–437.

Wilson ME, Spiegelhalter D, Robertson JA, et al. Predicting difficult intubation. Br J Anaesth. 1988; 61:211-216.

Related topics of interest

- Awake intubation (p. 13)
- Airway – difficult and failed intubation (p. 4)
- Airway – the emergency airway (p. 7)
- Airway – the shared airway (p. 10)

Airway – difficult and failed intubation

Key points

- Clear guidelines exist for difficult intubation, for example those produced by the Difficult Airway Society (UK)
- Thorough assessment of the airway allows for the anticipation of the difficult airway in most cases
- Prior preparation for the unexpected difficult airway may be life-saving
- There are a variety of devices available to manage the difficult intubation

Around 38% of general anaesthetics in the UK incorporate tracheal intubation. The incidence of difficult intubation ranges from 3% to 18% depending on the definition. In fact, definitions of difficult intubation vary from '2 failed attempts', 'use of additional equipment' such as a bougie to 'Cormack and Lehane grade 3–4 view'. Failure to intubate occurs in 1:2500 patients (1 in 300 in obstetrics).

Causes of difficult intubation

- Congenital, e.g. Pierre Robin syndrome (improves with age), Treacher Collins syndrome (worsens with age), Down's syndrome, and craniofacial dysostoses
- Anatomical. Variants of normal anatomy, e.g. prominent teeth, short thick neck, deep protuberant or receding mandible, pregnancy
- Acquired, e.g. trismus, soft tissue swelling, scarring, cervical rheumatoid arthritis, obesity and airway malignancy

Grading difficult laryngoscopy

Cormack and Lehane graded obstetric laryngoscopy but this classification is now widely used for nonobstetric intubations.
- Grade 1. Most of the glottis is seen
- Grade 2. Only the posterior extremity of the glottis is visible

- Grade 3. The epiglottis can be seen but no part of the glottis is visible
- Grade 4. Not even the epiglottis can be seen

Patients with grade 4 intubation are usually detected in advance, and appropriate precautions, techniques and skills are used to avoid morbidity and mortality. It is the unexpected grade 3 cases that give rise to the greatest risk. See Airway assessment topic.

Management of difficult intubation

Optimal patient positioning cannot be underestimated. The traditional 'sniffing' position is achieved by anterior flexion of the lower cervical spine and extension of the atlanto-occipital joint resulting in the axial alignment of the mouth, pharynx and larynx. Recently a 'ramped' or 'ear to sternal notch' head position has gained popularity, especially for the intubation of obese and obstetric patients. The external auditory meatus and sternal notch should be horizontally aligned. This can be achieved by pillow placement or purpose-built intubating pillows.

Attempts at intubating a patient known or predicted to be a difficult intubation should not be made without a suitably experienced anaesthetist with the skills to perform specialised techniques of intubation. Initially simple aids such as a gum elastic bougie may be used. Pressure on the cricoid cartilage can improve the view. More complex techniques may include use of specialised equipment such as follows.

Alternative intubating devices

- McCoy blade. A standard Macintosh blade with a hinged tip to allow for elevation of the epiglottis
- Airtraq. An anatomical-shaped optical laryngoscope with both an optical channel and a channel for passage of the endotracheal tube
- Video laryngoscopes. Examples include the GlideScope, McGrath video

laryngoscope and Pentax and Storz versions. All share the principle of displaying the 'view' of the larynx on a small video screen in real time from a camera positioned on the tip of the device. An anatomical curve in the blade allows for positioning of the ETT whilst the operator watches on the screen

- Bonfils laryngoscope. A thin stylet-type device designed for insertion using a retromolar approach. The ETT is railroaded into position under direct endoscopic vision
- Aintree airway catheter. The catheter lumen will allow passage of a fibreoptic bronchoscope. The catheter can be directed into the trachea and then an ETT railroaded over the top
- Intubating LMA. A specially designed bullet-tipped ETT is passed blindly into the trachea once the LMA is positioned. Success rates of 90% are reported following two attempts
- Flexible fibreoptic bronchoscope. Considered the gold standard, used for both awake and asleep fibreoptic intubation via the nasal or oral routes. The fibreoptic scope can also be used to railroad a small ETT or Aintree catheter through a conventional LMA under direct vision

'Front of neck' techniques

- Cricothyroid puncture. Large-bore airway cannulae such as the Quick Trach provide emergency access but are usually reserved for the 'can't intubate, can't ventilate' scenario (NAP4 reported a 60% failure rate in emergency use). Elective placement of smaller cannulae under local anaesthesia (e.g. the 13G Ravussin cannula) allows for transtracheal jet ventilation in head and neck surgery
- Surgical cricothyroidotomy. In extremis, this involves surgical placement of an ETT through the cricothyroid membrane
- Surgical tracheostomy. Best performed by an ENT surgeon; awake tracheostomy can be life-saving in severe upper airway obstruction provided there is time

Expired CO_2 should always be used to confirm successful intubation.

Failed intubation

The Difficult Airway Society (UK) has produced consensus guidelines on the management of failed intubation and the 'can't intubate, can't ventilate' scenario. The most up-to-date guidelines can be found on the Difficult Airway Society website; http://www.das.uk.com. There is a fundamental notion that repeated attempts at intubation using the same technique will fail and only serve to increase airway soiling and oedema, hence the concept of a 'plan A, plan B, plan C' approach. Following failed intubation, efforts should focus on achieving oxygenation, rather than intubation. In critical incidents, there is often failure of an active decision to wake the patient.

Major airway events are more likely in the emergency department or ICU setting and are frequently associated with complications resulting from rapid sequence induction. A number of high-profile catastrophes and NAP4 data highlighted the importance of human factors and prior planning in such situations. Failed intubation should be a well-rehearsed drill, which should be practiced regularly in a simulated environment.

Further readings

Cook TM, Woodall N, Frerk C. Fourth National Audit Project of the Royal College of Anaesthetists. Major complications of airway management in the United Kingdom. Royal College of Anaesthetists, 2011.

Difficult Airway Society (UK). Failed intubation, failed ventilation. London; Difficult Airway Society UK, 2004.

Related topics of interest

Airway – the emergency airway

Key points

- The airway is rarely the only factor which requires consideration in these cases
- Always involve senior colleagues early, including an experienced ENT surgeon
- Any patient likely to require a tracheostomy in this situation should have their airway management commenced in theatre with a surgeon prepared to perform that procedure

The emergency airway can be defined as that situation in which the patient is at imminent risk of potentially fatal airway obstruction. Causes of such an obstruction can be classified as follows:

- Intraluminal, e.g. blood, vomit, tumour, foreign body, soft tissue
- Mural, e.g. oedema, tumour, abscess
- Extramural, e.g. haematoma, oedema, abscess, tumour

These patients represent a particular challenge and have a high incidence of airway management difficulty. A senior anaesthetist and assistant and experienced ENT surgeon should be involved from an early point and good teamwork is key. Any patient who is likely to require surgical tracheostomy as part of their airway management should be moved to the operating theatre prior to induction of anaesthesia. Careful reassurance of a conscious patient is vital as extreme anxiety is typical and contributes to further airway compromise.

Problems

Patient factors:

- Anxiety
- Rapid desaturation
- Comorbidity, e.g. trauma, brain injury, pulmonary disease
- Inability to lie supine

Specific airway factors:

- Secretions, blood, vomit
- Airway reactivity
- 'Cork in bottle' effect
- Fixed airway tissues especially following radiotherapy
- Friable airway tissue
- Spinal immobility, i.e. trauma
- Airway injury – fractures, trismus, laryngotracheal collapse, loose teeth

Clinical features

The predominant three pathologies are trauma, infection and tumour. With trauma, the airway is seldom the only problem but is frequently compromised (fractures, loose teeth, blood, and vomit). It is rarely practical or appropriate to move the patient to theatre. Spinal immobilisation and agitation associated with a concomitant traumatic brain injury (TBI) add to problems. Nearly 50% of significant maxillofacial trauma is associated with TBI.

With airway infection the systemic effects, most notably hypotension, need consideration. Retropharyngeal and peritonsillar abscess affect any age but predominate in children. Presentation includes neck and retrosternal pain, fever, drooling, torticollis and stridor. Intubate carefully to avoid rupture of the abscess with airway soiling. Bacterial tracheitis is becoming more common than epiglottitis as a cause of life-threatening airway compromise (owing to *Haemophilus influenzae* Type B vaccination for the latter) and presents with cough, stridor and copious secretions. Unlike epiglottis, these patients (usually children) do not typically drool and can lie supine. Both diseases feature severe systemic toxicity. Croup, by contrast, rarely requires intubation; however, a persistently high Westley score (**Table 2**), despite medical treatment, may necessitate this. More common in adults are periodontal abscess and Ludwig's angina (severe, pustular cellulitis of the subglossal space). Both are complicated by trismus, which may be mechanical (due to pus and oedema) rather than pain-induced; anaesthesia and muscle relaxant may not improve airway malleability. Failure to protrude the tongue is highly suggestive of Ludwig's angina or other subglossal collection, e.g. haematoma.

Table 2 Westley croup score: mild <2, moderate 3–5, severe 6–11, prearrest >12						
Score	0	1	2	3	4	5
Breath sounds	Normal	Decreased	Markedly decreased			
Stridor	Not present	When agitated	At rest			
Cough	Not present	Hoarse cry	Bark			
Recession	Not present	Mild	Moderate	Severe		
Cyanosis	Not present				When agitated	At rest
Conscious level	Normal					Reduced

Acute, severe airway compromise is a common first presentation of ENT tumours. This is due in part to the absence of stridor before 50% occlusion and that these patients are usually smokers and may refute their diagnosis or attribute symptoms to chronic pulmonary disease. Gradual occlusion as the tumour grows tends to allow compensation unlike the acute compromise seen with infection; similar levels of respiratory distress from a tumour often represent a much more severe reduction in airway calibre. Stridor volume does not predict airway calibre and reducing noise may denote exhaustion or hypoxia-induced reduction in consciousness. Stridor at rest is common in these patients but postural exacerbation, particularly night-time choking, is worrying and should be noted. This suggests supine positioning for anaesthesia may also be problematic. Dysphagia and drooling are seen with supraglottic tumours. Similarly bleeding is often a feature, particularly with epiglottic tumours that are friable and can bleed profusely.

Investigations

There is rarely the time or need for any form of imaging in these scenarios. In the case of tumours, recent CT scans from clinic may provide useful information. Similarly, with these patients, an experienced ENT surgeon may be able to assess the airway at nasendoscopy in the cooperative adult patient. Inability to visualise the larynx usually predicts inability to visualise it laryngoscopically.

Anaesthetic management

Even in the most pressing emergency, some attempt must be made to assess the airway difficulty, systemic state of the patient and pertinent comorbidities to make appropriate plans. Wherever time allows, these patients should always be managed in conjunction with a senior anaesthetic colleague, assistant and, ideally, an ENT consultant.

Trauma airway

Reliable intravenous access is required and full monitoring should be applied whilst thorough preoxygenation is undertaken. The default mode of anaesthesia in these patients should be rapid sequence induction with a calculated dose of induction and relaxant agents. Cricoid pressure should be delegated to someone with experience of the technique; usually an operating department practitioner (ODP) can perform this and act as your airway assistant. Manual in-line stabilisation (MILS) of the cervical spine is required and you should decide if the C-spine collar is most safely removed before induction (co-operative patient) or immediately after induction (agitated patient). Blood, vomit and debris render fibreoptic intubation nearly impossible. Similarly, the need for rapid airway control and possibility of a full stomach preclude a gaseous induction. It is important to have rescue plans made, e.g. as seen in Difficult Airway Society (UK) guidelines.

Infection

Particularly in the paediatric population, minimal interference is key; distress increases respiratory effort, which may precipitate collapse and obstruction of a critical airway. Allow the patient to find their most comfortable position and apply pulse oximetry if possible. Escort to theatre and patiently achieve deep inhalational anaesthesia with the ENT surgeon scrubbed to provide surgical airway access if required. A similar approach would be suitable for airway foreign body; inhalational induction is followed by retrieval of the foreign body via rigid bronchoscope.

Tumour

If the larynx cannot be visualised at nasendoscopy, laryngoscopy is likely to be difficult. These patients are usually too distressed to tolerate awake fibreoptic intubation. Airway distortion, bleeding and obstruction of the narrow airway by the endoscope (cork-in-bottle) are also problems. Close liaison with the surgeon is vital and a low threshold for surgical tracheostomy under local anaesthesia should be adopted. Sedation in this instance is dangerous. Heliox has a role although consideration must be given to the low oxygen content of this mixture (21%).

Extubation

Guidance also exists for this phase of management which is frequently underestimated (again, see Difficult Airway Society (UK) for an example). Consideration should first be given to whether extubation is possible at that time; need for intravenous dexamethasone, no cuff leak, ongoing airway soiling. If extubation is undertaken, the patient must be fully awake and the surgical team should remain scrubbed in theatre until a spontaneous airway is well established.

Further reading

Cook TM, Woodall N, Frerk C. Major complications of airway management in the UK: results of the Fourth National Audit Project of the Royal College of Anaesthetists and the Difficult Airway Society. Part 1: anaesthesia. Br J Anaesth 2011; 106:617–631.

Maloney E, Meakin GH. Acute stridor in children. Br J Anaesth: Continuing Education in Anaesthesia, Critical Care & Pain 2007; 7:183–186.

Related topics of interest

Airway – the shared airway

Key points

- Communication with the surgeon at every phase is critical
- A wide range of airway techniques exist which can be employed in combination to achieve the desired effect
- Extubation is just as vital as intubation

Shared airway cases are commonplace in maxillofacial, ENT and thoracic surgery. They bring unique challenges for several distinct reasons:

- The surgical lesion is likely to interfere with the airway and its management
- Certain airway techniques may restrict surgical access
- Postoperative surgical complications are likely to compromise the airway
- Close communication between surgeons and anaesthetists is arguably more important than in other surgical specialties

The anaesthetic techniques for these procedures have evolved into a considerable variety of options, some of which are not encountered elsewhere, e.g. high- and low-frequency jet ventilation (HFJV and LFJV). Particular surgical techniques, e.g. laser surgery and rigid bronchoscopy, have specific considerations that must be taken into account.

Underpinning safe and successful management of these cases is a high dependency on teamwork between all members of the surgical and anaesthetic teams. There is also a degree of trust which the anaesthetist must have in their surgical colleague to communicate regarding such complications as accidental displacement of the airway device. This is best engendered through regular work with the same surgeon. An experienced assistant with particular expertise in these procedures is also invaluable; much of the equipment required is specialised.

These cases are often notable by the extent to which the anaesthetist is actively involved with the procedure itself. There may be points during induction or the procedure itself when surgical assistance is required to manage the airway and these must be recognised early. Similarly, the surgeon may require assistance or advice on how to maintain or adjust the airway device to facilitate surgery. An immobile surgical field is particularly important in some procedures. Smooth emergence without coughing but with swift return of airway reflexes is also desirable.

Problems

- Awareness
- Accidental loss of airway
- Airway soiling
- Dental/oral injury
- Tracheobronchial rupture (rigid bronchoscopy)
- Airway fires (laser surgery)
- Staff hazards from lasers – fire, eye damage, aerosolised carcinogens/viral particles
- Delayed post-op airway compromise (oedema, aspiration, haematomas, bleeding, residual airway anaesthesia)

Investigations

Routine preoperative assessment will dictate appropriate investigations (bloods, ECG, chest X-ray). Prior nasendoscopy may give important information particularly in prediction of airway difficulties. Blood group and save should be considered a minimum – the potential for bleeding particularly from tumours is high. Flow-volume loops may give information about airway dynamics. Static assessment with CT imaging is invaluable and should generally be requested and carefully reviewed by surgeon and anaesthetist during their planning of the case. Other imaging such as MRI and positron emission tomography may be available from malignancy assessment.

Certain procedures, particularly rigid bronchoscopy, are associated with an extreme sympathetic response. A careful preoperative assessment of the cardiovascular system with echocardiography and ECG is required in what is often an elderly and comorbid group of patients who are typically smokers.

Anaesthetic management

The choice of technique will often be made in conjunction with the surgeon. Thorough preoperative assessment and review of investigations is vital in these patients. A careful airway assessment is mandatory.

The airway can be topically anaesthetised and patients allowed to breath spontaneously, although the procedures suited to this are very limited and general anaesthesia is more commonly used. A variety of airway devices may be used including LMA, nasal, oral, laser-resistant and submental endotracheal tubes. Ring Adair Elwyn (RAE) and fleximetallic tubes often allow for better surgical access and reduce the chance of lumen occlusion. Where laryngeal access is important a cuffed microlaryngeal tube (MLT) and intermittent positive pressure ventilation (IPPV) offer a protected lower airway although the posterior glottis is poorly visualised. This may be more useful in those having examination of the upper oesophagus as opposed to the respiratory tract.

A spontaneous breathing technique may be undertaken via rigid endoscopes, although, in adult practice, muscle relaxation is typically administered. Ventilating or venturi bronchoscopes may be used. Both have considerations regarding considerable cardiovascular stress, particularly in the older, frail patient, e.g. using short-acting opiates such as remifentanil. The venturi bronchoscope requires LFJV with a Sander's injector (with an inherent risk of barotrauma). LFJV can either be undertaken in conjunction with an intermittent inhalational technique or with total intravenous anaesthesia (TIVA). HFJV is a useful alternative to an MLT and offers a near-unobstructed view of the larynx with jet entrainment occurring via a fine, subglottic catheter or a cricothyroid cannula. Both LFJV and HFJV have the inherent risks of an unprotected airway and the risks of awareness. Displacement of a cricothyroid cannula can lead to severe subcutaneous emphysema. Continuous waveform capnography cannot be used with either technique except as a qualitative estimate with certain types of subglottic HFJV catheters. Both also have a requirement for complex equipment for delivering TIVA and, for HFJV, the oscillator device.

Extubation should not be underestimated. The Difficult Airway Society of the UK has produced specific guidance on this. In general, most patients should be extubated in a semirecumbent position and, where experience and patient factors permit, under deep anaesthesia to prevent coughing and bleeding. Scrupulous aspiration of secretions, blood and clots, particularly from the postnasal space, is vital prior to waking. Following tonsillectomy, always evaluate the dryness of the tonsillar beds. Traditionally following this procedure, children should be extubated in the left lateral decubitus position slightly head down to drain secretions. Once awake, they should sit up to reduce venous engorgement of the tonsillar beds.

Postextubation, the recently instrumented airway remains at risk of intrinsic or extrinsic compromise, from oedema or haematoma in particular. Nebulised adrenaline 5 mg, intravenous dexamethasone 0.15 mg/kg or Heliox may all have a role. Clip removers to open neck wounds and evacuate expanding haematomas should be at the bedside at all times.

Further reading

Difficult Airway Society. Default strategy for intubation including failed direct laryngoscopy. London; DAS, 2007.

English J, Norris A, Bedforth N. Anaesthesia for airway surgery. Contin Educ Anaesth Crit Care Pain 2006; 1:28–31.

Related topics of interest

- Airway assessment (p. 1)
- Airway – difficult and failed intubation (p. 4)
- Human factors in patient safety (p. 86)
- Lasers in surgery (p. 98)

Awake intubation

Key points

- Intubation of the awake patient is an underused technique and can reduce morbidity and mortality in the presence of a challenging airway
- Local anaesthesia of the airway can be considered in three stages: the nasopharynx, the oropharynx and the larynx
- Sedation can improve the patient experience but should be used with caution in case of airway obstruction

Awake intubation is a useful technique for patients with a known difficult airway. This is most frequently achieved using a fibreoptic bronchoscope [awake fibreoptic intubation (AFOI)], although surgical tracheotomy in the awake patient is also possible in certain critical situations. The NAP4 audit found that AFOI was an underused technique in the UK, contributing to avoidable morbidity and mortality.

Even when local anaesthetic agents are used in the airway, the patient retains some ability to respond to a threat to the airway. Vomiting or regurgitation will produce coughing, retching or repeated swallowing despite the obtunded pharyngeal and laryngeal reflexes. The fibreoptic bronchoscope allows for direct visualisation of laryngeal anatomy and passage of the endotracheal tube under direct vision through either the nasal or oral route. The degree of disturbance to the patient will depend on the operator's skill, the psychological and pharmacological preparation and the advice that the patient has received.

Indications

- Potential upper airway obstruction. It is axiomatic to anaesthetic practice that muscle relaxants are not administered to patients with airway obstruction until it is clear that the airway can be maintained. Attempting intubation under deep inhalational anaesthesia in adults is difficult and can be hazardous, especially in the presence of a full stomach. An awake intubation offers an alternative. Topical anaesthesia of the airway and attempted awake intubation for upper airway obstruction can result in total obstruction. Tracheostomy under local anaesthesia is therefore recommended if there is severe stridor with markedly abnormal laryngeal anatomy. Placement of a transtracheal jet ventilation catheter through the cricothyroid membrane in the awake patient can provide a useful alternative
- Predicted difficult intubation. Intubation of patients who are known or suspected to be a difficult intubation may be achieved awake with the knowledge that if a particular technique fails the patient is still breathing and in control of their airway
- Previous difficulty in mask ventilation, rendering post-induction oxygenation problematic
- Avoidance of iatrogenic injury in patients with unstable cervical spine (e.g. rheumatoid arthritis). It also allows for neurological assessment post-intubation. AFOI requires the patient to lie still, however, which may be difficult in this situation
- Awake intubation has been suggested in patients with severe cardiovascular compromise to prevent the instability associated with induction of anaesthesia

Contraindications

- Patient refusal/unco-operation
- Bleeding disorders (due to obscuring of the view at fibreoptic laryngoscopy)
- Gross airway soiling, due to poor fibreoptic vision
- Children
- Advanced stenosing airway tumours (the 'cork-in-a-bottle' effect may lead to complete airway obstruction)
- Allergy to local anaesthesia

Anaesthetic management
Assessment and premedication

A full assessment of the upper airway is made. Stridor and positional airway changes are worrying signs. A simple, unhurried explanation of the anaesthetic plan will help allay patient anxiety and is essential to secure co-operation.

Antisialagogue premedication (glycopyrrolate 200 µg) is recommended. A dry oropharynx will improve the view, reduce the patient's desire to swallow and increase the effectiveness and duration of topical local anaesthetic agents.

Conduct of anaesthesia

Monitoring of the blood pressure, ECG and O_2 saturation should be standard. End-tidal CO_2 monitoring should be available to assist confirmation of tube placement. Oxygen should be administered, either via a cutaway facemask or nasal sponge positioned in the opposite nostril. Awake intubation may be performed orally or nasally. Blind techniques have now largely been superseded, although a blind lightwand-based technique has recently been described.

Local anaesthetic techniques

Topical anaesthesia

The airway can be anaesthetised topically in three separate stages:

Nasopharynx: The most patent nostril should be selected (although sometimes bony spurs prohibit the passage of the endoscope, forcing the use of the alternative nostril). Cocaine or phenylephrine are used as potent vasoconstrictors to reduce the risk of epistaxis. Surface anaesthesia of the nasal mucosae may be obtained by packing the nose with anaesthetic-soaked ribbon gauze or by using a 10% lignocaine via spray or mucosal atomiser device. An alternative approach is with serial dilation of the nares using Instillagel-coated nasopharyngeal airways of increasing size, which will prepare for passage of the endotracheal tube, but carries a risk of epistaxis.

Oropharynx: Options include amethocaine or benzocaine lozenges to suck prior to arrival in the operating department. An alternative is to use nebulised 4% lignocaine or 10% lignocaine spray delivered to the back of the oral cavity (note the dose delivered is 10 mg per actuation, thus maximum local anaesthetic doses can be rapidly exceeded without due care).

Larynx: Anaesthesia to the subglottic region may be provided using a cricothyroid injection. A narrow gauge needle is inserted through the cricothyroid membrane into the trachea. Correct placement is confirmed by the aspiration of air into the syringe. The patient is then asked to take a deep breath in. At the end of inspiration 2 mL of local anaesthetic are injected, producing an explosive cough, which results in coating the underside of the vocal cords and subglottic region. A 'spray as you go' method utilises the suction port of the fibreoptic scope to instil 2 mL local anaesthetic to the vocal cords under direct vision. An epidural catheter threaded through the suction port allows for deposition of local anaesthetic beneath the cords.

It is very easy to achieve the maximum toxic dose when anaesthetising the airway due to the volume and variety of anaesthetic agents used. Agents are readily systemically absorbed through mucosae that have a rich blood supply; however, absorption is variable due to the first pass effect of swallowed anaesthetic and incomplete absorption of nebulised anaesthetic. Up to 9 mg/kg lignocaine has been described when used topically. Intubating fibreoptic endoscopes are at least 25 cm long and are available with small diameters, e.g. 3 mm, although the field of view may be compromised.

Nerve blocks

Although these are described, most operators prefer topical anaesthesia as it provides good conditions with limited risk.

Anatomy:

- Sensation from the hard and soft palate, nasal mucosae and the nasopharynx is supplied by the second division of the trigeminal nerve (maxillary)
- The posterior third of the tongue, oropharynx and tonsillar area are supplied by the glossopharyngeal nerves
- The superior laryngeal nerve is a branch of the vagus and gives rise to an external and internal branch at the greater cornu of the hyoid bone. The external branch supplies the cricothyroid membrane, whilst the internal branch serves the mucous

membrane of the larynx down to the rima glottidis

- Sensation below the rima glottidis is supplied by the inferior laryngeal nerves, the terminal branch of the recurrent laryngeal nerve
  1. Maxillary nerve block. This is achieved by introducing a needle angled at 45° into the sphenopalatine canal via the greater palatine foraminae of the hard palate. A small volume of local anaesthetic (~2 mL) may then be deposited
  2. A glossopharyngeal nerve block may precipitate airway obstruction following loss of tone at the base of the tongue. It is helpful, however, in patients with an active gag reflex. It is achieved by inserting an angled tonsillar needle behind the posterior tonsillar pillar and injecting 3 mL of local anaesthetic agent.
  3. Superior laryngeal nerve block
     a. Krause's method. The superior laryngeal nerve lies just below the laryngeal mucosa in the piriform fossa. A dental pledget soaked in anaesthetic solution and firmly held by a pair of Krause's forceps is held in the piriform fossa for about 1 minute on each side
     b. Percutaneous block. The superior laryngeal nerve divides into internal and external branches at the greater cornu of the hyoid, a point at which it may be blocked. A skin weal is raised over the thyroid cartilage in the midline and a needle advanced in a lateral and cephalad direction onto the hyoid bone. The needle is walked off the hyoid at the greater cornu and 2 mL of local anaesthetic solution deposited. Passage to the cornu may be eased by gently pulling the hyoid bone to the left for a right nerve block and vice versa

Sedation

Sedative agents are appropriate in the nonobstructed airway. Remifentanil [0.05 µg/kg/min or 2–3 ng/mL target-controlled infusion (TCI)] provides excellent conditions with the added advantage of attenuation of the gag reflex and the ability to titrate if required. Midazolam or low-dose propofol TCI (1–2 µg/mL) are also well described techniques. It is important that patient safety is not compromised by the use of such agents and that verbal contact remains throughout.

Further reading

Rai MR, Parry TM, Dombrovskis A, et al. Remifentanil target-controlled infusion vs propofol target-controlled infusion for conscious sedation for awake fibreoptic intubation: a double-blinded randomised controlled trial. Br J Anaesth 2008; 100:125–130.

Sudheer P, Stacey MR. Anaesthesia for awake intubation. Br J Anaesth: Contin Educ Prof Develop Rev 2003; 3:120–123.

Related topics of interest

Awareness and depth of anaesthesia

Key points

- Awareness is a critical incident with potentially catastrophic consequences
- Avoiding awareness requires pre-, intra-, and postoperative strategies
- There is no gold-standard depth of anaesthesia monitor

We perceive our environment through the detection and interpretation of various sensory inputs (sight, smell, sound, taste, and touch) and memory is our ability to process, store, and retrieve such information. Usually both of these interlinked processes are abolished, or at least impaired, by general anaesthesia. Unintentional awareness is the perception and memory of events that have transpired during general anaesthesia.

General anaesthesia is not an all-or-nothing event, but exists as a continuum. Therefore, awareness too can be described as a spectrum:

- Conscious awareness with explicit recall – patient is awake (albeit undetected) and memories are later spontaneously recalled
- Conscious awareness with no explicit recall
- Subconscious awareness with implicit recall – patient is not awake and memories are not later spontaneously recalled, but may subconsciously affect mood or behaviour at a later date
- No awareness or implicit recall

Dreaming is an interesting scenario and two types of anaesthesia-related dream states are described in the literature:

- The near-miss, semiaware state
- The emergence/recovery state (in which the patient is semisedated)

It has been proposed that dreaming is common, unlikely to be related to depth of anaesthesia and mostly pleasant/harmless. Unsurprisingly awareness can potentially be catastrophic for the patient. Psychological sequelae include anxiety/depression, fear of subsequent anaesthesia/surgery, sleep disturbance and post-traumatic stress disorder. Awareness can also be distressing to the anaesthetist personally, professionally and financially.

Incidence

In the UK, the Royal College of Anaesthetists 5th National Audit Project (NAP5) is designed to evaluate the incidence of accidental awareness during anaesthesia.

Prior to the NAP5 study, the UK incidence of awareness was thought to be as follows:

- Explicit awareness with severe pain: 1 in 3000
- Explicit awareness without pain: between 1 in 142–1000

Baseline results from NAP5 put the incidence of awareness much lower at around 1:15,000 with around half of these occurring around the time of anaesthetic induction/prior to surgery.

Causes and risk factors

Awareness is caused by inadequate anaesthesia. The causes of this, however, are multifactorial and may include

- Patient factors
  - Normal variability in MAC
  - Resistance to anaesthetic agents, e.g. alcohol excess
- Situational factors
  - Tend to be related to the urgency of surgery (e.g. emergency caesarian section under GA) or unexpected difficulties (e.g. difficult intubation)
- Anaesthetic factors
  - Omission of anaesthesia or inadequate dose
    - Unintentional
    - Intentional – in order to avoid anaesthetic side effects
  - Use of muscle relaxants roughly doubles the incidence of awareness
  - Use of total intravenous anaesthesia
  - Inability to monitor vapour concentration

- Use of drugs that may mask the clinical signs of awareness
- Equipment factors
  - Malfunction or disconnection
  - Other, e.g. sequestration of anaesthetic drugs in cardiopulmonary bypass circuit

Assessment and management

The evaluation of awareness is continuous across the perioperative period.

Preoperative

- The preoperative visit also presents the opportunity to identify risk factors, elicit anxieties and provide reassurance
- Premedication with an amnesic agent (e.g. benzodiazepines) may help to reduce the incidence of awareness

Intraoperative

- Assessment of depth of anaesthesia using both clinical markers and equipment can be useful, although there is no single gold standard

Clinical markers
- Guedel's stages of anaesthesia
  - First described in 1937, using spontaneous respiration and ether
  - Transition is too rapid with modern agents to be reliably observed
  - Stage 1 – Induction (ends with loss of consciousness) → normal pupils, normal respiration
  - Stage 2 – Excitement → dilated + divergent pupils, irregular respiration, active airway reflexes, and loss of eyelash reflex
  - Stage 3 – Surgical anaesthesia
    - Plane 1 – central pinpoint pupils + regular, large volume respiration + loss of eyelid reflex
    - Plane 2 – Reduced intercostal respiration + loss of corneal reflex
    - Plane 3 – Normal pupils, diaphragmatic respiration, reduced laryngeal reflexes
    - Plane 4 – Reduced diaphragmatic respiration and reduced carinal reflex
  - Stage 4 – Overdose and coma, large dilated pupils, apnoea and hypotension
- Evans scoring system (PRST)
  - Based on clinical signs associated with sympathetic stimulation, i.e. blood **P**ressure, heart **R**ate, **S**weating and **T**ears
  - However, they are not specific and can also be affected by a number of drugs used in anaesthetic practice, e.g. remifentanil

Equipment
- End-tidal monitoring and MAC
  - Can be used for patients receiving inhalational anaesthetics
  - Unfortunately, MAC values are based on an expected requirement and that there are many different factors that may alter a patient's required MAC
  - Also the definition of MAC does not take account of awareness
- Tunstall's isolated forearm technique
  - Tourniquet placed on arm before induction of anaesthesia which isolates it from any muscle relaxants that may have been administered – i.e. the patient can move their hand to alert any problem
- Lower oesophageal contractility
  - Oesophageal contractions are triggered by stress and emotion in awake patients. Under general anaesthesia, a balloon catheter can be used to detect such contractions
- Evoked potentials
  - Operates on the theory that auditory perception is the final sense to disappear under anaesthesia
  - Clicks are delivered to the anaesthetised ear and the EEG is monitored for a response
- EEG-based
  - Several different monitors are available that incorporate various algorithms to either modify the EEG waveform or produce a dimensionless number that 'correlates' with depth of anaesthesia
  - Such methods include BIS, entropy and spectral edge frequency
  - Several studies (e.g. B-Aware and B-Unaware) have tried to confirm the validity of these methods. Unfortunately

none to date have been able to do so in entirety

The NAP5 project recorded that, although depth-of-anaesthesia monitoring was available in 62% of UK institutions, <2% of anaesthetists routinely used it.

Postoperative

- Visit the patient with a witness as soon as possible
- Awareness is usually assessed with the structured modified Bryce interview
  - What was the last thing you remember before going to sleep?
  - What was the first thing you can remember after waking up?
  - Can you remember anything in between?
  - Did you have any dreams during your operation?
  - What was the worst thing about your operation?
- Attempt to confirm the cause (if able)
- Acknowledge the patients feelings and give an apology
- Give a full explanation of events including
  - That awareness may not be through any particular fault of the anaesthetist
  - That they can safely receive further general anaesthetics
- Offer follow-up, including psychological assessment/support
- Aim to make an accurate and contemporaneous record of what occurred, the patient's exact memory of events and any subsequent interactions (keep your own copy)
- People to notify
  - Hospital administration
  - Patient's GP
  - Your medical defence organisation

Legal situation

It is largely accepted that patients expect to be unaware and that a reasonable effort to ensure this is part of an anaesthetist's duty of care. A review of NHS Litigation Authority claims between 1995 and 2007 showed 79 claims related to awareness and 20 claims related to brief awake paralysis with average awards of £32,680 and £24,364 respectively.

Further reading

Griffiths D, Jones JG. Awareness and memory in anaesthetised patients. Br J Anaesth 1990; 65:603–606.

Leslie K, Skrzpek H, Paech MJ, et al. Dreaming during anesthesia and anesthetic depth in elective surgery patients: a prospective cohort study. Anesthesiology 2007; 106:33–42.

Pandit JJ, et al. A national survey of anaesthetists (NAP5 Baseline) to estimate an annual incidence of accidental awareness during general anaesthesia in the UK. Br J Anaesth 2013; 110:501–509.

Sandin, et al. Awareness during anaesthesia: a prospective case study. Lancet 2000; 355:707–711.

Related topics of interest

Blood physiology

Key points

- The oxygen-carrying capacity of blood is affected by abnormal haemoglobins, which may require modification of the anaesthetic technique
- Coagulation is a complex process involving initiation, amplification and propagation of thrombus at the endothelium
- Pharmacological agents affecting coagulation target particular molecules and pathways in the clotting system
- Thromboelastography (TEG) allows for rapid assessment of the whole coagulation process through near-patient testing

The haematological system is a complex life-support system with multiple functions.

Red blood cells and haemoglobin

Haemopoesis starts in the yolk sac and continues in the liver and spleen in the first few months of life before the bone marrow takes over. It is controlled predominantly by the glycoprotein erythropoietin (EPO), produced in the kidney. EPO is produced in response to hypoxia, anaemia and a raised metabolism and is mediated by corticosteroids, androgens, thyroxine and growth hormone.

The predominant form of haemoglobin in humans is HbA, comprising 2α and 2β chains. Pathological haemoglobins usually result from genetic variation in these chains, e.g. HbC, HbD, HbS (sickle cell, abnormal β) or thalassaemia (variations in α or β chains). Abnormal haemoglobins usually result in reduced oxygen-carrying capacity and haemolytic anaemia with an associated iron deficiency. Treatment of thalassaemia with chronic transfusion risks iron overload. Iron-chelating agents are often co-administered to prevent this.

Due to Mendelian genetics, most haemoglobinopathies present in a milder (or asymptomatic) form when heterozygous with limited implications for the anaesthetist. Fetal blood (85% HbF, 15% HbA) has a greater affinity for oxygen than adult blood (97% HbA, 2.5% HbA2, 0.5% HbF).

Oxygen carriage

Haemoglobin increases the oxygen capacity of the blood 50 times. The molecule 'breathes' during oxygen uptake and release, shifting the oxygen dissociation curve as it circulates.

Factors affecting the oxy-haemoglobin dissociation curve:

- Right shift: acidosis, hyperthermia, hypercapnoea and raised 2,3-diphosphoglycerate (2,3-DPG). O_2 is bound less avidly at a given ambient Pao_2, promoting release into tissues
- Left shift: HbF, methaemoglobin, carbon monoxide poisoning. O_2 is bound more avidly, promoting fetal uptake

By enclosing Hb within the red blood cell (which also contains 2,3-DPG), a low plasma viscosity and oncotic pressure can be preserved, whilst allowing for maximum oxygen carriage (red cells normally carry over 98% of the oxygen in arterial blood). Very little oxygen dissolves in the plasma, which explains the tissue hypoxia seen in severe anaemia despite increases in inspired oxygen.

CO_2 carriage

Carbon dioxide may be dissolved (5%), incorporated as bicarbonate (90%) or carried by carbamino groups (5% of carriage). The Haldane effect describes the increased carriage of CO_2 by deoxygenated blood due to the increased buffering effects of deoxy-Hb.

Coagulation

Clot formation and dissolution is a complex process involving proteolytic enzymes (coagulation factors). The end point is the formation of a fibrin clot. Venous thrombosis is predominantly fibrin based, whilst arterial thrombus has a higher platelet content. Traditional models of factor-based intrinsic and extrinsic clotting cascades, although useful for laboratory diagnosis, do not account for the whole picture, hence the development of a cell-based model of coagulation in vivo.

The cell-based model considers clot formation in three overlapping phases:

- Initiation. A cell (e.g. vessel wall endothelium) exposes tissue factor, which activates factor VIIa, which in turn leads to activation of factors IX and X. This generates a small amount of thrombin. Circulating inhibitors, such as anti-thrombin, inactivate any factor Xa that leaves the surface of the cell thus localising activity
- Amplification. Platelets are activated and stick to the site of injury, clad in cofactors in preparation for massive thrombin production
- Propagation. Occurs on the surface of the platelets; a burst of thrombin is produced by the platelet prothrombinase complex of sufficient magnitude to generate fibrin deposition

Abnormal coagulation inhibitors:

- Factor V Leiden (autosomal dominant, prevalence 5% Caucasians) is a mutation rendering factor V less sensitive to activated protein C. It is associated with venous rather than arterial thrombosis and is present in 20% deep vein thrombosis (DVT) presentations. Most carriers do not get DVT though and prophylaxis (even in pregnancy) is not advocated
- Protein C/S deficiency (prevalence <0.5%) increases the risk of venous thrombosis as activated protein C inactivates factors V and VIII, thus halting thrombin production. Protein S is a cofactor for protein C

Platelets: biconcave discs, with a lifespan of 7–14 days. Granules within contain coagulation factors, von Willebrand factor (essential for platelet adherence) and growth factors. Platelet aggregation is a key target for anticoagulant medication, especially when inhibiting arterial thrombus.

Measurement of coagulation

Laboratory-based:

- Prothrombin time/international normalised ratio (INR). Tests the extrinsic pathway and is prolonged by warfarin, heparin, liver disease, disseminated intravascular coagulation (DIC), reduction in factors V, VII and X

- Activated partial thromboplastin time: Tests intrinsic pathway and is prolonged by heparin, liver disease, DIC, coagulation inhibitors
- Fibrinogen and platelet level

Thromboelastography (TEG) measures the whole clotting process by measuring changes in the torque of a pin placed in a rotating cuvette of whole blood. Liquid blood has no torque, so the rotation of the cup is not transmitted to the pin (ROTEM uses the same principle). As the blood clots, the torque transmission increases. Characteristics of clot formation and strength, including platelet aggregation and fibrinolysis, can be inferred from the graph produced.

Advantages of TEG include real-time assessment of coagulation function allowing better targeting of blood products and measurement of intervention effect, heparinase modification to assess for heparin excess and fibrinolysis activity.

Pharmacological haemostatic agents

- Tranexamic acid: competitively inhibits the formation of plasmin. The CRASH-2 study recorded a reduction in mortality when used in trauma patients
- Desmopressin: induces von Willebrand factor release and factor VIII activation, but of limited use outside of congenital coagulopathies
- Recombinant factor VII: initial promising trial results have been marred by an increase in arterial thrombosis. Use is limited by cost and it remains off-licence for use outside of haemoglobinopathy treatment
- Aprotinin: a proteolytic agent that inhibits fibrin breakdown, it was commonly used until use was suspended following the BART study (2008), which suggested an increase in mortality. The European Medicines Agency has since lifted the ban

Immune function

Immune function can be divided into innate (prevention of organism entry or elimination before they can cause damage) and adaptive, which may be cell mediated or non-cell mediated.

Cell-mediated functions

- B cells: manufacture antibodies and evolve into plasma cells under the influence of T-cell cytokines
- T cells: TH (helper) cells express the CD4 glycoprotein on their surface and secrete cytokines, which activate B cells, Tc (cytotoxic) cells and macrophages etc. Tc cells eliminate cells displaying foreign antigen. HIV infects TH cells, hence the use of the CD4 cell count to track viral activity
- Neutrophils: first line of defence, they contain granules containing cytotoxic substances and enzymes and migrate to sites of inflammation
- Macrophages: part of the reticuloendothelial system, alongside other phagocytes, these have multiple functions, including antibody-mediated cytotoxicity, action as antigen presenting cells and regulators of the inflammatory response

Non-cell-mediated functions

- Cytokines: produced by neutrophils, macrophages and lymphocytes, these soluble proteins regulate the host response. They may be proinflammatory (interleukins 1,6 and tumor necrosis factor alpha) or anti-inflammatory (IL4, IL10, IL13)
- Antibodies: bind to antigen to label the foreign substance, thus allowing phagocytosis
- Complement: these are circulating inflammatory mediators, which attach to foreign cells. They function to label the foreign cell (opsonisation), activate phagocytes and can directly cause cell lysis

Further reading

Ruseva AL, Dimitrova AA. A new understanding of the coagulation process – the cell based model. J Biomed Clin Res 2011; 4:17–22.

Related topics of interest

Blood transfusion and salvage

Key points

- Collection and transfusion of homologous blood is highly regulated around the world. For example, in the UK the annual serious hazards of transfusion (SHOT) report reviews serious incidents
- Autologous blood carries lower risk to the patient and has a higher oxygen carrying capacity when transfused
- There are a number of therapeutic options to manage preoperative anaemia. This should be corrected prior to surgery where possible
- Careful and early management of intraoperative blood loss improves surgical outcomes

The regulation and management of blood transfusion services including the processing of blood products vary according to individual countries and healthcare systems. This chapter describes the current systems in place in the UK. In recent years, blood transfusion has become less hazardous due to advances in the preservation of blood and advancing knowledge of immunohaematology. However, there remain significant hazards, scarcity and financial costs of blood transfusion, leading to a re-evaluation of the indications, risks and benefits for each individual patient.

Autologous blood is a suitable alternative to allogeneic blood. Cell salvage is the most effective mechanism for obtaining autologous blood (in the UK it is a key component of the Department of Health 'Better Blood Transfusion Initiative').

Types of blood transfusion

- Homologous/allogeneic blood transfusion: blood and blood components collected from donors, intended for transfusion to other individuals
- Autologous blood transfusion: a transfusion in which the donor and the recipient are the same person and in which predeposited blood or blood components are used

Homologous blood transfusion

- Screening: First-time donors must be aged between 17 and 66 years. The donor health check questionnaire is a fundamental requirement
- Testing: Direct antiglobulin testing is used to determine ABO group and rhesus status. An immediate spin cross-match to check for agglutination will take around 5 minutes. A full cross-match involves incubation of donor cells and recipient sera for at least 15 minutes, followed by a Coombs test to detect antibody on donor cells. Every blood donation is tested for immunodeficiency virus (HIV 1 and 2), hepatitis B and C, human T-cell lymphotropic virus (HTLV) and syphilis. Selected cases are tested for malaria and *Trypanosoma cruzi* (Chagas disease)
- Emergency administration: Group O blood can be used; however, premenopausal females should be given group O-negative blood to avoid sensitisation to the rhesus D antigen

At present, there is no specific test for variant Creutzfeldt–Jakob disease (vCJD). For this reason, any person considered at increased risk of vCJD on screening and anyone who has had a previous blood transfusion is currently excluded from donation. In the UK, all donated blood is leukodepleted and children under the age of 16 years are given methylene blue virally inactivated fresh-frozen plasma (FFP) imported from outside UK.

Collection and storage media

Short-term storage

- CPD-A (citrate, phosphate, dextrose, adenine) preserves blood for 35 days
- SAG-M (saline, adenine, glucose, mannitol) preserves blood for 42 days

Saline is used to adjust osmotic pressure, adenine maintains ATP levels, glucose/dextrose provides an energy source, whilst mannitol prevents haemolysis. The haematocrit is around 0.6–0.7. Blood should be stored at an ambient temperature of 2–6°C.

Maintenance of the 'cold chain' is critical in preventing bacterial growth.

Long-term storage   Cryopreservation of red blood cells (RBCs) is used to store rare units, or by the armed forces, for up to 10 years by adding in a glycerol solution which acts as a cryoprotectant ('antifreeze') within the cells.

Effects of storage

- Reduced pH
- Reduced levels of 2,3-DPG and ATP
- Increased potassium level, due to cell rupture and Na⁺/K⁺ ATPase pump failure
- Reduced viability of blood constituents, hence the freezing of stored plasma
- Formation of microaggregates

Blood components (Figure 1)

Whole blood is separated by centrifuge to packed RBCs and platelet-rich plasma. This is separated further into platelets and plasma, containing clotting factors (this becomes FFP). FFP can be separated further into cryoprecipitate (containing factor VIII and fibrinogen) and the supernatant that is rich in albumin, immunoglobulins and factor IX.

Broadly speaking, a unit of red cells will raise the haemoglobin level in a nonbleeding recipient by around 10 g/L and the haematocrit by 3–4%. FFP should be ABO compatible. As a general rule, 4 units of FFP increase the main coagulation factors by 10% with an associated improvement in coagulation status.

Cryoprecipitate contains fibrinogen (approximately 350 mg per donation), von Willebrand factor, factor VIII, factor XIII and fibronectin. It is administered as a pool of units from four to six donations in a single bag, which can be expected to increase the plasma fibrinogen level by around 450 mg/L.

Serious hazards of blood transfusion

SHOT is a haemovigilance scheme funded by the UK transfusion services; it was the

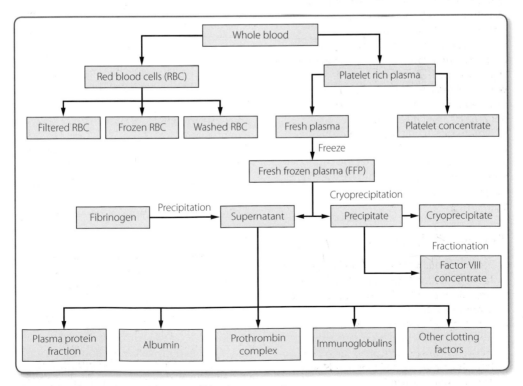

Figure 1 Diagrammatic representation of blood components.

first scheme of this type to be set up in the world and will be used as an example in this topic. The scheme collates reported adverse events and produces an annual report with recommendations. Pathological reactions can be reported under the following headings:

- Acute transfusion reactions. Febrile or hypotensive reactions and allergic reactions occurring at any time up to 24 hours following a transfusion of blood or components
- Haemolytic transfusion reactions. May be acute (<24 hours) or delayed (>24 hours): fever and clinical features of haemolysis such as a drop in Hb, positive cross-match, rise in lactate dehydrogenase or bilirubin. Also includes alloimmunisation, which is the presence of new clinically significant antibodies
- Post-transfusion purpura. Thrombocytopenia occurring within 5–12 days post-transfusion associated with the presence of antibodies against the human platelet antigen system
- Transfusion-associated graft-versus-host disease. Fever, rash, liver dysfunction, diarrhoea, pancytopenia and bone marrow hypoplasia occurring within 30 days of transfusion due to cloning of viable donor lymphocytes in a susceptible host
- Transfusion-associated circulatory overload (TACO). Defined as any four of the following occurring within 6 hours of transfusion: acute respiratory distress, tachycardia, high blood pressure, pulmonary oedema and evidence of positive fluid balance. All ages are at risk
- Transfusion-related acute lung injury (TRALI). Acute dyspnoea with hypoxia and bilateral pulmonary infiltrates during or within 6 hours of transfusion, not due to circulatory overload
- Transfusion-associated dyspnoea. Dyspnoea within 24 hours of blood transfusion, which is not TRALI or TACO
- Transfusion transmitted infection. Low risk in many countries (e.g. UK), but may include bacterial, prion or virus transmission. *Yersinia enterocolitica* is most often associated with stored red cell contamination and is related to duration and condition of storage

Autologous blood transfusion options

- Cell salvage (autotransfusion). Collection of blood from operative sites (intraoperatively) or wound sites (postoperatively), for reinfusion to the patient
- Preoperative autologous donation. A process whereby blood is removed from the patient prior to surgery, stored within the blood bank ready for reinfusion during or after surgery as required (e.g. a patient may give a unit each week for up to 6 weeks prior to surgery). It is often wasteful and cannot be used if there is systemic infection, unstable angina or preoperative anaemia. Preoperative iron supplementation is usually required
- Acute normovolaemic haemodilution. A technique whereby blood is removed from a patient immediately prior to surgery. Circulating volume is replaced with crystalloid or colloid fluid and the collected blood is reinfused once any ongoing blood loss has ceased. The patient starts their operation with a relative anaemia. The process has the advantage of minimal risk of administrative error, but is expensive and rarely used

Hyperthermic/hypotensive reactions are still possible with autologous blood use.

Cell salvage

Cell salvage is the most commonly used method for autologous transfusion in the UK. Indications:

- Anticipated intraoperative blood loss >1 L or 20% of blood volume
- Preoperative anaemia or increased risk factors for bleeding
- No consent to allogeneic blood transfusion, e.g. Jehovah's witness

Cell salvage process (Figure 2)
Perioperative blood from the surgical field is mixed with heparinised saline and collected in a reservoir. The contents are then macrofiltered to remove clots and debris and the remaining volume is drawn into a centrifuge and processed. Photo-optics detect the maximum cell density and then initiate a washing process with a selected volume of

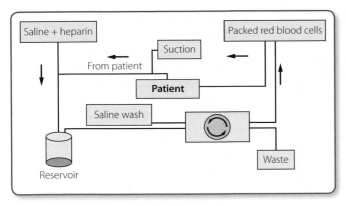

Figure 2 Cell salvage process.

saline. RBCs are collected in a bag and the waste is discarded. The collected RBCs can be reinfused up to 4 hours after processing.

Advantages:
- Immediate transfusion is near body temperature
- High levels of 2,3-DPG give improved and immediate oxygen delivery, compared with stored blood
- No incompatibility reactions
- Adverse transfusion reactions unlikely
- Lower overall costs compared with allogeneic blood (which requires an expensive haemovigilance system)
- Usable in many Jehovah's witnesses and those with rare blood groups or antibodies

Disadvantages:
- Initial equipment costs and costs of disposables
- Cell salvage systems require trained staff immediately available
- Some red cell loss due to 'skimming'
- Air/fat embolism and a theoretical risk of amniotic fluid embolism in obstetrics

Anaesthetic management in patients requiring blood transfusion

Preoperative measures

- Treatment of anaemia if detected at preassessment clinic. Preoperative anaemia is a major predictor for perioperative transfusion
- Erythropoietin. There is evidence that recombinant human erythropoietin

therapy can reduce perioperative allogeneic transfusion but, partly due to cost, it is yet to become common practice
- Iron supplements – oral or intravenous. Intravenous iron therapy will raise haemoglobin by 20–30 g/L in 5–10 days if the patient is iron deficient

Intraoperative and postoperative measures

- Restrictive versus liberal transfusion policies. There has been a move towards minimal transfusion in recent years with mounting evidence that patients who are transfusion restricted have lower morbidity, fewer infections and a reduced length of stay with fewer readmissions. The TRICC trial found overall reduced mortality using a threshold Hb of 70 g/L in the ICU setting
- Reduce blood loss: surgical techniques, such as laparoscopic surgery and equipment such as the harmonic scalpel have seen a reduction in perioperative blood loss. The CRASH-2 study supports tranexamic acid in major trauma to reduce transfusion requirements
- Perform standard safety checks for safe blood transfusion
- Consider cell salvage early
- Point-of-care testing; for example, thromboelastography can provide a real-time assessment of coagulation status and allow for targeted administration of appropriate blood products
- Aggressive correction of coagulopathy during massive blood transfusion. Recent evidence from the battlefield suggests a

ratio close to 1:1:1 for RBCs:FFP:platelets may be optimal. Although there is some controversy over whether this data can be extrapolated to the civilian operating theatre, it is currently accepted that FFP/platelets have historically been under-used in acute major haemorrhage

- Normothermia and treatment of metabolic acidosis, hyperkalaemia and hypocalcaemia (due to citrate toxicity) are essential for the optimum functioning of coagulation enzyme systems. Hypothermia will shift the oxygen dissociation curve to the left
- Early involvement of haematology department and consultant haematologist in massive haemorrhage management

Future trends

Haemoglobin substitutes such as perfluorocarbon emulsions and haemoglobin-based oxygen carriers (e.g. MP4) have been extensively researched for many years with some promising results. Limitations include anaphylaxis, undesirable vasoactive effects, accumulation in reticuloendothelial system and short half-lives. Despite ongoing phase 3 trials, there are, as yet, none approved for clinical use. More favourable results may be found in the future with biochemically engineered and stem-cell-derived red cells.

Further reading

The Association of Anaesthetists of Great Britain and Ireland. Blood transfusion and the anaesthetist Red cell transfusion. London; The Association of Anaesthetists of Great Britain and Ireland, 2008.
Carson JL, Terrin ML, Noveck H, et al. Liberal or restrictive transfusion in high-risk patients after hip surgery. N Engl J Med 2011; 365:2453–2462.

Serious Hazards of Transfusion (SHOT). Annual SHOT Report 2012. Manchester; SHOT, 2012.

Related topics of interest

- Blood physiology (p. 19)
- Obstetrics – emergencies (p. 160)

- Polytrauma (p. 217)

Burns

Key points

- Early burn mortality is usually due to inhalational injury or shock
- The principles of management of a major burn follow the ABC approach
- Particular care should be given to fluid balance. Potential massive redistribution and hypovolaemia require careful management
- Early intubation in the presence of airway burns is essential before airway oedema causes obstruction

In England and Wales, out of a total population of 56 million, 140,000 people present to emergency departments each year with burns injuries. Around 8000 are admitted to hospital, of whom 400 die.

The majority of early deaths are due to inhalational injuries or burn shock (a combination of hypovolaemic and distributive shock due to capillary leak and massive tissue damage). Delayed mortality is commonly due to sepsis or multiorgan failure. Risk factors of death include advanced age, larger surface area burn, inhalational injury and concurrent comorbidities. A significant improvement in mortality and morbidity can be achieved by prompt resuscitation, early surgical debridement and wound closure with an emphasis on prevention of complications.

Definition of a burn

- First-degree burn: affecting the epidermal layers; red, painful and dry without blisters
- Second-degree burn: involves the epidermal and dermal layers; divided into superficial or deep depending on the extent of damage to the dermis. Skin is red, blistered, oedematous and painful
- Third-degree (full thickness) burn: destruction of all layers of the skin, can reach into the underlying tissues. It appears white or leathery and is painless

A major burn is defined as follows:
- Full-thickness burn involving >10% total body surface area (TBSA)
- Partial-thickness burn involving >25% TBSA in adults or >20% in children or elderly

- Burns to the face, hands, perineum or feet
- Burns affecting a major joint
- Inhalational, chemical or electric burns

Initial assessment and resuscitation

The initial management of a burns patient should be approached using an ABCDE approach. Certain aspects are unique in burns patients:
- Airway. Patients should receive 100% oxygen. The airway should be managed with cervical spine immobilisation unless direct trauma can be excluded. Signs of inhalational burns include:
  - Burns to the face, lips or tongue
  - Singed facial hair
  - Swollen lips, tongue or pharynx
  - Signs of upper airway irritation or obstruction, e.g. coughing, wheezing or stridor
  - Soot in the nose, mouth or sputum

If present, early intubation with an uncut tracheal tube should be strongly considered. An awake fibreoptic or inhalational technique should be considered if evidence of airway oedema.

Pulse oximetry can be inaccurate even in severe hypoxia as standard pulse oximeters cannot distinguish between oxyhaemoglobin (HbO) and carboxyhaemoglobin (HbCO). Co-oximeters are available which use different light wavelengths to differentiate between HbO and HbCO. Arterial blood gas analysers may be required if a co-oximeter is not accessible. Haemoglobin binds carbon monoxide 250 times stronger than oxygen, leading to oxygen displacement from haemoglobin, a left shift in the oxygen dissociation curve and tissue hypoxia. Treatment with 100% oxygen will decrease the half-life of CO from 4 hours to <1 hour.

Inhalation of toxic substances, e.g. cyanide, ammonia or phosgene can cause severe airway irritation and swelling or act as specific poisons. Cyanide blocks mitochondrial aerobic respiration resulting in histotoxic hypoxia and a persistent lactic acidosis. Specific treatments include thiosulphate, dicobalt edetate or amyl nitrate.

- Breathing. This should be assessed clinically for equal chest movement and tracheal position. Blast injuries can cause lung contusions, tension pneumothoraces or diffuse alveolar trauma. Circumferential full-thickness burns to the chest may require escharotomy
- Circulation. Massive fluid shifts can occur with burn injuries leading to organ hypoperfusion. Adequate intravenous fluid resuscitation through large-bore peripheral cannulae is required for all burn victims with TBSA >15%. Venous access may be difficult to achieve using traditional access sites and lower extremity or femoral access is frequently required

The Parkland formula is used to estimate the fluid requirements for the initial 24 hours after the incident. The total amount of crystalloid required is calculated as follows:

$$4 \times TBSA \text{ burnt (in \%)} \times \text{patient weight (kg)}$$

The first half of this should be given during the first 8 hours, and the second half over the following 16 hours (as calculated from the time of the burn, rather than from the start of rehydration). Adequacy of fluid resuscitation should be assessed by hourly urine output of 30–50 mL/h in adults. Hartmann's solution is the fluid of choice.

Over-resuscitation can lead to devastating complications including acute lung injury, abdominal and peripheral compartment syndromes, multiorgan failure and death. Presence of concurrent injuries may necessitate a higher intravenous fluid requirement. It is unusual for hypovolaemic shock to be due to the burn itself and, if present, other causes such as bleeding or fractures should be sought.

There is now a significant body of evidence to suggest that use of colloid solutions (e.g. hydroxy-ethyl starches) carries a higher mortality than crystalloids.

- History. The pattern of expected injuries, the possibility of inhalational burns and the time elapsed since the burn. Location is important as inhalational injuries almost exclusively occur in enclosed spaces. The presence of noxious or flammable chemicals can create a safety risk for the medical personnel involved. This might be the only time when a full medical history is obtainable in a critically injured patient
- TBSA burn. The Wallace 'Rule of Nines' (**Figure 3**) is used to estimate the TBSA burn. This is then used as a guide to fluid resuscitation and an assessment of burn severity. It is important to expose the patient completely to ensure full assessment
- Analgesia. Burn injuries are painful. Opioid analgesia should be titrated to effect. Full-thickness burns are painless, but a mixture of partial- and full-thickness injury is common. NSAIDs are controversial due to possible renal hypoperfusion
- Metabolic changes. The euthermic body temperature is reset to 38.5°C after a major burn due to changes in the hypothalamic–pituitary–adrenal axis. Patients become hypermetabolic with an increase in oxygen consumption and carbon dioxide production. Early enteral feeding will maintain gut integrity and reduce bacterial translocation

Secondary management

Burn injuries should be managed by a multidisciplinary team in a dedicated burns unit.

- Debridement and skin grafting. Recent trends have focused on early debridement of the devitalised tissue and wound coverage. This aims to re-establish an effective barrier to infection and so prevent sepsis. Coverage is achieved using partial-thickness grafting from healthy skin or skin substitutes if healthy skin is unavailable. Novel therapies such as cultured epithelial autografts may, in the future, allow for grafting large surfaces without harvesting skin from healthy donor areas. The decision to perform early surgery can be difficult when faced with a patient with deteriorating physiology. Severe burns may be debrided in stages

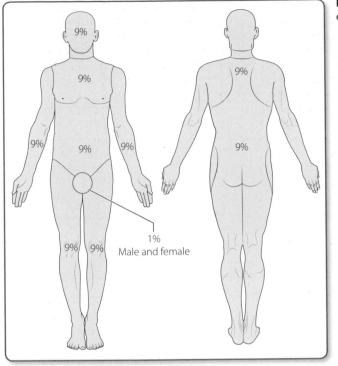

Figure 3 Wallace's rule of nines for estimation of percentage burn area.

according to the tolerance of surgical procedures. Escharotomy may be needed for full-thickness circumferential burns to maintain perfusion in distal compartments. The burnt skin constricts and acts as a tourniquet, especially as the underlying soft tissue becomes oedematous from the resuscitation efforts

- Management of infection and sepsis. Sepsis with multiorgan failure is the leading cause of death in burns patients. Diagnosis is problematic, as the usual diagnostic parameters are already raised by the inflammatory response. The routine culturing of sputum aspirates, wound swabs or urine samples can aid in the timely diagnosis of infections. The pharmacokinetics of many antibiotics are altered; e.g. the clearance of meropenem and vancomycin is increased

Anaesthetic management

Monitoring can be difficult due to lack of access to healthy skin. The ECG can be attached by crocodile clips to skin staples or subcutaneous needles. Pulse oximeters can be applied to alternative sites like earlobes, lips, tongue or the nose. Arterial lines are essential for major burns, as insidious and/or significant bleeding can be expected during debridement and skin grafting. Central venous access may only be possible by femoral or long lines. Burns patients are hypermetabolic and often require vasoactive support, thus assessment of haemodynamic changes is difficult.

Multiple procedures are the norm, and it is helpful to review previous anaesthetic charts. Patients often require escalating doses of analgesics. Morphine or mixed morphine/ketamine infusions are used in critical care to provide analgesia and neuropathic pain agents such as pregabalin should be considered. Regional anaesthesia can be helpful in smaller burns. A ketamine-based anaesthetic is ideal for dressing changes as it provides sufficient long-acting analgesia, whilst preserving airway reflexes.

Hypothermia is a constant hazard during surgical procedures. Careful maintenance of core body temperature can be achieved by warming theatre to 30–32°C and maintaining a high ambient humidity. The use of suxamethonium is contraindicated due to the massive potassium flux caused by extrajunctional acetylcholine receptors. This sensitivity is present from 24 hours up to a year after the injury.

Further reading

Bishop S, Maguire S. Anaesthesia and intensive care for major burns. Br J Anaesth: Contin Educ Anaesth, Crit Care Pain 2012; 12:118–122.

Kearns RD, Cairns CB, Holmes JH, et al. Thermal burn care: a review of best practices. EMS World 2013; 42:43–51.

Rex S. Burn injuries. Curr Opin Crit Care 2012; 18:671–676.

Related topics of interest

Cardiac anaesthesia – congenital heart disease

Key points

- The proportion of congenital heart disease patients surviving to adulthood is increasing
- Lesions are categorised into simple, moderate and severe – all but simple should be managed with specific tertiary centre input
- Those with pulmonary hypertension are at a markedly higher risk under anaesthesia than other patients in this group
- Congenital cardiac lesions are frequently associated with other congenital malformations

Approximately 7 per 1000 live births are complicated by congenital cardiac lesions, accounting for around one-third of all congenital abnormalities. The majority of these are corrected in infancy or early childhood but 10–15% are not diagnosed until adulthood. Even those who undergo repair have excess morbidity and mortality; requirements for revision surgery, heart failure, arrhythmias and persisting or residual defects may complicate anaesthesia for the grown-up congenital heart disease (GUCH) patient. Only the simplest procedures (e.g. ligation of patent ductus arteriosus) are associated with near-normal life expectancy (around a fifth of all GUCH patients); nearly half of patients have a significant reduction with 20% dying from sudden adult cardiac death (SACD) at an average age of 39 years and a further 25% dying on average at age 51 through heart failure.

Irrespective of this, the prognosis is much better than in the past and GUCH patients are an increasingly common population presenting for surgery.

Problems

- Cardiac
  - Lesion specific
  - Nonlesion specific
    - Heart failure
    - Arrhythmias including sudden arrhythmic cardiac death (SACD)
    - Pulmonary hypertension including Eisenmenger's syndrome
    - Systemic hypertension
    - Infective endocarditis
    - Factors surrounding implanted pacemakers/defibrillators
    - Effects on cardiac function related to IPPV
    - Effects relating to inotropic or vasoactive drugs
- Noncardiac
  - Issues surrounding anticoagulants and antiplatelet agents
  - Renal and urate metabolism abnormalities (in noncorrected cyanotic disease)
  - Concurrent abnormalities, e.g. features of trisomy 21
  - Depression and anxiety

Classification

To categorise lesions according to their broad management, they can be classified as simple, moderate or severe complexity (**Table 3**).

Investigations

These patients should undergo standard anaesthetic preassessment. This should include ECG and routine blood tests; full blood count, electrolytes and biochemistry and coagulation tests. Echocardiography should be considered and, where atrial thrombus is a risk, special consideration should be given to transoesophageal echocardiography. Permanent pacemakers and defibrillators should be checked within 3 months. Noncardiac comorbidities and other congenital malformations are common and must be elicited and further considered.

Anaesthetic management

For all but simple disease, consultation with the patient's specialist cardiologist is recommended prior to anaesthesia outside a tertiary centre. Those with severe disease should be considered for transfer to tertiary

Table 3 Classification of GUCH lesions		
	Examples	**Management**
Simple	Small VSD or ASD PFO Repaired PDA, ASD or VSD Congenital aortic stenosis	Should have adult cardiology review at least once following transition from paediatric care General Hospital anaesthesia care if discharged by cardiology
Moderate	Tetralogy of Fallot Ebstein's anomaly Coarctation of aorta Anomalous pulmonary venous drainage	Discuss with patient's tertiary specialist prior to General Hospital anaesthesia care
Complex	All cyanotic lesions All univentricular hearts All with duct or conduit repairs Pulmonary hypertension MV, TV or PV atresia Transposition of great vessels Eisenmenger's syndrome	Discuss with patient's tertiary specialist prior to General Hospital anaesthesia care Transfer to tertiary centre for most nonemergency procedures, especially with pulmonary hypertension

GUCH, grown-up congenital heart disease; MV/TV/PV, mitral/tricuspid/pulmonary valves; PDA, patent ductus arteriosus; PFO, patent foramen ovale; VSD/ASD, ventricular/atrial septal defect.

care for any surgical procedure except emergencies. These include those with a balanced circulation and univentricular or Fontan systems. In particular, those complicated by pulmonary hypertension are at very high risk (50% mortality risk). An appreciation and understanding of the anatomy of the underlying condition and, where applicable, of any repair is crucial to caring for these patients.

Special considerations

Pulmonary hypertension

- Can result in terminal right heart failure
- Results from increased PVR; therefore exacerbated by hypoxia, acidaemia, hypercarbia and high intrathoracic pressure
- Acute exacerbation resulting from suboptimal anaesthetic technique can obstruct Fontan/total cavopulmonary connections (TCPC), reverse left-right shunts (Eisenmenger's syndrome) or cause severe right ventricular failure
- 20% of Eisenmenger's syndrome mortality occurs during a medical procedure

Infective endocarditis

- Incidence is 15–140 times greater than in the noncongenital heart disease population (all age groups)

- 2009 European Society of Cardiology guidelines on infective endocarditis suggest prophylaxis only for GUCH patients with
  - Cyanotic lesions (unrepaired or repaired but with residual defects or prosthetic shunts/conduits)
  - Lesions repaired by any means employing prosthetic material within the last 6 months
  - Any lesion repaired with prosthetic material where there is a residual defect adjacent to the material
  - A history of infective endocarditis
- The only procedures now qualifying for prophylaxis in these groups are dental procedures involving gingival/periapical manipulation of a tooth or perforation of oral mucosa

Bleeding

- Patients are often taking antiplatelet agents and this may impact on regional anaesthesia possibilities and the likelihood of perioperative bleeding
- Decision to interrupt antiplatelet therapy and commencement of heparin bridging therapy should be made in conjunction with the surgeon and cardiologist; conduit/valvular obstruction or embolus may be catastrophic

- Platelet count is often reduced particularly in those with metal valves or associated chronic renal dysfunction

Fluids and heart failure

- High incidence of chronic heart failure with risk of acute decompensation
- Exacerbated by arrhythmias particularly atrial fibrillation
- Previous right ventriculotomy predisposes to arrhythmias
- Antiarrhythmic agents such as amiodarone should be used carefully (negative inotropy)
- Fluid must be titrated with careful assessment of filling status
- Fontan or TCPC for univentricular hearts depend on high CVP for entirely passive pulmonary inflow; PVR and left-sided pressures must be minimised and sinus rhythm maintained. CVP monitoring is mandatory

Shunt

- Prior to anaesthesia, establish the direction of any shunt present
- Prevent reversal of a left-to-right shunt or worsening of right-to-left shunt
- Maintain SVR and minimise increases in PVR
- Regional anaesthesia offers analgesia and reduced catecholamine release but risks SVR decrease
- Left-to-right shunt will delay intravenous induction onset, whilst a right-to-left shunt will delay the onset of inhalational anaesthesia

- Paradoxical embolus (clot, air, bone cement etc.) must be considered in light of the specific anatomy

Obstetric patients

- Cardiac disease is among the key causes of maternal death. In the UK, for example, it is both the highest indirect and overall cause of death. However, only around 10% of these deaths are amongst GUCH patients and this proportion has fallen steadily in the last 20 years
- Aortic stenosis (<1.5 cm^2 valve area), LVEF <40% and aortic root >4.5 cm carry up to 30% maternal mortality
- Arterial Spo_2<85% carries >88% risk of foetal loss
- Pulmonary hypertension carries the same mortality risk in labour as under anaesthesia (50%) and counselling against pregnancy as well as recommending termination are usual
- Early epidural use and assisted delivery avoid cardiac stress of pain, anxiety and 'pushing'
- Vaginal delivery is preferable but if indicated, caesarean may be undertaken with regional or general anaesthesia with appropriate monitoring and control of pulmonary and systemic vasculature
- Bleeding is a particular risk especially with antiplatelet therapy
- Avoid ergometrine or bolus-dose oxytocin
- Postpartum cardiomyopathy may necessitate extended inpatient monitoring

Further reading

Cove Point Foundation. Congenital heart disease, list of topics. http://www.pted.org/?id=list#4.

Kelleher A. Adult congenital heart disease (grown-up congenital heart disease). Br J Anaesth: Contin Educ Anaesth, Crit Care Pain 2012; 12:28–32.

The Task Force on the Prevention, Diagnosis, and Treatment of Infective Endocarditis of the European Society of Cardiology (ESC). Guidelines on the prevention, diagnosis, and treatment of infective endocarditis. Eur Heart J 2009; 30:2369–3413.

Related topics of interest

Cardiac anaesthesia – valvular heart disease

Key points

- Echocardiography is important to assess type and severity of the valvular disorder
- Important issues include cardiac rhythm and rate, circulatory control, anticoagulation and antibiotics
- Screening echocardiography may be warranted in some patient groups

Although less common than ischaemic heart disease, valvular heart disease has a reported prevalence of 2.5% in developed countries. It is predominantly a disease of the elderly with >13% of those over the age of 75 having moderate or severe disease. In the developing world, where rheumatic fever is still widespread, younger adults are at increased risk. Increasingly, patients treated for congenital heart lesions in childhood are presenting for noncardiac surgery later in life and associated valvular problems may then need to be considered.

Problems

- Lesion-specific cardiovascular ramifications (see below)
- Risk of infective endocarditis (IE)
- Anticoagulation: if and when to stop preoperatively and implications for regional anaesthesia
- Regional anaesthesia considerations directly related to valve lesion

Clinical features

A full cardiovascular history should be taken with particular reference to symptoms of cardiac failure, syncope and angina.

Examination should include cardiac auscultation and other stigmata of valvular disease should be actively sought, e.g. the malar flush of mitral stenosis (MS) or the collapsing pulse of aortic regurgitation (AR). In one study of patients presenting for emergency hip fracture surgery, 70% of those with clinically detected murmurs had proven lesions on echocardiography. Furthermore, 30% of patients with no clinically detectable murmur at initial assessment were subsequently shown to have valve lesions on echo. Lesions can be graded echocardiographically (e.g. **Table 4** for stenotic lesions). Specific features of individual lesions are discussed later.

Investigations

An ECG should be performed to look for signs of ventricular hypertrophy and rhythm abnormalities. In general, new murmurs, or murmurs associated with symptoms, merit echocardiological assessment and subsequent referral to the cardiology service for further treatment where necessary. Murmurs associated with cardiac failure are of particular concern and are associated with higher surgical mortality. Routine preoperative testing (blood tests, pulmonary function tests) should be ordered according to usual criteria. A coagulation screen is essential for those on warfarin or other such agents.

Anaesthetic management

The details of perioperative management are dependent on the type of valvular lesion

Table 4 Echocardiological criteria for definition of severe stenotic disease			
	Aortic stenosis	Mitral stenosis	Tricuspid stenosis
Valve area (cm²)	<1.0	<1.0	<1.0
Indexed valve area (cm²/m²)	<0.6	–	–
Mean gradient (mmHg)	>40	>10	≥5
Maximum jet velocity (m/s)	>4.0	–	–
Velocity ratio	<0.25	–	–

present. In the case of mixed valve lesions, the predominant lesion should be prioritised. It is useful to consider the intraoperative management in terms of control of the patient's preload, contractility, afterload, cardiac rate and cardiac rhythm.

Aortic stenosis (AS)

This is usually degenerative in aetiology and classically presents with angina, syncope and symptoms of left ventricular failure. In moderate or severe disease, invasive arterial pressure monitoring should be instituted prior to induction of anaesthesia. The primary aim of cardiovascular management is to maintain systemic vascular resistance within tight limits in order to maintain the aortic root pressure. For this reason, central neuroaxial blockade should be approached with extreme caution in severe AS. Adequate preload is needed to maintain stroke volume, and maintenance of sinus rhythm capitalises on the contribution of atrial kick to ventricular filling. Tachycardia should be avoided to allow for diastolic coronary artery perfusion as well as adequate ventricular filling. Bradycardia may also be catastrophic as with a limited ventricular ejection, patients are often reliant on heart rate to preserve an adequate cardiac output.

Aortic regurgitation (AR)

AR is often secondary to a bicuspid aortic valve and usually presents as left sided heart failure. A regurgitant fraction of >60% represents severe AR. The principle of anaesthetic management of AR is to maintain forward flow through the aortic valve by minimising the regurgitant fraction. To this end, systemic vascular resistance may be allowed to fall, and heart rate is best maintained in the range 80–100 beats per minute (bpm) to reduce the time for regurgitation. Adequate preload should be ensured and sinus rhythm should be maintained to optimise ventricular filling.

Mitral stenosis (MS)

This lesion is becoming less frequent in developed countries as the incidence of rheumatic fever decreases but is still common in the developing world. It is associated with other valvular lesions in >50% of cases (often MR, but also AS). In severe MS, maintenance of sinus rhythm is key as ventricular filling is more reliant on active atrial contraction. Maintaining adequate preload is important as is the avoidance of tachycardia to ensure time for flow from left atria to ventricle.

Mitral regurgitation (MR)

MR most commonly results from dilated cardiomyopathy (causing dilation of the valve annulus) or ischaemic damage to the papillary muscles. In common with MS, it is also sometimes seen following rheumatic fever. As in AR, the main haemodynamic aim is to avoid increased afterload and aim for a heart rate of 80–100 bpm to reduce time for diastolic filling and reduce overfilling of the left ventricle (and the subsequent annular dilatation).

Other valvular lesions

Pulmonary valve lesions are usually congenital in nature, whilst tricuspid regurgitation is almost always functional (i.e. secondary to right ventricular dilatation or pulmonary hypertension). It is worth considering that patients with pulmonary and tricuspid lesions will very commonly have associated pulmonary pathology. This may be as a result of the valve lesion itself, or the valve lesion may be secondary to a primary lung pathology. In all such cases, a comprehensive respiratory history and examination should be performed and lung function tests arranged.

Replacement valves

Valve replacements may be broadly defined as tissue or metallic. Careful assessment should be made of the patient's functional status, and the reason for the replacement should be sought. Given that these valves have a limited lifespan, the results of a recent echo should be available. It is also important to consider any anticoagulants the patient may be taking. Patients with metallic valves often have high target INRs (3–4), and will need bridging heparin anticoagulation therapy around the time of surgery. Consultation with the patient's cardiologist is strongly advised.

Antibiotic prophylaxis for infective endocarditis (IE)

There are specific guidelines for antibiotic prophylaxis against IE, for example the UK NICE guidance (CG64) which characterises the following groups as being 'at risk':

- Acquired valvular heart disease with stenosis or regurgitation
- Valve replacement
- Structural congenital heart disease, including surgically corrected or palliated structural conditions, but excluding isolated atrial septal defect, fully repaired ventricular septal defect or fully repaired patent ductus arteriosus, and closure devices that are judged to be endothelialised
- Previous IE
- Hypertrophic cardiomyopathy

Antibiotic prophylaxis for IE is not recommended for mitral valve prolapse. Prophylaxis is not recommended for patients undergoing upper or lower GI endoscopies, bladder procedures or childbirth. Despite these recommendations, many patients will expect antibiotic prophylaxis based on previous guidelines and a degree of pragmatism is needed in their management.

Further reading

Frogel J, Galusca D. Anesthetic considerations for patients with advanced valvular heart disease undergoing noncardiac surgery. Anesthesiol Clin 2010; 28:67–85.

Mittnacht AJC, Fanshawe M, Konstadt S. Anesthetic considerations in the patient with valvular heart disease undergoing non-cardiac surgery. Semin Cardiothorac Vasc Anesth 2008; 12:33–59.

National Institute for Health & Care Excellence. Prophylaxis against infective endocarditis. London: NICE, 2008.

Related topics of interest

- Cardiac surgery (p. 43)
- Coronary artery disease (p. 47)
- Venous thromboembolism – prevention and treatment (p. 320)

Cardiac dysrhythmia

Key points

- Dysrhythmia is common during anaesthesia and may be due to patient, surgical or anaesthetic factors
- Treatment of malignant arrhythmias should centre on eliminating the cause, terminating the arrhythmia and maintaining organ perfusion
- Synchronised direct current (DC) cardioversion may be required in the compromised patient

Although most dysrhythmias occurring during anaesthesia require little intervention, serious arrhythmias can occur and need urgent treatment. Certain stimuli tend to cause specific arrhythmias.

Types of dysrhythmia

- Supraventricular. Sinus bradycardia (usually due to vagal stimulation or drugs), sinus tachycardia, ectopic beats, atrial flutter, atrial fibrillation (AF), junctional tachycardia
- Ventricular. Ventricular ectopics, idioventricular rhythm (the ventricular muscle underlying rhythm, around 40 bpm), ventricular tachycardia, ventricular fibrillation
- Conduction problems. Sick sinus syndrome, sinus arrest, first- and second-degree heart blocks (Wenckebach/Mobitz 1; progressively longer PR intervals followed by a nonconducted P-wave. Mobitz 2; regular failure of A-V conduction, e.g. 2:1 or 3:1. Mobitz 2 block is more likely to progress to complete heart block). Third-degree heart block, bundle branch blocks. Trifascicular block (long PR, left axis deviation, RBBB) may progress to third-degree block necessitating perioperative pacing
- Asystole
- Pulseless electrical activity (PEA) (formerly electromechanical dissociation)

Preoperative causes

- Pre-existing cardiac lesions, ischaemic heart disease (IHD), valvular heart disease, cardiomyopathy
- Endocrine disorders, e.g. hyperthyroidism (AF or sinus tachycardia), phaeochromocytoma
- Drugs, e.g. beta-blockers, digoxin and tricyclics
- Acid–base disorders and electrolyte disturbance, e.g. hypokalaemia (ventricular ectopics), hyperkalaemia (asystole)
- Anxiety (endogenous catecholamine driven)
- Raised ICP (bradycardia indicates end-stage disease)

Perioperative causes

- Anaesthetic causes
  - Depth of anaesthesia (too light or deep)
  - Hypoxia (especially in children) or hypercarbia
  - Hypo/hyperthermia
  - Hypo/hypertension
  - Laryngeal stimulation (vagal response)
  - CVP line insertion
  - Drugs: volatile agents, suxamethonium, local anaesthetics with epinephrine, remifentanil. Effects are often compounded by polypharmacy
- Surgical causes
  - Stimulation, especially of the eye (oculocardiac reflex), carotid body, throat, peritoneum (especially pneumoperitoneum), anus and cervix. All generally lead to vagus-mediated bradycardia
  - Diathermy and pacemakers
  - Manipulation of endocrine tumours (phaeochromocytoma and carcinoid)
  - Intraoperative crises, e.g. air embolism (usually PEA), pulmonary embolism, myocardial infarction, intracranial bleeding and pneumothorax
- Postoperative causes
  - Hypoxia
  - Pain
  - Residual effects of perioperative drugs

Perioperative management

Prior to elective surgery, stabilisation or correction of the arrhythmia should be undertaken if possible. Antiarrhythmic therapy is continued until surgery. This is not possible with urgent surgery, where a more pragmatic approach must be taken and risk–benefit decision made with some attempt at rate control. As with all perioperative crises, an initial ABC approach should be taken.

Treatment should centre on elimination of the cause (stop surgical stimulation, check electrolytes, correct hypercarbia etc.) and specific treatment of the arrhythmia. Immediate treatment, such as DC cardioversion, is required if there are signs of circulatory compromise or cardiac ischaemia (e.g. tachyarrhythmia with IHD). The resuscitation council regularly updates its guidelines on the management of tachyarrhythmia and advanced cardiac life support. The most recent guidelines can be found at www.resus.org.uk.

Invasive monitoring should be considered, although some cardiac output monitors perform badly in the presence of arrhythmia. Beta-blockers and calcium antagonists can interact with volatile agents with a resultant hypotension and reduced cardiac output. Cardiology advice should be sought for complex arrhythmias, e.g. Wolf-Parkinson-White syndrome with AF.

Postoperative care

A new serious rhythm disturbance may necessitate admission to a critical care or coronary care bed and further investigation, e.g. cardiac enzymes, ECG and echocardiography.

Cardioversion

Although commonly performed semielectively to convert AF to sinus rhythm, DC cardioversion may be required in the emergency setting for atrial or ventricular dysrhythmias. Chronic AF carries a yearly stroke risk of up to 5% dependent on other cardiac risk factors. Anticoagulation reduces the risk by 60%, but increases the risk of intracranial haemorrhage, especially in the elderly.

DC cardioversion causes depolarisation of a proportion of cardiac cells, rendering them refractory, thus allowing the sinoatrial node to regain control as the pacemaker. Cardioversion is more likely to be successful if acidosis and hypokalaemia are corrected and AF is of new onset. Success can also be increased by administration of antiarrhythmic medication. The patient should be anticoagulated or within 48 hours of AF onset to minimise the risk of emboli.

Anaesthetic management for elective cardioversion

- Preoperative: elicit a detailed cardiac history and correct electrolytes and coagulation status
- Conduct of anaesthesia: careful titration of induction agent is more important than the choice of agent itself. Small doses of midazolam have minimal effect on cardiac output, but will prolong sedation beyond the procedure. Ketamine should be avoided. Etomidate provides cardiac stability, but there is overwhelming evidence regarding adrenocortical suppression, even with single doses. Propofol, either by infusion or judicious bolus doses, can provide a relatively cardiac stable course and a rapid emergence. Opiates are generally not required
- Countershock should be delivered at the end of expiration (lowest thoracic impedance) and synchronised with the R-wave as delivery at the peak of the T-wave can induce VF/VT. Low-energy shocks are less likely to succeed, thus an energy level of 200 J should be selected. Success is unlikely following two failed attempts. Post-shock myocardial depression may occasionally be seen but tends to resolve with the increase in cardiac output. Respiratory acidosis should be avoided as it may provoke arrhythmia

Further reading

Resuscitation Council (UK). The resuscitation guidelines 2010. London; Resuscitation Council, 2010.

Related topics of interest

Cardiac pacemakers

Key points

- Electromagnetic interference (EMI), especially the use of surgical diathermy, can cause changes in pacemaker behaviour, inappropriate pacing or defibrillation
- Use of magnets to modify pacemaker function can be unpredictable
- The implanted cardioverter defibrillator (ICD) function of a pacemaker should be disabled preoperatively
- Backup external pacing should always be available

Implanted cardiac pacemakers and ICDs are increasingly common devices found in patients presenting for surgery. Technological advances have led to an increasingly wide range and complexity of implants, although the generic 5-letter coding system helps classify their function (**Table 5**).

In the elective setting, it is essential for a clear plan to be made in advance of surgery, tailored to the individual and proposed operation. This will include clarification of a number of factors (**Table 6**). In the emergency setting, however, some of this information may not be available and so it is important that all anaesthetists are familiar with basic pacemaker technology and are able to provide safe perioperative care to these patients.

The main issues in managing patients with these devices relate to the underlying cardiac condition and the potential for EMI in the operative environment (**Table 7**). EMI can affect the pacemaker's function and, where an ICD is present, can potentially trigger inappropriate defibrillation. Surgical diathermy poses the greatest risk of EMI, although advances in pacemaker technology have reduced their vulnerability to EMI. The effect of a clinical magnet over the pacemaker varies between different devices and should not be relied upon as the sole management strategy (**Table 5**).

Table 5 British Pacing and Electrophysiology Group (BPEG) pacemaker code				
Pacing	**Sensing**	**Response**	**Rate modulation**	**Multiuse pacing**
A = atrium V = ventricle D = dual (A and V)	A = atrium V = ventricle D = dual (A and V) O = none	I = inhibited T = triggered D = dual O = none	R = rate modulating O = none	A = atrium V = ventricle D = dual (A and V) O = none

Table 6 Preoperative clarification of pacemaker and ICD status
Date and indication for implant
Degree of pacemaker dependency
Presence or absence of ICD functionality
Implant complexity (bradycardia control, cardiac resynchronisation therapy)
Most recent battery and device functionality check
Determining whether significant electromagnetic interference will be present intraoperatively
Determining whether reprogramming of device functionality is required (e.g. rate modulation function)
ICD, implanted cardioverter defibrillator.

Table 7 Potential sources for intraoperative EMI
Surgical diathermy (particularly monopolar)
Nerve stimulator and evoked potential monitors
Lithotripsy
Fasciculation and shivering
Electroconvulsive therapy
Magnetic resonance imaging
EMI, electromagnetic interference.

Problems

- Effects of EMI: EMI can cause the pacemaker either to inhibit its pacing function (if the interference is sensed as cardiac activity) or may revert the pacemaker to its backup fixed-rate mode (if the interference is seen as background noise)
- EMI with an ICD: Where an ICD is present, EMI may result in inappropriate cardiac defibrillation, thus the ICD function should be deactivated perioperatively
- Tissue heating at lead tips: EMI energy can be introduced into the pacemaker lead systems, causing tissue heating at the lead tips and subsequent tissue damage. This risk is increased with increasing duration of EMI and its proximity to the device leads
- Factors affecting pacemaker capture: Hypoxaemia, hypo/hypercarbia, acidosis, electrolyte abnormalities and drugs may influence pacemaker capture and so it is important to control against these during anaesthesia

Anaesthetic management

Preoperative

In the elective setting, it is essential that patients who have a permanent pacemaker or ICD are identified in advance. Many organisations now include a specific question regarding pacemakers in the preoperative checklist. Careful planning with the surgical team should address the need for equipment that may cause EMI, in particular surgical diathermy and lithotripsy. As a minimum, a detailed preoperative evaluation should clarify the factors listed in **Table 6**. Most guidelines recommend the pacemaker should be checked within 3 months of surgery for function and battery life.

Routine investigations should include a 12-lead ECG (to look for underlying rhythm and pacing capture), a chest X-ray (which will show lead placement and may indicate lead damage) and blood tests, including electrolyte levels.

Most pacemakers will not need reprogramming preoperatively but the following points should be noted:

- Pacemaker-dependent patients who will be exposed to significant EMI should have their device reprogrammed to an asynchronous mode prior to surgery
- Rate modulation should be suspended for devices that use the minute ventilation method of physiological pacing
- Devices with an ICD function should be reprogrammed to a 'monitor only' mode to prevent inappropriate shock delivery due to EMI
- Devices with a 'sleep mode' should have this deactivated if late surgery is planned (**Table 6**)

Intraoperative

There must be a backup source of pacing and defibrillation immediately available for all these patients. In addition to routine monitoring, the use of direct invasive arterial blood pressure monitoring has the added benefit of giving beat-to-beat evidence of mechanical capture. Care should be taken when using central venous and pulmonary artery catheters due to the risk of dislodging the pacemaker electrodes.

Most anaesthetic drugs and techniques are appropriate, and it is not thought that modern anaesthetic agents affect the capture threshold. However, physiological disturbances, such as hypoxaemia, hypo- or hypercarbia, acidosis and high concentrations of local anaesthetic agents can do so. The use of succinylcholine should be avoided to reduce the chances of inappropriate sensing from fasciculation.

Potential sources for EMI should be considered (**Table 7**). The most common issue arises from the use of electrical diathermy. If required, bipolar diathermy is preferable to monopolar. If this is not possible, the diathermy ground plate should be placed as far away from the pacemaker as possible (**Table 7**).

Use of pacemaker magnets is unpredictable and advice for their use remains controversial. Regarding ICDs, a magnet will generally suspend the ICD function (whilst the magnet is present over the device), although some pacemakers can be programmed to ignore magnet application. For pacemakers, magnet application will not necessarily guarantee asynchronous (nonsensing) pacing.

Postoperative

After surgery, the patient needs to be monitored with immediate backup pacing available until the device has been restored to baseline.

A formal postoperative check is required if there is

- Preoperative reprogramming of the device
- Intraoperative use of a magnet
- Significant haemodynamic instability
- Perioperative external pacing or defibrillation
- Emergency surgery where preoperative checks were not possible

Further reading

Diprose P, Pierce T. Anaesthesia for patients with pacemakers and similar devices. Br J Anaesth: Contin Educ Prof Develop Rev 2001;166-170.

MHRA: Guideline for the perioperative management of patients with implantable pacemakers or implantable cardioverter defibrillators, where the use of surgical diathermy/electrocautery is anticipated. London; Medicines and Healthcare Products Regulatory Agency, 2006.

Stone ME, Salter B, Fisher A. Peri-operative management of patients with cardiac implantable electronic devices. Br J Anaesth 2011; 107:i16–i26.

Related topics of interest

- Cardiac dysrhythmia (p. 37)

Cardiac surgery

Key points

- Increasingly comorbid patients are presenting for cardiac and repeat cardiac surgery due to advances in care
- Risk stratification is vital in case selection
- Cardiopulmonary bypass (CPB) has important physiological and pathophysiological consequences

There are a large number of cardiac surgeries performed in different countries every year. For example, approximately 35,000 cardiac operations are performed each year in the UK. Over the last 10 years there has been an overall improvement in mortality for cardiac surgery (**Table 8**). The proportion of patients >75 years has increased to >20% and a greater number have significant comorbidities increasing surgical risk and mortality for some specific procedures. Many cardiac patients now present for revision or second surgery. Most of these changes reflect an increase in the quality of surgical and anaesthetic in-patient care given to these patients.

Risk stratification and informed consent are important components of cardiac surgery. The EUROSCORE-2 is used in European countries to establish expected mortality rates.

Problems

Cardiovascular

The underlying cardiovascular disease can lead to changes in the electromechanical and electrophysiological function of the heart. Ventricular function can be compromised due to chronic disease processes (e.g. valvular disease) or acute changes (e.g. ischaemia/infarction). Electrical conduction may be impaired, leading to arrhythmias.

Respiratory

Pre-existing respiratory problems can be compounded by the effects of surgery and CPB. The large mediastinal wound and presence of pericardial, mediastinal and pleural drains can all hinder return of normal respiratory function in the postoperative period. Poor postoperative myocardial function, combined with increased fluid loads, can lead to pulmonary oedema and a need for prolonged respiratory support. Patients can develop acute respiratory distress syndrome as a result of the inflammatory response to CPB.

Neurological

Type of surgery, increasing age, hypotension and pre-existing cerebrovascular disease all contribute to the risk of stroke (2–9%). Minor complications such as confusion and behavioural changes are common. Significant events may relate to cerebral hypoxia or embolic events (plaque rupture, air or debris). Intraoperative ultrasound can help to identify aortic plaques prior to aortic cannulation. Transoesophageal echocardiography (TOE) can be used to look for gas emboli prior to coming off CPB. Transcranial near-infrared spectroscopy can be used to monitor cerebral oxygenation during CPB.

Table 8 Mortality for cardiac surgery		
Operation	2002 Mortality (%)	2011 Mortality (%)
All cardiac surgery	3.58	2.97
Isolated first time CABG	1.92	1.41
Isolated first time AVR	2.91	1.49
Isolated first time MV repair	1.3	1.21
Isolated first time MV replacement	5.09	3.94
Mitral valve replacement and CABG	10.7	12.03
CABG, coronary artery bypass grafting; AVR, aortic valve replacement; MV, mitral valve.		

Endocrine

Diabetes increases mortality risk in EUROSCORE-2. Blood sugars should be controlled perioperatively to decrease the risk of infection, poor wound healing, myocardial infarction, stroke and arrhythmias.

Renal

Acute kidney injury affects 50% of patients following surgery, especially those with chronic kidney disease. Its pathophysiology is unclear but probably relates to hypoperfusion, nephrotoxins (haemolysis on CPB) and the inflammatory response to CPB. Approximately 2–4% will require renal replacement therapy postoperatively.

Antiplatelet therapy

Patients with previous stents or critical left main stem disease may remain on antiplatelet therapy up to the time of surgery. Use of thromboelastography and platelet mapping will help direct blood product use post-CPB.

Cardiopulmonary bypass

Although some procedures are now performed 'off-pump' to reduce the associated risks and complexities, CPB remains the commonest way to perform most procedures. Blood is drained from the venous circulation, passes through a heat exchanger and oxygenator and finally returns to the arterial circulation directly into the aorta (or femoral artery), thus bypassing the heart and lungs (**Figure 4**). Exposure of the blood to the roller pumps and air interfaces of the bypass machine leads to a systemic inflammatory response and can also affect platelet function. Newer, mini-CPB circuits have centrifugal pumps, smaller priming volume and minimal blood air interfaces which theoretically limit the inflammatory response and platelet dysfunction.

Cooling reduces the metabolic rate and oxygen demand of the cells. In addition to this, cold cardioplegia (all types being rich in potassium but vary significantly in other respects) is infused into the coronary circulation to arrest the heart in diastole providing further myocardial protection. In aortic arch surgery, deep hypothermic circulatory arrest (DHCA) may be employed to offer maximal organ protection from hypoperfusion during the fall in cardiac output. Adjuvant drugs such as thiopentone

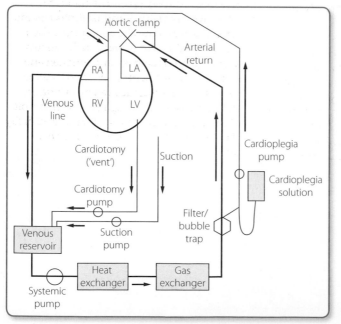

Figure 4 Conventional cardiopulmonary bypass circuit.

may also be given during DHCA to maximise cerebral protection.

Anaesthetic management

Preoperative

Cardiac preassessment clinics are now commonplace in many hospitals. This allows coordinated investigation into the cause and significance of coronary, cardiac and valvular disease. Investigations include MRI, CT and chest X-rays, angiography, echocardiography and pulmonary function tests. A thorough understanding of the severity of the disease is essential to providing appropriate monitoring and drug therapy during induction of anaesthesia.

Intraoperative

Blood pressure and oxygen supply and demand can all be affected by induction. Most patients will have had been premedicated with a benzodiazepine and supplemental oxygen prior to leaving the ward for surgery. This helps reduce the effects of anxiety on heart rate and blood pressure. Monitoring is established with 5-lead ECG, pulse oximetry and noninvasive blood pressure. Large-bore intravenous access and arterial lines are inserted. Patients with poor cardiac function may require a central line for inotropes or vasopressors prior to induction. There is no definitive opinion of which induction agent to use and no current evidence to prove any one agent is superior. However, desflurane and ketamine should be avoided due to increased risk of myocardial ischaemia. A clear understanding of the effect the induction agent will have on the cardiovascular system is vital. Most techniques combine a medium-to-high dose opiate (e.g. fentanyl, 10–100 µg/kg) with another agent such as propofol, thiopentone or etomidate.

Following induction, the inevitable fall in systemic vascular resistance (SVR) can be reversed with small doses of vasopressors such as metaraminol or phenylephrine. Valvular lesions require specific management to minimise the effects of regurgitant or stenotic valves in order to maintain the cardiac output. In general, regurgitant lesions require SVR reduction and a heart rate 80–100, whilst stenotic lesions require maintenance of SVR and heart rate 60–80.

TOE is an increasingly common technique for intraoperative management. It is valuable for ventricular assessment, visualisation of residual air towards the end of CPB and, particularly, assessment of the success of valvular procedures allowing intraoperative adjustment. In theatre, there are key stages that are summarised in **Table 9**.

Postoperative

Following surgery the patient is transferred to the cardiac intensive care unit (CICU) for ongoing support. Once the patient is warm (>36ºC), cardiac output is adequate and stable, respiratory function is satisfactory with adequate gas exchange, there is no ongoing bleeding, the haemoglobin is stable, the electrolytes are within normal limits and the patient is neurologically appropriate, then extubation should be considered. Patients with good preoperative heart function and uncomplicated surgery may be considered 'fast-track' patients; they can be extubated and transferred to the high dependency unit within 6 hours. This maximises the availability of CICU beds and throughput of cardiac cases.

Table 9 Intraoperative phases of open cardiac surgery		
Stage	Surgical activity	Anaesthetic consideration
Pre-bypass	Sternotomy Opening of pericardium. Dissection of arterial graft (e.g. left internal mammary, radial artery) Venous graft harvesting Cannulation of the aorta (or femoral artery) and vena cava Handling the heart	Ensuring all IV lines are accessible and patent Ensure ventilation and maintenance of anaesthesia Maintain oxygen supply and minimise demand Deflation of lungs to reduce the risk of damage to the pericardium/right ventricle during sternotomy Transoesophageal echo Heparin (300 IU/kg) to achieve an activated clotting time (ACT) of >400 seconds Systolic blood pressure <100 mmHg during cannulation of the aorta
Bypass	Revascularisation using artery or vein graft Replacement or repair of valve Other surgical procedure	Maintain anaesthesia with propofol infusion Set monitors and alarms to CPB mode Discuss with surgeons a plan for weaning from bypass
Post-bypass	Haemostasis Insertion of temporary pacing wires Insertion of drains to pericardium/mediastinum/pleura Closure of chest	Prior to coming off bypass check: Temperature Electromechanical activity (+/− pacing) Ventilation on 100% oxygen Haemoglobin Potassium/electrolytes within normal range Vasopressors (e.g. noradrenaline), vasodilators (e.g. GTN), inotropes (e.g. adrenaline, dopamine, dopexamine) Consider intra-aortic balloon pump augmentation if unable to wean from CPB Communicate clearly with the surgeons and perfusionist regarding performance of the heart and fluid filling once off bypass Monitor for arrhythmias, e.g. AF or VF Slowly give 1 mg of protamine for every 100 IU heparin used (risk of hypotension, especially with fast injection). Inform the perfusionist when giving (pumps must be turned off to prevent clots in the bypass system). On occasion, the patient will need to go back on to bypass due to bleeding, hypotension, low cardiac output, graft occlusion Reassess ACT Thromboelastogram to assess clotting function and target blood product use

CPB, cardiopulmonary bypass; AF, atrial fibrillation; VF, ventricular fibrillation; GTN, intravenous nitrate

Further reading

National Confidential Enquiry into Patient Outcome and Death (NCEPOD). Death following a first time, isolated coronary artery bypass graft; The heart of the matter. London: NCEPOD, 2008.

Preisman S, Kogan A, Itzkovsky K, et al. Modified thromboelastography evaluation of platelet dysfunction in patients undergoing coronary artery surgery. Eur J Cardiothorac Surg 2010; 37:1367–1374.

Roques F, Michel P, Goldstone AR, et al. The logistic EuroSCORE. Eur Heart J 2003; 24:882–883.

Society for Cardiothoracic Surgery in Great Britain & Ireland. Blue Book Online. [Online]http://bluebook.scts.org [2014].

Related topics of interest

Coronary artery disease

Key points

- Ischaemic heart disease is a frequent cause of perioperative morbidity and mortality
- Coronary artery disease is considered as an inflammatory process
- Cardiac risk continues well into the postoperative period with significant events commonly occurring in the days following surgery
- Perioperative care should centre on minimising surgical stress and optimising oxygen supply and demand

Ischaemic heart disease is the single largest cause of death worldwide according to 2012 WHO mortality data. It represents 12.7% of global mortality. Risk factors include increasing age, male gender, smoking, hypertension, diabetes, hypercholesterolaemia and a positive family history. Coronary events include angina, unstable angina, non ST-elevation myocardial infarction (NSTEMI) and ST-elevation myocardial infarction (STEMI); each has an increasingly worse prognosis.

Sixty per cent of patients who die within 30 days of surgery have evidence of coronary artery disease. Broadly speaking, stable angina, effectively treated, carries a relatively small perioperative risk; however, unstable or new angina carries a much greater risk of morbidity.

Pathology

Atherosclerosis is now recognised as an inflammatory disease with macrophages and T-lymphocytes playing a key role. Atheromatous plaques in the coronary arteries may cause sufficient stenosis of the artery lumen to reduce flow, often presenting as stable angina. Acute coronary syndrome (ACS) results from plaque rupture or erosion often in previously nonobstructing plaque. The ruptured plaque provides a stimulus for thrombosis and platelet aggregation. Myocardial damage will ensue if the vessel is occluded by thrombus. ACS may also be precipitated by an increase in circulating prothrombotic or antifibrinolytic mediators in the blood (e.g. as seen in the stress response to surgery).

Myocardial oxygenation is a product of arterial oxygen content and coronary blood flow and oxygen extraction. Arterial oxygen content is dependent on haemoglobin and its saturation. Coronary perfusion pressure is dependent on the difference between systemic diastolic pressure and the left ventricular end-diastolic pressure (LVEDP). Oxygen extraction is dependent on heart rate, contractility, muscle mass and wall tension.

Coronary blood flow at 250 mL/min, occurs mostly in diastole. Myocardial oxygen consumption is high, even at rest (10 mL/100g/min) and, despite an oxygen extraction ratio of 75%, any increased demand can only be met by an increase in flow. Perioperative ischaemic events may be due to reduced flow through a pre-existing stenotic lesion (e.g. due to systemic hypotension), or due to primary plaque rupture exacerbated by a prothrombotic haematological state.

Problems

- Coexisting morbidities such as diabetes mellitus and peripheral vascular disease
- Myocardial oxygen supply may be affected by other noncardiac factors such as haematocrit, systemic blood pressure or lung disease
- Anaesthesia and surgery may alter the myocardial supply:demand ratio with an increase in sympathetic drive, increase in arrhythmia and reduction in body temperature
- Antianginal medications may exacerbate the cardiovascular effects of anaesthetic agents or interact with coadministered drugs
- Previous myocardial infarction within the last 3 months is associated with a high risk of reinfarction
- Previous coronary grafts usually carry a low risk of myocardial infarction, although systemic hypotension should be avoided to prevent graft thrombosis
- Coronary angioplasty and stents. Cardiac risk remains high in the early post-stent

period (<6 months). In fact one study revealed a 42% risk of perioperative cardiac event if operated on within 6 weeks of stenting. Dual antiplatelet therapy is mandatory after placement and discontinuation requires careful consideration. Bare-metal stents carry a higher in-stent restenosis rate and require a minimum of 4-week antiplatelet therapy. Drug eluting stents are less likely to restenose but require up to 12 months antiplatelet therapy (due to delayed stent endothelialisation). Elective surgery should be deferred during these time periods and antiplatelet therapy should be continued where possible. Overall perioperative stent thrombosis rate is around 2%

Anaesthetic management

- Preoperative risk stratification. Cardiac risk should be defined prior to surgery. Exercise or dobutamine stress echocardiography is useful screening tool for coronary ischaemia and may necessitate angiography. Use of scoring systems allows for informed consent and more rational risk assessment. The Lee cardiac index generates a percentage risk, based on the following factors: high-risk surgery, ischaemic heart disease, insulin-treated diabetes, history of congestive cardiac failure (history of stroke and renal impairment. The surgical procedure itself significantly affects cardiac risk, e.g. vascular surgery conferring a >5% risk of cardiac morbidity
- Preoperative therapy. Current recommendations support the continuation of beta-blocker therapy in patients already taking them. However, there is controversy over perioperative beta-blocker use following publication of the POISE trial in 2008, which suggested that, although cardiac events were fewer, beta-blocker therapy was associated with a higher stroke rate and overall mortality. Revised American Heart Association guidelines recommend starting therapy cautiously in high-risk patients weeks prior to surgery, titrating the dose to heart rate and blood pressure

- Arrhythmias, especially tachyarrhythmias, should be controlled prior to surgery. Optimum metabolic control, especially normoglycaemia in diabetic patients, and normothermia improve cardiac outcome
- Evidence suggests that pre-op revascularisation is generally only indicated in unstable disease or left main stem disease
- Management of antiplatelet therapy in patients post-stenting requires careful management in conjunction with a cardiologist. The risk of significant surgical bleeding is increased by 50% with dual antiplatelet therapy, but there is no increase in mortality. Recent evidence suggests that continuation of therapy may not mitigate against major adverse cardiac events

Anaesthetic technique

Aims include:
- Maintenance or improvement of oxygen supply:demand ratio
- Avoidance of extremes of blood pressure
- Avoidance of tachycardia, which increases oxygen demand and reduces diastolic flow
- Avoidance of high preload, which can increase LVEDP and oxygen demand
- Balance afterload to maintain coronary perfusion whilst minimising cardiac workload

In addition to routine monitoring, invasive arterial monitoring and ECG ST analysis should be considered. Use of a 5-lead ECG or the CM5 configuration will increase sensitivity for left ventricular ischaemia. Cardiac output monitoring is controversial, although oesophageal Doppler is now supported by NICE for high-risk surgery following trial evidence of a reduction in perioperative morbidity.

Evidence of pulmonary flotation catheters and other methods is less clear. Regional anaesthesia will reduce the surgical stress response, reduce preload, improve peripheral circulation and can reduce pain-related sympathetic activation; however, the MASTER trial (2002) was unable to show benefit of epidural use to high-risk patients.

Volatile use confers pharmacological preconditioning, in a manner similar to short periods of ischaemia (ischaemic preconditioning). This biomolecular phenomenon gives a cardioprotective effect attenuating the effects of future periods of myocardial ischaemia. Despite strong evidence of an improvement in disease markers, there is little evidence of outcome benefit as yet.

For general anaesthesia, periods of intense stimulation, such as laryngoscopy, skin incision and extubation, require attenuation. Short-acting opiates, such as remifentanil or fentanyl in adequate doses, are often used. Induction agents require slow titration due to a prolonged arm-brain circulation time and the sparing effects of coadministered opiates. Maintenance with an inhalational agent may improve cardiac outcomes over total intravenous anaesthesia. The agent used does not appear to be important, although desflurane will cause tachycardia, which is best avoided. Intraoperative ischaemia should be promptly treated with 100% oxygen and normalisation of cardiovascular parameters using GTN, beta-blockers and fluids. Level 2/3 care should be considered.

Postoperative care

Postoperative ischaemia (particularly silent ischaemia) is present in up to 48% of at-risk patients in the first 48 hours after surgery. It is the most important indicator for serious cardiac event. Risk continues for many weeks following major surgery. Silent ischaemia is common and may be due to peri/postoperative cardiac instability, coagulation disorder, proinflammatory mediators or hypoxaemia. More than 2 hours of ischaemia is likely to result in a serious cardiac event.

Adequate analgesia and use of α_2-agonists can reduce ongoing sympathetic activation.

Treatment of myocardial ischaemia

Suspicion should be high in the postoperative period. Hypoxia, especially at night, increases the risk of ischaemia and oxygen therapy should be administered as required to ensure oxygen saturations >92% for the first 5 days following major surgery. The diagnosis of an acute coronary event is made on history, ECG changes (most are non-Q-wave infarctions), and cardiac enzyme elevation.

Treatment of an acute coronary event should be similar to standard medical practice, including aspirin, other platelet inhibition agents (e.g. ticagrelor, prasugrel, clopidogrel), antithrombotic agents (e.g. fondaparinux) and nitrates. Angiography and revascularisation may be required and early referral to a cardiologist is warranted. Significant myocardial damage may precipitate cardiogenic shock, requiring inotropic support and intra-aortic balloon counterpulsation.

Abnormal cardiac rhythms should be managed with antiarrhythmics such as amiodarone. ACE inhibitors are of clear benefit if left ventricular function is impaired. NICE have published guidelines (2010) on the management of acute chest pain and NSTEMI including the use of antiplatelet agents such as glycoprotein IIb-IIIa inhibitors and clopidogrel, now a mainstay of therapy. Risks of postoperative bleeding are often overemphasised compared with those of a cardiac event and there does not appear to be an increase in major bleeding following the use of these agents in the postoperative period.

Further reading

Fleisher LA. Cardiac risk stratification for noncardiac surgery. Cleve Clin J Med 2009; 76:S9–15.
Libby P, Theroux P. Pathophysiology of coronary artery disease. Circulation 2005; 111:3481–3488.

More C, Leslie S. Coronary artery stents: management in patients undergoing noncardiac surgery. In: Johnston I, Harrop-Griffiths W, Gemmell L, Eds. AAGBI Core Topics in Anaesthesia 2012. Oxford; Wiley, 2012.

Related topics of interest

- Cardiac dysrhythmia (p. 37)
- Cardiac pacemakers (p. 40)
- Cardiac surgery (p. 43)
- Cardiac anaesthesia – valvular heart disease (p. 34)
- Elderly patients (p. 64)
- Hypertensive disease (p. 89)
- Preoperative assessment – risk evaluation (p. 236)
- Preoperative assessment – risk modification (p. 239)

Day surgery

Key points

- Consider day surgery as the default – ask 'why not?' rather than 'why?'
- Day surgery is optimised by effective preoperative assessment and preparation (nurse delivered, consultant supported), protocol-driven nurse led discharge and rigorous audit and patient follow-up
- Anaesthetic techniques should maximise recovery, minimise postoperative discomfort (pain, nausea, vomiting) and promote early safe discharge
- Surgical advances – minimally invasive techniques have increased day surgery scope of procedures

Definition

In the UK, day surgery is defined as a patient being admitted for a planned surgical procedure and also being discharged home on the same calendar day. This contrasts with some other countries including America, where stays of up to 23 hours may be considered as day surgery.

National guidelines and targets

Day surgery is a continually evolving concept. In the UK, for example, over the years it has broadened to include increasingly complex surgical procedures and a wider case mix of patients. The following list of initiatives demonstrates the complexity of setting targets or creating guidelines in this area.

- Department of Health's NHS Plan (2000) – 75% of all elective surgery in the UK to be performed as day case procedures
- Audit Commission (2001) – 25 procedures identified to form a 'basket'. The aim was to provide focus for units to target achievement in day surgery rates and benchmark themselves nationally
- British Association of Day Surgery (BADS) – 'Trolley of procedures' (extra 17 procedures on top of the 'basket'). Continually updated and expanded. Now a 'Directory of procedures' providing aspirational day surgery rates for 200 procedures (4th edition, 2012)
- Department of Health: Day Surgery Operational Guide (2002) – aimed to guide efficiency improvements when planning and managing elective surgical services
- NHS Modernisation Agency: 'Ten High Impact Changes' document (2004) – recommendation to 'treat day surgery (rather than inpatient surgery) as the norm for all elective surgery'. Politically raised the profile of day surgery
- NHS Better Care, Better Value Indicators – trusts report quarterly on day surgery rates for selected day surgery procedures to reflect productivity and identify areas for efficiency improvements and cost savings

Advantages of day surgery

- Clinical outcomes
  - Shorter hospital stay and early mobilisation reduce rates of hospital acquired infection and venous thromboembolism
  - Many principles of day and short stay surgery can be applied to reducing length of stay for in-patient procedures and for enhanced recovery programmes
- Service delivery
  - Increased productivity, lower incidence of nonclinical cancellation and reduced waiting times from better utilisation of hospital capacity
  - Cost savings and reduced in-patient workload
- Patient experience
  - Patient acceptability and psychological benefit – most prefer their own surroundings with less disruption
- Staff benefits
  - Flexible working, less antisocial hours
  - Involvement in all aspects of patient pathway

Controversies regarding day surgery

- Reduced period of postoperative monitoring to detect potential complications

- Greater care burden on patient and their supporting family/friends
- Patient may deteriorate at home and need to access emergency out-of-hours medical support (primary/secondary care)
- Unplanned admissions may suddenly produce pressure on in-patient bed states
- Patients commonly have reduced cognitive abilities after general anaesthesia with impaired recall of information. Lack of awareness of important postoperative information they may have been given; hence it is vital to supplement information in written format

Organisational issues

- Dedicated day surgery lists in an autonomous unit provide the best model of care and avoid tension from competing interests of mixed in-patient and day case lists
- Equipment, monitoring and staffing in theatres and recovery areas should be of the same standard as in-patient facilities
- Application of industrial models, 'lean' thinking and process mapping contribute to building effective patient pathways, e.g. laparoscopic cholecystectomy pathway (NHS Institute for Innovation & Improvement)
- Organising efficient patient flow is vital for success
- Staffing levels should have flexibility to match peak activity periods
- Each day surgery unit should have a clinical lead, unit manager and administration support
- Local policies should be developed and clinical governance processes must be in place

Patient selection

- Published successful outcomes for patients with multiple comorbidities have changed previously stringent limitations on patient groups (e.g. ASA3, BMI >35, age >70)
- Age: Full-term infants over 1 month old (or if ex-premature >60 weeks postconceptual age; increased risk of postoperative apnoea). No upper age limit

- Social requirements
  - Responsible adult to escort patient home and be available for carer support
  - Access to telephone
  - Geographical proximity to hospital; travelling time >1 hour may be contraindication for certain procedures (e.g. day case tonsillectomy)
  - Patient motivation; need to engage, understand and trust the day surgery process
- Medical requirements
  - Comorbidities should be assessed and patients optimised for day surgery on an individual basis. Avoid arbitrary limitations such as BMI
  - Stable chronic medical conditions, e.g. diabetes are often best managed by patient. Day surgery management therefore minimises disruption
  - Obesity – morbidly obese patients may still be suitable. Most complications are intraoperative or early stage recovery thus would have been attended to before day surgery discharge. Appropriate resources and experienced surgical and anaesthetic personnel required
- Surgical requirements
  - There should be no significant risk of major postoperative complications necessitating immediate medical intervention
  - Pain controllable with oral analgesia +/− regional anaesthesia technique
  - Patient able to rapidly resume normal functions (oral intake, mobilisation)
  - Urgent procedures can also be performed via a semi-elective day case pathway, e.g. incision and drainage of abscess

Principles of perioperative care

- Preoperative assessment
  - Nurse-delivered, consultant-supported service
  - Structured questions to assess the patient's medical and social fitness for day case surgery

- Optimisation of patient's health; patient education (weight loss, exercise, smoking cessation)
- Collection of patient-specific information to help plan for surgical procedure
- Opportunity to provide patient with key verbal and written information about their day surgery care
- Anaesthetic management
  - Techniques to promote rapid emergence with good recovery profile following general anaesthesia, e.g. total intravenous anaesthesia
  - Multimodal analgesia including prophylactic oral analgesia and use of local anaesthetic infiltration/regional anaesthetic techniques where appropriate
  - Postoperative nausea and vomiting (PONV) risk assessment to guide use of antiemetics
  - Routine administration of intravenous fluids to enhance patient well-being and reduce PONV
  - Aggressive early management of postoperative pain, nausea and vomiting
- Postoperative
  - Variable length of postoperative observation depending on patient factors and specific procedure requirements, e.g. paediatric tonsillectomy mandating a minimum period of observation

- Protocol-driven, nurse-led discharge
- Provision of analgesics, postoperative instructions and discharge advice (supplemented in written form), including emergency contact details
- Routine day 1 telephone call follow-up is best practice. Provides support to patients as well as generating auditable data on postoperative pain, PONV and degree of patient satisfaction

Role of audit

- Data should be collected to monitor and drive improvements in efficiency and quality of patient care
- All sections of the patient pathway should be routinely audited, including
  - Booking processes
  - Cancellation rates
  - Theatre utilisation
  - Unplanned admissions
  - Patient satisfaction
  - Indicators on quality of care (postoperative pain scores, PONV rates, surgical symptoms and unplanned contact with primary care/out of hours services)

Results should then be analysed and disseminated to staff.

- Good leadership to support and motivate the day surgery team and empower individuals to drive change is key

Further reading

Association of Anaesthetists of Great Britain and Ireland. Day case & short stay surgery (2). London; AAGBI Publications, 2001.

Lemos P, Jarret P, Phillip BK. (eds). Day surgery: development and practice. Porto; International Association for Ambulatory Surgery, 2006.

Smith I, McWhinnie D, Jackson I (Eds). Oxford Handbook of Day Surgery. Oxford; Oxford University Press, 2011.

www.bads.co.uk

Related topics of interest

Dental anaesthesia

Key points

- General anaesthesia for dental surgery requires the same standards of safety and preparation as other surgeries
- Procedures are commonly performed under local anaesthesia, sedation and general anaesthesia
- Consideration should be given to the shared airway and airway soiling
- There are a number of possible airway devices that are suitable for dental anaesthesia

Anaesthesia in dental surgeries, once commonplace in the UK, has all but vanished in the last 20 years. Serious and preventable morbidity and mortality led to restrictions imposed by the General Dental Council and Royal College of Anaesthetists in the 1990s.

General anaesthesia is not warranted for the majority of dental interventions. Indications for general anaesthesia may include some paediatric patients, dentoalveolar infection, learning difficulties, severe dental phobia and failure/contraindication to local anaesthesia.

Problems

- Those of day case surgery
- The shared airway, especially perioperative airway soiling
- High proportion of paediatric patients
- Dental surgery units may be isolated as they are often geographically distant to other operating theatres
- Many patients have special educational needs or physical disability requiring particular experience and expertise

Techniques

Local anaesthesia

Usually administered by the dental practitioner. Agents with or without adrenaline are injected into the buccal fold of the gum adjacent to the affected tooth. The inferior alveolar nerve block and a variety of lingual and mental nerve blocks may also be used to provide more extensive anaesthesia to the teeth and gums. Infraorbital nerve blocks will anaesthetise the upper jaw.

Sedation

Procedural sedation and analgesia (previously known as 'conscious sedation') may be provided by the nonanaesthetist with specific training in the correct environment. A key feature is the maintenance of verbal contact throughout.

Deeper levels of sedation and general anaesthesia should only be provided by an anaesthetist. This may be achieved via the following routes

- Oral, e.g. benzodiazepines
- Inhalational. N_2O/O_2 combinations and low-dose sevoflurane (end tidal 0.3–0.5%) provide conscious sedation. Both have some mild amnesic and analgesic effect
- Intravenous. Small aliquots of midazolam (0.5–1 mg) provide suitable conditions for surgery. Multiple dosing will lead to accumulation and prolonged sedation, however, which may delay discharge. There is a potent synergy with opiates tending towards oversedation. Propofol sedation, ether by judicious intermittent bolus (10–20 mg) or infusion (0.5–1.5 μg/mL TIVA), provides excellent sedation and is titratable. It may be combined with small doses of short-acting opiate, such as fentanyl
- The key to sedation in dentistry is getting the depth right. Oversedation results in a noncompliant patient who refuses to open their mouth or worse. If this occurs, options are to either wait until consciousness and co-operation are regained or conversion to general anaesthesia. AAGBI minimum monitoring standards should be observed.

General anaesthesia

Anaesthetic management

The same principles apply to dental anaesthesia as for day case anaesthesia. All sites should be fully equipped with resuscitation and monitoring equipment. Oral premedication is not usually required. Inhalational induction with sevoflurane may be considered for severely needle phobic patients or children. Inhalational induction is associated with an increased incidence of arrhythmias, particularly with halothane.

Tracheal intubation, if required (e.g. extensive molar work), may be achieved with a small dose of nondepolarising neuromuscular blocker or under deep-plane anaesthesia. Short-acting opiates such as alfentanil (up to 30 µg/kg) or remifentanil (1–2 µg/kg) can also be used, although these techniques require experience and bradycardia may be profound. Full, unobstructed surgical access to the airway can be provided by nasal intubation. Nasal patency should be determined with preoperative questioning. A prewarmed soft endotracheal tube can be positioned with the assistance of McGills forceps and a laryngoscope. Prior topical phenylephrine will reduce epistaxis and ease the passage of the tube. It is not without complication and carries an epistaxis rate (sometimes severe) of 5%.

Maintenance of anaesthesia during dental anaesthesia requires the provision of a clear airway. The most commonly used airway options are a nasal mask (e.g. Goldman or McKesson) or flexible LMA. A mouth pack is usually placed to prevent mouth breathing/lightening anaesthesia and airway soiling if a nasal mask is used. Close cooperation and vigilance are required by dental surgeon and anaesthetist to ensure unobstructed respiration. Flexible LMAs commonly become dislodged as they are often not tied or taped to allow operator manoeuvrability. The pharynx should be cleared of secretions and debris by suction at the end of surgery and the patient recovered in the lateral position. A head-down tilt will ensure blood drains away from the vocal cords.

Learning difficulties

Patients with learning difficulties can be particularly challenging. Issues include poor dental hygiene (often unknown until after induction), communication difficulty and heightened anxiety. Adult patients are often physically strong. There may be associated syndromes or physical problems such as cardiovascular abnormalities, epilepsy or trisomy 21.

Patients with severe learning disabilities will require a carefully prepared admission plan. Many organisations have a learning disabilities team who liaise with the parent, GP, dental surgeon, anaesthetist and nursing staff prior to admission. Particular areas of consideration include premedication – what, when and where – ensuring minimal disruption to the daily routine, transport to and from hospital, location of preop and postop periods and specific discharge criteria.

Extraction of impacted molars

This is commonly performed on a day case basis. A flexible LMA is usually suitable to maintain a clear airway. As with all day surgery, control of postoperative symptoms (pain and swelling) is essential to permit patient discharge. Perioperative intravenous dexamethasone (4–8 mg) is both analgesic and reduces tissue oedema with the added benefits of antiemesis. There is a small reported increase in bleeding. Analgesia may be provided by Paracetamol and NSAID premedication, intravenous short-acting opiate and local anaesthesia infiltration.

Further reading

Cantlay K, Williamson S, Hawkings J. Anaesthesia for dentistry. Br J Anaesth: Contin Educ Anaesth, Crit Care Pain. 2005;5:71–75.

Related topics of interest

Diabetes

Key points

- Diabetes is a multisystem disorder
- Diabetes results in end-organ injury, which presents significant comorbidity
- Type 2 diabetes is more prevalent and is associated with an ageing population and increases in population BMI

Diabetes is a disease of rapidly increasing prevalence and affects 1 in 20 adults in the UK. The greatest rise is amongst the type 2 group who represents 90% of UK diabetics. This is due to a combination of increasing obesity, sedentary lifestyle, an ageing population and migration of susceptible populations. The disease is due to an absolute deficiency of (type 1) or insensitivity to (type 2) insulin. Type 2 may also feature insulin deficiency. Pregnancy may also precipitate diabetes (gestational diabetes) and, although most recover at delivery, up to 50% go on to develop true type 2 diabetes later in life. Poor control of gestational diabetes is associated with neonatal macrosomia, congenital cardiac and central nervous system lesions and placental vascular insufficiency.

All forms of diabetes have the commonality of being a multisystem illness by virtue of the widespread micro- and macrovascular damage which results. This produces a surgical patient with often extensive comorbidities. In addition, all diabetic patients are at risk of acute diabetic emergencies such as ketoacidosis and the hyperosmolar hyperglycaemic state.

Problems

- Respiratory
  - Stiff joints syndrome (mainly type 1) – implications for airway manipulation
  - Associated respiratory complications of obesity
- Circulatory
  - Hypertension
  - Ischaemic heart disease (including asymptomatic ischaemia)
  - Autonomic dysfunction (orthostatic hypotension, reduced heart rate variability)
  - Peripheral vascular disease
  - Aneurysmal disease and dissection
- Gastrointestinal
  - Autonomic gastroparesis
- Renal
  - Diabetic nephropathy
  - Susceptibility to urinary tract infection
- Ophthalmic
  - Diabetic retinopathy
  - Cataracts
  - Vitreous haemorrhage and retinal detachment
- Neurological
  - Cerebrovascular disease
  - Verterbrocarotid atherosclerosis
  - Peripheral sensory neuropathy
  - Autonomic neuropathy
- Dermatological
  - Ulceration
  - Poor wound healing
- Endocrine
  - Hyperlipidaemia
  - Association with hyperpituitarism, hyperadrenalism, hyperthyroidism and phaeochromacytoma

Clinical features

The classical first presentation of type 1 diabetes is either as an episode of ketoacidosis (Kussmaul's breathing, dehydration, abdominal pain, depressed consciousness, profound acidaemia, ketotic foetor, tachycardia, hypotension, ketonuria) or as the triad of tiredness, polyuria and polydipsia. The latter results from the diuretic effects of excess renal tubular glucose.

Type 2 diabetes is more likely to present as an incidental finding at health screening or at the presentation of end-organ damage.

Investigations

In the preoperative context, all diabetics require full blood count, urea and electrolytes and blood sugar testing. In addition, HbA_{1C} (glycosylated haemoglobin) assay gives an indication of the adequacy of glucose control in the preceding 2–3 months. This is a useful test as recent poor control has been linked to poorer surgical outcomes. All type 2 diabetics should have an ECG and consideration should be given to more detailed cardiology workup in those with severe disease or who are undergoing more major surgery. All patients should have urinary screening for microalbuminuria (heralds the onset of new diabetic nephropathy) and ketonuria.

Further blood sugar testing should be performed hourly in the perioperative period.

Treatment

Type 1 diabetics are managed with insulin and this is typically with a basal-bolus regimen, using a longer-acting insulin to provide background levels and short-acting insulin 15–20 minutes prior to meals.

Type 2 diabetics usually undergo a trial of nonmedical management in the initial phase (weight loss, exercise, diet modification). Around 60% progress to requiring oral antihyperglycaemic agents (see **Table 10**). Around 1 in 6 progresses to requiring insulin in addition to other therapy.

Anaesthetic management

A thorough preoperative assessment must actively seek the features listed above but particularly those relating to airway problems, renal disease, autonomic dysfunction and cardiovascular morbidity; presence of these, as well as retinopathy and neuropathy, also denotes advanced disease. Consideration should then be given specifically to glucose management: patients should omit oral agents on the morning of surgery. Some recommend continuation of long-acting insulin to maintain the basal component of the regimen. Diabetic patients should, wherever possible, be operated on first on the theatre list to minimise the fasting period and time without their usual antihyperglycaemic therapy. Scrupulous perioperative care should aim to facilitate a prompt return to oral intake, particularly without nausea and vomiting. Dexamethasone can increase blood glucose slightly but in all but the most brittle diabetics, the powerful antiemetic benefit outweighs this risk.

All those normally taking insulin and those who do not but are undergoing major surgery should be managed with intraoperative insulin dextrose 'sliding scale' infusion. Hourly blood sugar measurement should guide this, although it must be understood that manufacturing tolerances permit ±20% error on blood glucose test strips at levels above 5.5 mmol/L. Serum potassium levels should also be monitored every 2 hours in this context.

There is no evidence that regional anaesthesia offers a better alternative to

Table 10 Oral antihyperglycaemia agents			
Class	Example	Mechanism	Comments
Biguanides	Metformin	Increases sensitivity to insulin	Does not cause weight gain but may cause lactic acidosis especially in renal disease
Sulphonylureas	Gliclazide	Increase insulin secretion	Can cause weight gain and hypoglycaemia
Thiazolidinediones	Pioglitazone	Increases sensitivity to insulin	Can cause weight gain (leptin suppression) and oedema with heart failure exacerbation
GLP-1 agonists	Exenatide	Delays gastric emptying, provides satiety, stimulates pancreatic insulin release, reduces glucagon release	Nausea, vomiting and diarrhoea especially on starting treatment
DPP-4 inhibitors	Vildagliptin	Prevents GLP-1 agonist breakdown.	No appetite suppression but less gastrointestinal side effects than GLP agonists
α-Glucosidase inhibitors	Acarbose	Delays starch and sucrose digestion and absorption	Flatulence

GLP, glucagon-like peptide; DPP, dipeptidyl peptidase.

general anaesthesia in terms of mortality or morbidity. Careful assessment of neurological function should be performed prior to any regional technique as direct nerve injury may worsen neurological function (as with any block). If general anaesthesia is selected, consider the airway carefully and assess the risk of aspiration if gastric paresis is evident. Regional techniques also have a role in mitigating the stress response and its deleterious influence on glucose control; they can usefully be employed in conjunction with general anaesthesia.

Postoperative blood sugar measurement can extend to 2 hours as oral intake and usual diabetic therapy is reinstated as soon as feasible. Intravenous fluids and the continuing insulin-dextrose infusion should be prescribed where applicable and the patient should be discharged from the theatre suite to the care of suitably trained ward staff.

Further reading

Dhatariya K, Levy N, Kilvert A, et al. NHS diabetes guideline for the perioperative management of the adult patient with diabetes. Diabet Med 2012; 29:420–433.

McAnulty GR, Robertshaw HJ, Hall GM. Anaesthetic management of patients with diabetes mellitus. Br J Anaesth 2000; 85):80–90.

Nicholson G, Hall GM. Diabetes and adult surgical inpatients. Contin Educ Anaesth Crit Care Pain 2011; 11:234–238.

Related topics of interest

- Airway assessment (p. 1)
- Endocrine disease (p. 72)
- Preoperative assessment – risk evaluation (p. 236)
- Renal disease – chronic kidney disease (p. 253)
- Vascular surgery – occlusive disease (p. 316)

Drug allergy and adverse reactions

Key points

- Perioperative anaphylaxis is either immunological [immunoglobulin E (IgE) mediated or other immunological mechanism] or nonimmune, such as direct mast cell activation
- Diagnosis is difficult due to multiple drug administration, confounding anaesthetic techniques, fluid shifts and comorbidity
- Referral to an allergy centre along with full documentation is essential
- In practice, the underlying mechanism is irrelevant as clinical severity may be the same and the management is identical. The distinction is important in terms of testing, prevention and prognosis

Adverse drug reaction (ADR)

These are defined as an unintended, undesired, noxious effect of a drug and fall into two types:

- Type A reactions are predictable from pharmacological effects. Can occur in anyone given sufficient dose and exposure. Account for 90% of ADRs, e.g.
  - NSAIDs and adverse cardiovascular events infarction and strokes
  - Tricyclic antidepressants potentiate indirect sympathomimetic effects of ephedrine and metaraminol
- Type B reactions are unpredictable, hypersensitivity reactions (10% of ADRs). Divided into:
  - Exaggerated sensitivity to known drug toxicity:
    - Halothane hepatotoxicity – anaerobic cytochrome P450 reductive metabolism in poorly perfused liver causing lipid peroxidation
  - Idiosyncratic drug reactions unrelated to properties of a drug:
    - Malignant hyperpyrexia in response to suxamethonium and volatile anaesthesia due to Ryanodine receptor gene defects on chromosome 19

- Plasma cholinesterase variants causing suxamethonium apnoea
- Porphyria-triggering drugs induce 5-aminolevulinic acid synthetase upon metabolic stress or haemorrhage
- Sevoflurane or halothane hepatitis – trifluoroacetate binds to liver cell proteins stimulating antibody production. Subsequent exposure results in hepatic necrosis
  - Immunologic reactions account for 8% of all ADRs

Perioperative allergic drug reactions are now around 1:13,000. There is a large range in denominator due to under-reporting and variable usage of drugs. French, Danish and Australian database reports dominate the literature.

The current World Allergy Organization definition for anaphylaxis is a severe, life-threatening, systemic, hypersensitivity reaction. Sixty per cent of perioperative anaphylaxis occurs due to IgE-mediated reactions usually within minutes of intravenous administration and, by definition, within 1 hour (**Figure 5**). Whatever the mechanism, the final common pathway is the same:

- Degranulation of mast cells and basophils to release biologically active products (histamine and tryptase), which act directly on tissues to cause allergic symptoms
- Cytokines (tumor necrosis factor and interleukins) and lipid-derived mediators (platelet activating factor, prostaglandin-D_2 and leukotrienes) are generated and alter the sensitivity of target cells to influence the severity of anaphylaxis. These chemotactic substances attract other inflammatory cells such as eosinophils as well as involving serum components of the complement, coagulation and kallikrein–kinin pathways to propagate the inflammatory reaction

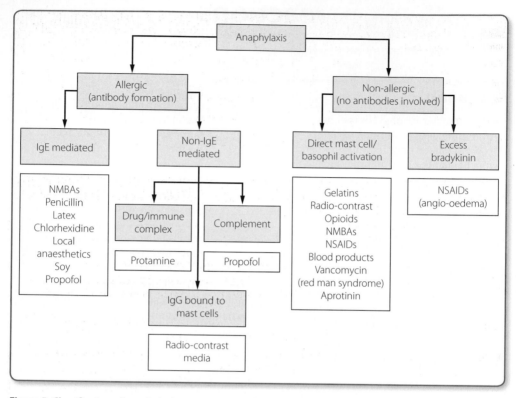

Figure 5 Classification of anaphylaxis.

Other allergic reactions occurring later are type 4 hypersensitivity reactions and are tested for by patch testing normally performed by dermatologists.

Clinical features

Recognition may be hampered by:
- Hypotensive interactions from both volatiles and sympatholytic effects of regional blockade
- Skin changes hidden by surgical drapes
- Delayed onset due to tourniquets, massive fluid shifts or large vessel clamping

Thus, perioperative anaphylaxis is often more severe and mortality higher. Biphasic reactions may occur in 20%.

Single-system presentation may occur but the majority are generalised involving respiratory or cardiovascular compromise. Redistribution with reduced venous tone also exacerbates hypovolaemic shock with massive fluid extravasation. It may induce profound myocardial depression, ischaemia and conduction defects. Recent estimates of mortality are 1.4 % with fatalities divided between circulatory collapse and respiratory arrest. Two per cent of survivors suffer from brain injury (**Table 11**). Culprit agents are wide ranging (**Table 12**).

Treatment

This is clearly laid out in the AAGBI 'Anaphylaxis Drill' guidance and involves an ABC approach with administration of oxygen, fluid and adrenaline. Steroids and antihistamines form the second phase of management.

Risk factors

Genetic factors play a role in atopy and multiple hypersensitivity. Risk factors for anaphylaxis include asthma, atopy, multiple

Table 11 Presenting features of anaphylaxis			
Initial presenting symptoms	Patients (%)	Frequency of symptoms involved	Patients (%)
Pulseless	26	CVS collapse	54
Difficulty ventilating	25	Bronchospasm	44
Flushing	18	Erythema/urticaria	70
Desaturation	11	Angio-oedema	12
Cough	7	Cardiac arrest	4

Table 12 Features and incidence of anaphylaxis for different culprit agents		
Cause	Proportion of all anaesthesia anaphylaxis caused by agent (%)	Features
Relaxants	58	65% cross-reactivity amongst neuromuscular blocking drugs
Latex	17	Onset ~30 minutes (visceral surface absorption from gloves, drains and catheters). 50% sensitisation with repeat catheters and operations. Anaesthetic staff 15% sensitisation
Antibiotics	15 (50% USA)	Penicillin allergy due either to β-lactam ring or R-group side chain. Cross-sensitivity ranges from 2% to 10%
Hypnotics	3	Mainly thiopentone. No evidence for cross-reactivity between soybean (in propofol) and egg or soy
Colloids	3	Associated with known food gelatin allergy
Opioids	<2	Codeine and morphine cause direct histamine release with urticaria and pruritus but IgE-mediated allergy very rare
Alanine dyes Patent blue Isosulphan blue Methylene blue	<2	Patent blue dye has 1% incidence of anaphylaxis with significant cross reactivity with isomer isosulphan blue. Methylene blue incidence lower
Chlorhexidine		Increasing exposure within health care: 4/14 healthcare workers in UK DGH had positive skin (at-risk of anaphylaxis) Increasing reports with skin decontamination, Venflon insertion, mouthwashes, Savlon, hair-dyes, contact lens solutions and toothpaste
Local anaesthetics		IgE-mediated anaphylaxis extremely rare but delayed-type reactions can occur. Reactions to sulphite preservatives found in solutions containing vasoconstrictors
Protamine Insulin		Link with salmon allergy
Povidine iodine		
Heparin		Associated pork allergy. Extremely rare
Sterilising agents Ethylene Cidex		Repeat procedures with sterilised equipment, e.g. cystoscopy

exposures and past history of anaphylaxis. Antibiotic allergy is increased in smokers. Environmental exposure is more influential:

- Anaphylaxis 3x commoner in women – sensitisation to allergens in cosmetics
- Quarternary ammonium structures in personal products accounts for anaphylaxis on first exposure to muscle relaxants
- Pholcodeine in cough medication increases the incidence of NMBA allergy via higher prevalence of IgE antibodies to succinylcholine

Investigations

Contemporaneous documentation on theatre and anaesthetic charts of all drugs, skin preparations, local anaesthetic and plastic catheters/cannulas inserted is vital.

Blood tests

Three samples for mast cell tryptase (MCT) should be taken as soon as possible, at 2 hours and 24 hours as clotted serum (yellow-top Vacutainer). Raised baseline levels >15 ng/mL may mean mastocytosis and increased risk of anaphylaxis.

High MCT occurs in 68% of IgE-mediated reactions and 4% of non-IgE-mediated reactions. Therefore, a normal MCT does not exclude anaphylaxis. Tryptase may be measured retrospectively in frozen samples for up to 1 year. The ImmunoCAP-specific IgE blood test (**Figure 6**) can also be used to quantify IgE antibodies. Allergens available include penicillin determinants, chlorhexidine, suxamethonium and latex.

Skin tests

Patients should also be referred to an allergy centre with relevant charts and documentation for skin-prick testing (at 4–6 weeks to allow replenished histamine levels in mast cells). The AAGBI maintains an online list of suitable centres. Antihistamines should be stopped for 5 days prior to testing.

Undiluted drugs on the volar aspect of forearm are pricked with lancets to deliver controlled dose into outer layer of dermis to determine presence of allergen-specific

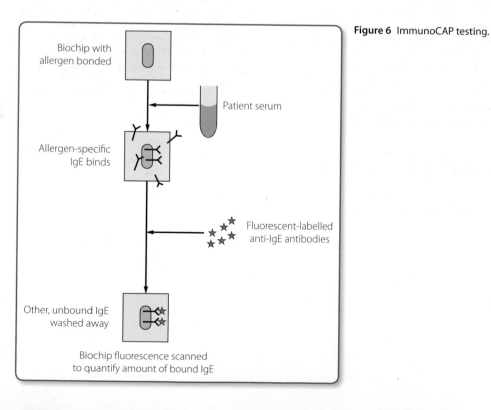

Figure 6 ImmunoCAP testing.

Biochip with allergen bonded

Patient serum

Allergen-specific IgE binds

Fluorescent-labelled anti-IgE antibodies

Other, unbound IgE washed away

Biochip fluorescence scanned to quantify amount of bound IgE

IgE on cutaneous mast cells. Degranulation results in a positive wheal and flare response read at 15 minutes which is 3 mm larger than negative control (saline). Histamine is used as a positive control.

Intradermal tests starting at 1:1000 dilutions can verify negative skin-prick tests where a high index of suspicion exists. Risks of sensitisation and high rate of false-positives preclude screening, but it is important to test for cross-reactivity between classes, especially neuromuscular blocking agents.

Challenge testing for opiates, antibiotics and NSAIDs should only be performed if clinically imperative due to significant risk of reaction. Continuously vigilant, senior personnel with full resuscitation equipment and adrenaline immediately available are required at all times.

Follow-up

Test results and recommendations for future anaesthesia should be documented in the notes and copied to the patient, GP and dentist. Pretreatment of non-IgE-mediated reactions may reduce severity and risk of further reactions. After IgE-mediated reactions avoid all identified agents and drugs of similar class and all neuromuscular blocking agents if cross-reactivity is demonstrated. A medic-alert bracelet inscribed with allergy details is recommended. The reaction should be reported via the MHRA Yellow Card System and to the AAGBI anaphylaxis database.

Further reading

Association of Anaesthetists of Great Britain & Ireland. Management of a patient with suspected anaphylaxis during anaesthesia safety drill. London: AAGBI, 2009.

Ewan PW, Dugue P, Mirakian R, et al. BASCI guidelines for the investigation of suspected anaphylaxis during general anaesthesia. Clin Exp Allergy 2010; 40:15–31.

Hughes R. Anaphylaxis. Critical Incidents. [Online] https://e-learningforhealthcare.org.uk/data/scorm/decompressed/ANA_01_075_server2_275992700/d/ANAE_Session/358/session.html#overview.html [2013].

Mills ATD, Sice PJS, Ford SMS. Anaesthesia-related anaphylaxis: investigation and follow-up. Br J Anaesth: Contin Educ Anaesth, Criti Care Pain 2013;doi:10.1093/bjaceaccp/mkt034.

Nagendran V, Wicking J, Ekbote A, et al. IgE-mediated chlorhexidine allergy: a new occupational hazard? Occup Med 2009; 59:270–272.

Sadleir PHM, Clarke RC, Bunning DL, et al. Anaphylaxis to neuromuscular blocking drugs: incidence and cross reactivity in Western Australia from 2002 to 2011. Br J Anaesth 2013; 110:981–987.

Related topics of interest

Elderly patients

Key points

- As the population ages, the issues affecting elderly patients are seen with increasing frequency
- Safe delivery of anaesthesia in elderly patients requires careful consideration of all organ systems· Physiological reserve is reduced with advancing age

Due to changes in demographics and longer survival, more elderly patients are presenting for more complex surgery than in previous times. Specific challenges are presented by aging body systems, often due to a decline in functional reserve with age. Specific diseases also become more prevalent with advancing age. Chronological age does not equate with physiological age. Multidisciplinary input during preparation for surgery has been shown to improve operative outcome including preoperative review and optimisation by a geriatrician, e.g. allowing for correction of anaemia, improving nutritional state and the placement of adequate social support. A clinical lead for elderly anaesthesia should be nominated in each anaesthetic department.

It is often difficult to accurately quantify risk to surgery due to multiplicity of risk factors. Decision to operate should involve the patient and their family and centre upon improvement in quality of life as perceived by the patient and relief of suffering.

Problems

- Cardiovascular system. Decreasing vessel elasticity leads to a less compliant vascular tree (a raised systemic vascular resistance) with systemic hypertension, left ventricular strain and hypertrophy, and a stiff, noncompliant ventricle. Cardiac conduction time is increased and stroke volume is reduced. Conduction defects may necessitate pacing. Cardiac output falls by 3% per decade, and arm/brain circulation time is increased. Baroreceptor sensitivity, sympathetic tone and the ability to increase the heart rate when required are reduced. Anaemia will reduce oxygen availability for the ischaemic heart
  - Diseases: Hypertension, heart failure, IHD, valvular disease (especially mitral regurgitation and aortic stenosis), atrial fibrillation (present in 18% of >85 years olds) and peripheral vascular disease
- Respiratory. Pulmonary elasticity, lung and chest wall compliance, FEV_1, FVC, vital capacity and inspiratory reserve are all reduced. The closing volume exceeds functional residual capacity (FRC) in the supine position after the age of 45 years with resultant V/Q mismatch and hypoxaemia. The residual volume is increased. There is a reduced response to hypoxaemia and hypercarbia, and protective airway reflexes decrease in old age
  - Diseases: Chronic obstructive airflow and emphysema
- Central nervous system. Neuronal density (30% loss by 80 years), brain transmitters, cerebral blood flow, and cerebral metabolic rate are all reduced. This lowers the dose of induction and volatile agents, sedatives, opioids and local anaesthetics. Reduced peripheral nerve function leads to a reduction in afferent flow and less sensitive sensory input. Autonomic neuropathy may occur. Postoperative cognitive dysfunction is more common. The mechanism is not fully understood, but is likely to be multifactorial. There is evidence that prophylactic haloperidol therapy can reduce postoperative delerium.
  - Diseases: cerebral vascular disease, dementia, Parkinsonism and depression. Deafness and poor vision may make communication difficult
- Renal. Renal blood flow, GFR and concentrating ability are all reduced. There is a 1% loss in function per year after 30 years. This leads to reduced renal clearance of drugs, a raised blood urea but a stable blood creatinine until function has diminished by around 50%. Renal impairment will contribute to hypertension
  - Diseases: Transitional cell malignancy, prostatic hypertrophy and malignancy

- Hepatic. Hepatic blood flow and drug clearance are reduced. There is a 1% loss in function per year after 30 years
- Metabolic/endocrine. Adipose tissue increases whilst muscle bulk and total body water are reduced. The BMR falls by 1% per year after 30 years, and thermoregulation is impaired
  - Diseases: Diabetes (in 25% of over 85 years olds), thyroid disease, osteoporosis and nutritional disorders
- Pharmacology. Altered drug absorption, protein binding, metabolism and excretion in combination with ageing body systems make drug effects more variable in the elderly. Minimal alveolar concentration drops by 5–6% per decade after 40 years. One-third of over 75 years olds take three or more drugs each day
- Social issues. There is a wide variation in social support in the elderly, ranging from full care in a residential home to complete independence or as sole carer for an invalid spouse. Such issues affect ability to get to hospital and suitability for discharge, especially if day case surgery is anticipated. An alteration in surroundings or routine can be particularly distressing for an elderly patient
- Manual handling. Skin loses elasticity and becomes thin and easily bruised. Care is required when using adhesive dressings/tape and small wounds can take months to heal. Special attention with patient positioning and lifting is required to ensure that skin tears and pressure areas do not develop
- Airway. Dentition is often poor with loose incisors particularly at risk. Reduced neck movement and mouth opening will increase difficulty with intubation. Gastro-oesophageal reflux is more common. Conversely, the edentulate airway is usually easier to manage

Anaesthetic management

Assessment and premedication

History and examination should be system specific and may lead to other investigations as indicated. Depending on surgery, it is typical in most institutions to take baseline FBC, urea and electrolytes and ECG in over 65 years olds. Anaemia is often iron deficient and may be corrected with intravenous iron. A social history should be taken to ensure adequate home support. Reduced cognitive ability will require careful assessment to ensure the patient fully understands their procedure.

Anxiolytic premedication can reduce perioperative sympathetic drive/cardiac stress but should be considered carefully as it carries the risk of postoperative confusion and delayed discharge. NSAIDs should also be given careful thought due to the increased risk of renal damage and gastric irritation in the elderly. If used, duration of treatment should be limited to the initial perioperative days. The decision to operate may be difficult and should be made at consultant-level with the patient and their relatives where possible.

Conduct of anaesthetic

Monitoring is as indicated by the systems pathology and planned surgery. Depth of anaesthesia monitoring is recommended to allow more accurate titration of anaesthetic agents. Regional anaesthesia avoids the problems of a GA and should be used where possible although there is currently little evidence of outcome benefit for regional anaesthesia over GA. Due to a poorly compliant vascular tree and reduced autonomic control, hypotension is common with neuroaxial block. All patients should receive supplementary O_2. Hypotension and hypoxaemia may lead to perioperative confusion.

Propofol is the induction agent of choice due to its rapid elimination and minimal side-effect profile. Intravenous agents should be given slowly and in small doses, being wary of a slow arm/brain circulation time. Synergy with opiates and other agents can quickly lead to overshoot of the desired anaesthetic depth. Dentition is often poor and IPPV may cause a marked fall in blood pressure. Special care should be taken with respect to pressure points when positioning the patient. Patient warming from the anaesthetic room onwards will prevent hypothermia. Operating times should be kept to the minimum. Glycopyrrolate should be used in preference to atropine, as it does not cross the blood/brain barrier to cause confusion. Intravenous fluids should be used judiciously as both dehydration and fluid overload are easy to achieve and carry significant morbidity. Generally preop elderly patients are more often under filled than over.

Pressure areas should be carefully padded. Advancing age is a risk factor for DVT and prophylaxis should be used, although graduated compression stockings are contraindicated in PVD or leg ulceration.

Postoperative care

Supplementary O_2, intensive physiotherapy, nutrition and early mobilization will reduce postoperative sequelae. Thromboembolic events are frequent and prophylaxis should be used. Analgesia is titrated to effect when using opioids. PCA or regional techniques may also be used. Fluid balance, including the use of charts, is again crucial in the postoperative period to maintain renal and cardiac perfusion. Pressure-relieving air mattresses should be used postoperatively for major surgery to prevent pressure injury. Perioperative nutritional status should be optimised and early post-operative nutritional support instigated at the earliest opportunity. There should be a low threshold for HDU admission, which may improve the long-term outcome.

Further reading

Griffiths R, Beech F, Brown A, et al. Peri-operative care of the elderly. Anaesthesia 2014;69 (Suppl. 1):81-98.
Kelly F. Anaesthesia for the elderly patient. Update in Anaesthesia 2009. http://update.anaesthesiologists.org/wp-content/uploads/2009/08/Elderly-Patients-and-Anaesthesia.pdf

Related topics of interest

Electroconvulsive therapy

Key points

- Electroconvulsive therapy (ECT) remains an important treatment option for severe psychiatric disorders
- Physiological changes produced by the therapy can be marked
- ECT almost invariably occurs in remote locations with all the inherent issues of that setting

ECT still has a place in modern psychiatric therapy although the role is quite narrowly defined. For example, UK NICE recommendations confine use to 'acute treatment of severe depression that is life-threatening and when a rapid response is required, or when other treatments have failed'. It may rarely be used to treat mania and catatonia. ECT consists of delivery of an electrical current to the cerebral hemispheres with the aim of inducing a generalised seizure of between 10 and 120 seconds. The electrodes may be either bilateral (more effective, but more likely to produce cognitive deficits) or unilateral, applied to the nondominant hemisphere. Courses of ECT are usually between 6 and 12 treatments. The precise mechanism of effect is unknown.

Problems

Physiological effects of ECT

ECT stimulates the autonomic nervous system, initially parasympathetic (with transient hypotension, bradycardia and possible asystole), then sympathetic discharge. The latter results in hypertension, tachycardia and increased myocardial oxygen demand. Oxygen consumption by skeletal muscle also increases during fits, and thus myocardial ischaemia may occur. Left ventricular dysfunction may last up to 6 hours post-procedure. Recent MI (<3 months) is a relative contraindication to ECT.

Cognitive deficits including disorientation, agitation and amnesia occur in up to 50% of patients receiving ECT. Most resolve within 6 months. Cerebral blood flow and intracranial pressure (ICP) increase during treatment, and recent stroke or raised ICP are relative contraindications.

Skeletal muscle contraction may be marked during seizure activity. Prior to the routine use of muscle relaxants, fractures were common. Presence of unstable fractures or severe osteoporosis are relative contraindications.

Remote site anaesthesia

The Royal College of Anaethestists' (UK) guidance on remote site anaesthesia specifies that, wherever possible, care should be consultant delivered. This recognises the higher risk associated with providing anaesthesia outside of the normal theatre environment.

Specific guidance and standards also exist regarding provision of remote site anaesthesia for ECT. For example in the UK, the ECT Accreditation ECT Accreditation Service (ECTAS) is a standards committee affiliated with the Royal College of Psychiatrists. Approximately 80% of UK ECT clinics are accredited. The anaesthesia standards have been set in conjunction with the AAGBI and the Royal College of Anaesthetists.

Consent issues

Patients receiving ECT may be inpatients or outpatients. If inpatients, they may be there voluntarily, or detained under mental health legislation ('sectioned'). If their psychiatrist believes ECT to be in the patient's best interests and the patient lacks capacity to consent, a second opinion must be sought from an independent doctor (appointed by the CQC in England). Very occasionally, this process may be omitted in an emergency, e.g. patient refusing to eat or drink with a serious threat to life.

Patients may have an advance directive specifying that they would not accept ECT. Provided that this is a valid directive (applicable to the scenario in question, made when the person had capacity, properly witnessed), this cannot be overruled.

Anaesthetic management

Preoperative

As for any elective case, patients should have had appropriate investigations including ECG, and be fasted. The risk:benefit ratio of anaesthetising ASA >3 patients in a remote site should be carefully considered. The presence of qualified anaesthetic assistance and recovery staff and pretreatment safety checklists is essential. In addition to standard minimum monitoring, seizure activity is monitored with a limited EEG to guide titration of the stimulation dose. Equipment and drugs should be available as stated in ECTAS guidelines (**Table 13**).The anaesthetist must be satisfied that consent is either present, or the correct processes have been followed to proceed without it.

Intraoperative

All currently available intravenous induction agents are suitable for use in ECT; however, propofol is used most frequently. All agents, with the possible exception of etomidate, raise the seizure threshold. Use of a short-acting opioid, such as alfentanil 10–20 µg/kg, may help to offset the anticonvulsant properties of the induction agent by dose reduction. Propofol doses of 0.75–2.5 mg/kg are used.

In early ECT treatments, stimulus magnitude may be altered until acceptable seizure duration is seen. This may require further doses of induction agent. Once treatment is well established, it is preferable to keep the dose of induction dose relatively constant to allow the psychiatrist to adjust the stimulus as necessary (seizure threshold usually increases during the treatment course).

In order to reduce the risk of musculoskeletal injury, it is common to attenuate the seizure with a small dose of muscle relaxant. This is usually suxamethonium 0.5 mg/kg but if contraindicated, then mivacurium 0.15 mg/kg is acceptable.

The patient should be preoxygenated. After induction, hyperventilation can help to reduce the seizure threshold. Bite blocks are routine to avoid tongue biting. Advanced airway management is not usually required. Post-seizure, ventilation can be assisted until spontaneous ventilation returns.

Postoperative

During recovery, the patient should be monitored as normal. Emergence agitation can be reduced by familiar staff, a quiet environment and very occasionally by small doses of midazolam. Cardiovascular disturbance may still occur at this stage.

Table 13 Standards for provision of anaesthesia for ECT	
Standard type	Standard
1	Comply with 'Recommendations for standards of monitoring during anaesthesia and recovery', Association of Anaesthetists of Great Britain and Ireland (2007) minimum monitoring standards
1	The anaesthetist checks all anaesthetic equipment, including suction. Also personally prepares anaesthetic drugs
1	There is a consistent use of anaesthetic agents and dosing
2	Any reason for a change in anaesthetic induction agent is discussed with the ECT team and documented
1	Oxygen should typically be delivered before ECT in order to maintain suitable oxygen saturation
1	Anaesthesia is administered on a trolley or bed that can be swiftly tipped to a head down position
1	Before induction, a member of the anaesthetic team ensures dentures are either secure or removed
2	The clinic should maintain and adhere to up-to-date guidelines for ECT anaesthesia
2	The anaesthetist explains what he/she is doing and why
2	The anaesthetist ensures that the patient is protected during the seizure
2	When the patient is induced, a member of the anaesthetic team inserts a bite block if required

Adapted from ECTAS guidelines.
Type 1, infringement would compromise patient safety; Type 2, expected of an accredited ECT clinic; Type 3, expected of an excellent ECT clinic. ECT, electroconvulsive therapy; ECTAS, ECT Accreditation Service.

Further reading

National Institute of Health and Care Excellence. Depression in Adults (CG 90). London: NICE, 2009.

The Royal College of Anaesthetists. Anaesthetic services in remote sites. London: RCoA, 2011.

Royal College of Psychiatrists' Centre of Quality Improvement. ECTAS Standards for the administration of ECT. London: RCPCQI, 2012.

Uppal V, Dourish J, Macfarlane A. Anaesthesia for electroconvulsive therapy. Br J Anaesth: Contin Educ Anaesth, Crit Care Pain 2010; 10:192–196.

Related topics of interest

- Day surgery (p. 51)
- Ethics and consent (p. 76)
- Neurological disease – epilepsy (p. 140)

Emergency anaesthesia

Key points

- Time pressures prevent full preoptimisation of the emergency patient
- Emergency surgery carries a significantly higher mortality than elective procedures
- The time-critical nature of surgery needs to be balanced against time spent in preoperative resuscitation and optimisation
- Critical events are more likely during emergency surgery

Despite an increase in consultant presence out of hours in UK hospitals, emergency procedures are still often undertaken by less experienced clinicians at night or weekends. Management of high-risk patients out of hours by junior anaesthetists is associated with worse outcome.

Problems

- Limited time to prepare the patient for surgery and anaesthesia
- Hypovolaemia. This is common and may be related to poor fluid intake, haemorrhage (covert or overt), diarrhoea, vomiting, sweating or abnormal fluid shifts. There may be associated electrolyte disturbance, especially related to potassium
- Aspiration risk. Stomach emptying is unreliable in emergency patients and depends on the volume and content of the last meal, pain, analgesia administered and emotional state of the patient. Gastric motility is reduced by fear, pain and opioids. Controversy exists as to when it is safe to assume the stomach is empty. A 6-hour rule is often applied from the ingestion of food to anaesthesia, but trauma patients have been found to have substantial food residues after 24 hours. The time from food ingestion to time of trauma is useful in deciding likelihood of gastric emptying (a solid meal taking < 6 hours). The NAP4 audit found aspiration to be the commonest cause of anaesthesia-related death, particularly in emergency

procedures and (those undertaken by) junior anaesthetists. Risk of aspiration was generally understated with failure to perform rapid sequence induction (RSI) and overuse of supraglottic devices a clear factor
- Pain. Preoperative regional anaesthesia, such as femoral nerve block, can provide significant relief
- Premedication is often not possible
- Coexisting disease. Uncontrolled medical conditions may present at the same time as a surgical emergency, e.g. diabetes, hypertension, cardiac failure or atrial fibrillation. The urgency of surgery will require balancing against time spent optimising such conditions. Preoptimisation may be best undertaken in the HDU setting where even a short period of time can improve the clinical picture and reduce perioperative morbidity

Anaesthetic management

All patients must be assessed prior to anaesthesia and emergency patients are no exception to this. The risk of pulmonary aspiration and anticipated ease of intubation should be noted. The results of relevant investigations and the availability of blood and blood products should be checked (autologous or fully cross-matched blood should be used where possible). Results of necessary investigations should be available prior to anaesthesia unless there is an immediate threat to life, e.g. ruptured aortic aneurysm. Near-patient testing, such as HemoCue, arterial blood gas measurement and thromboelastography, can provide rapid results in a time-pressured setting.

Fluid resuscitation should be initiated and hypovolaemia and electrolyte disturbance treated prior to the induction of anaesthesia. Anaesthetic induction in the presence of severe hypovolaemia is extremely high risk and often results in cardiac arrest.

Diabetes, cardiac failure and other acute medical conditions should be managed where possible in a pragmatic manner, although full optimisation may not be possible in a reduced time span. Preoperative assessment may be limited to an 'AMPLE' history (Allergies, Medications, Past medical history, Last food/drink, recent Events), timely examination, an explanation of the proposed anaesthetic procedure and the control of pain.

Antibiotic prophylaxis and thromboembolism prevention are easily forgotten in the emergency setting. The planned management of the case should be discussed with senior staff and appropriate help requested. Measures to empty the stomach (postpone operation, fasting, gastric suction, prokinetic agents) should be considered.

Standard equipment, emergency drugs (including vasopressors, atropine, suxamethonium) and minimal monitoring standards should always be available. Ensure adequate intravenous access with a large-bore cannula. Preoxygenate the patient with 100% oxygen for 3 minutes (or 4 vital capacity breaths). A RSI with thiopentone, cricoid pressure and suxamethonium (unless contraindicated) has traditionally been the method of choice for general anaesthesia. However, propofol and rocuronium 1-1.2 mg/kg (with the availability of sugammadex) are now alternative agents gaining greater acceptance for use in rapid sequence induction. Most anaesthetists are now more familiar with the characteristics of propofol than thiopentone, and rocuronium has a favourable side-effect profile to suxamethonium whilst producing similar intubation conditions.

Induction agents should be administered with care in patients who are hypovolaemic or septic. Ketamine, (often the drug of choice in severe hypovolaemia) and etomidate are associated with less hypotension following administration. Etomidate has other undesirable side effects.

A technique should be chosen which guarantees rapid return of protective airway reflexes. The aspiration risk is still present at extubation and this should only be performed after full return of these reflexes, when the patient is awake. Regional anaesthesia can be particularly effectual for emergency surgery, obviating the need for definitive airway control. In fact, 'rapid sequence spinal' anaesthesia has recently been described for emergency caesarean section. Postoperatively, HDU or ICU should be considered if the patient remains unstable or requires further resuscitation.

Further reading

Campling EA. Who operates when? A report of the National Confidential Enquiry into perioperative deaths. London; NCEPOD, 1997.

Cook TM, Woodall N, Frerk C. Fourth National Audit Project. Major complications of airway management in the UK: results of the Fourth National Audit Project of the Royal College of Anaesthetists and the Difficult Airway Society. Part 1: anaesthesia. Br J Anaesth 2011; 106:617–631.

Kinsella SM, Girgirah K, Scrutton MJ. Rapid sequence spinal anaesthesia for category-1 urgency caesarean section: a case series. Anaesthesia 2010; 65:664–649.

Related topics of interest

Endocrine disease

Key points

- Endocrine disease frequently complicates surgery for unrelated conditions
- Adrenal disease requires careful consideration and management of volume and electrolyte status
- The principal aim of anaesthesia in carcinoid syndrome is to provide stable, smooth anaesthesia and chemical suppression of vasoactive substances

The endocrine system is a complex autoregulatory messenger system of glands secreting messenger chemicals into the bloodstream (as opposed to exocrine glands, which secrete substances directly into ducts).

Adrenal disease

The adrenal cortex produces glucocorticoid, mineralocorticoid and sex hormones (mainly testosterone). Cortisol, the principal glucocorticoid, modulates stress and inflammatory responses. It is a potent stimulator of gluconeogenesis and antagonises insulin. Aldosterone is the principal mineralocorticoid. It causes increased sodium reabsorption, and potassium and hydrogen ion loss at the distal renal tubule. Adrenal androgen production increases markedly at puberty, declining with age thereafter. Androstenedione is converted by the liver to testosterone in the male and oestrogen in the female. Cortisol and androgen production are under diurnal pituitary control (adrenocorticotropic hormone – ACTH). Aldosterone is released in response to angiotensin II (produced following renal renin release) and subsequent pulmonary angiotensin I conversion. Clinical diseases result from relative excess or lack of hormones.

Adrenocortical excess

Cushing's syndrome

This may result from steroid therapy, adrenal hyperplasia, adrenal carcinoma or ectopic ACTH.

Cushing's disease

This is due to an ACTH-secreting pituitary tumour. Clinical features of adrenocortical excess include moon face, thin skin, easy bruising, hypertension (60%), hirsutism, obesity with a centripetal distribution, buffalo hump, muscle weakness, diabetes (10%), osteoporosis (50%), aseptic necrosis of the hip and pancreatitis (especially with iatrogenic Cushing's syndrome).

Problems

- Control of blood sugar (insulin may be required)
- Hypokalaemia resulting in arrhythmias, muscle weakness and postoperative respiratory embarrassment
- Hypertension, polycythaemia, congestive heart failure. The patient may require cardiac output monitoring
- Atrophic skin and osteoporosis demand care when positioning the patient during anaesthesia and with vessel cannulation

Adrenocortical deficiency

Acute

This may follow sepsis, pharmacological adrenal suppression or adrenal haemorrhage associated with anticoagulant therapy. Critical illness usually triggers mineralocorticoid release; however, critical illness or prior chronic high-dose steroid therapy can result in adrenocortical suppression. Clinical features include apathy, hypotension, coma and hypoglycaemia.

Chronic

Chronic deficiency may follow surgical adrenalectomy, autoimmune adrenalitis (Addison's disease), adrenal infiltration with tumour, leukaemia, infection (TB, histoplasmosis), amyloidosis, or secondary to pituitary dysfunction. Clinical features include fatigue, weakness, weight loss, nausea and hyperpigmentation. Hypotension, hyponatraemia, hyperkalaemia, eosinophilia and occasionally hypoglycaemia may also be found on further investigation. A short

Synacthen test is used to assess the adrenal gland's ability to produce cortisol.

Problems

- Hypotension, a low intravascular volume and a small heart may precipitate circulatory collapse with minor fluid overload
- Hypoglycaemia
- Hyperkalaemia – potential risk with suxamethonium
- Steroid replacement therapy

Hyperaldosteronism

Primary (Conn's syndrome)

This is caused by an adenoma in the zona glomerulosa secreting aldosterone. Clinical features include hypokalaemia, muscle weakness and hypertension.

Problems

- Hypokalaemia may result in cardiac arrhythmias, postoperative muscle weakness and respiratory embarrassment
- Hypertension
- Hypernatraemia, metabolic alkalosis
- Hormone and sodium replacement following adrenalectomy

Anaesthetic management

Assessment and premedication

The state of the disease must be assessed preoperatively and electrolyte and glucose disorders corrected. Steroid supplementation will be required for patients with Addison's disease, or if pituitary ablation or adrenalectomy is to be performed. Supplementary perioperative steroids should be given if the patient takes >10 mg prednisolone/day or has done so regularly within the last 3 months. The patient should take their usual steroid dose with additional hydrocortisone supplementation, ranging form a single 25 mg perioperative dose (minor surgery) to 100 mg/day in divided doses for the 72 hours following surgery (major surgery). Patients taking high-dose steroids to produce immunosuppression should remain on the same doses perioperatively. Excess supplementation can cause immunosuppression, glucose intolerance and delayed wound healing.

Conduct of anaesthesia

A single dose of etomidate may interfere with cortisol synthesis for at least 24 hours in the critically ill patient. A meta-analysis in 2012 concluded that there was a 1.2 increase in relative mortality risk following a single dose. Epidural anaesthesia may reduce the stress response, providing the level of block is adequate and it is continued into the postoperative period. Blood volume, glucose and potassium should be monitored regularly. Pneumothorax may occur following adrenalectomy. Steroid replacement will be required after adrenalectomy and is usually started preop.

Pituitary disease – acromegaly

Usually due to a pituitary adenoma, this is due to oversecretion of growth hormone. Physical characteristics include large hands and feet, splayed teeth and multinodular goitre. There is an increased risk of malignancy. It may be diagnosed by glucose tolerance test and pituitary imaging. Primary treatment is usually surgery. Medical options are more limited but include octreotide and dopamine agonists (bromocriptine).

Problems

- Cardiovascular disease. Hypertension, hypertriglyceridaemia and cardiomyopathy. Patients have double the rate of cardiac-related death compared with the general population
- Diabetes mellitus
- Airway. The large jaw and tongue make intubation more difficult. There may be epiglottic hypertrophy, vocal cord thickening and subglottic stenosis. Sleep apnoea is common (70%)
- Myopathy – usually proximal
- Hypercalcaemia

Anaesthetic management

Likelihood of difficult intubation should be assessed and a history of sleep apnoea explored. Coexisting diabetes should be managed. Echocardiography should be considered to assess cardiomyopathy/hypertrophy. Nerve compression is frequent and particular care should be taken with patient positioning.

Postoperative care should be in the HDU/ICU setting. Noninvasive ventilation should be considered for obstructive sleep apnoea.

Carcinoid syndrome

Carcinoid tumours may secrete 5-hydroxytryptamine (5HT), bradykinin, histamine, substance-P or prostaglandins. Various clinical manifestations may therefore be seen. Tumours arise in enterochromaffin (argentaffin) cells and produce symptoms when peripheral levels of 5HT, etc. reach high levels. In 36%, the tumour is of the small bowel (metastasising to the liver before causing the carcinoid syndrome); however, other sites such as the lung, pancreas, large bowel and stomach are described. They are often multiple in number and generally slow growing, utilising dietary tryptophan (causing nicotinamide deficiency manifesting as pellagra). The classic syndrome is of diarrhoea, flushing with hypotension, telangiectasia and bronchospasm. Less commonly, hypertension and right-sided valvular lesions (endocardial fibrosis) occur. The $5HT_2$ receptor mediates vasoconstriction. Attacks may be precipitated by exercise, anxiety and alcohol. Diagnosis is confirmed by a raised urinary 5-hydroxyindole acetic acid on a low serotonin diet. The incidence is 1:12,000.

Problems

- Right ventricular or biventricular heart failure due to excess hormone release. Cardiac lesions especially pulmonary stenosis and tricuspid regurgitation
- Haemodynamic effects of tumour products may manifest as hyper- or hypotensive crises in the perioperative period, even in the asymptomatic patient
- Bronchospasm
- Electrolyte imbalance and malnutrition (diarrhoea)
- Of the primary tumour, e.g. bleeding and gastrointestinal obstruction

Anaesthetic management

Assessment and premedication

A careful cardiac assessment, including echocardiography and possibly exercise testing/angiography, will determine the extent of cardiac involvement. Standard investigations should include FBC, urea and electrolytes, blood sugar, liver function tests, clotting, ECG and chest X-ray, with more specific tests as indicated by the symptoms and signs.

It is important to determine what substance the tumour is predominantly secreting, as this will allow prediction of the likely effects. The preoperative assessment should include a search for all the features of the syndrome. Treatment is aimed at blocking the release or effects of vasoactive substances. Preoperative octreotide therapy (a somatostatin analogue) blocks gastroenteropancreatic peptide release as well as growth hormone, glucagon and insulin. Side effects include QT prolongation, hypoglycaemia, bradycardia, abdominal cramping and nausea. An octreotide infusion (100 μg/h) should commence at least 12 hours prior to surgery. Additional 5HT antagonists such as methysergide, ketanserin or cyproheptadine may be used.

Premedication may be with an oral benzodiazepine, H_1 and H_2 antagonists. Patients who have received steroids will require further supplementation.

Conduct of anaesthesia

Regional anaesthesia. Thoracic epidural is considered a reasonable approach to minimise stress-induced carcinoid crises. However, epidural-related hypotension can cause release of bradykinin with associated cardiovascular instability, which can be extremely difficult to control. On balance, careful placement and judicious use of an epidural is probably the safest approach.

General anaesthesia. Monitoring should include arterial pressure (preinduction) and invasive cardiac monitoring, with central venous access and/or oesophageal Doppler or similar to guide fluid management. Large-bore intravenous (IV) access should be available. Blood sugar should be monitored.

The principal aim is for smooth, stable anaesthesia and surgery. Avoid histamine releasing and drugs prone to cardiac instability (including suxamethonium, morphine, atracurium). Judicious dosing of propofol and remifentanil will provide smooth intubating conditions. Rocuronium or vecuronium are suitable neuromuscular blocking drugs. Total intravenous anaesthesia or sevoflurane/isoflurane is recommended maintenance agent. Infusion of octreotide should be given during the procedure.

Management of perioperative stressors and tumour manipulation:

- Hypertension should be treated with magnesium (0.5–1 mg IV), octreotide (20–50 µg IV), phentolamine (0.5–12 mg IV), GTN infusion or labetalol (5 mg IV). Careful titration of these agents is required to prevent overshoot

- Hypotension should be managed with IV fluid bolus, octreotide (20–50 µg) or metaraminol/phenylephrine
- Sympathomimetics are conventionally avoided as they may precipitate release of peptides by a-adrenergic stimulation leading to paradoxical rebound hypotension
- Note that octreotide can be given for perioperative hyper- and hypotension

Postoperative care

ITU/HDU care should be used for the immediate postoperative period, as cardiovascular instability is likely. Good analgesia, careful fluid management and octreotide infusion should be continued for 24–48 hours.

Further reading

Davies M, Hardman J. Anaesthesia and adrenocortical disease. Br J Anaesth: Contin Educ Anaesth Crit Care Pain Med 2005; 5:122–126.

Related topics of interest

Ethics and consent

Key points

- There are a number of ethical principles that can be applied to medicine, which may not always be compatible with each other
- There are ethical, practical and legal considerations when taking consent
- Legislation (e.g. in England and Wales, the Mental Capacity Act, MCA) may be used to assist in gaining consent where patients may lack the capacity

Ethics involves the development of ideas about right and wrong in relation to human intentions, decisions and actions. Biomedical ethics is a practical application of this discipline, which seeks to provide professional guidance to health workers and scientists, and influences the development of medical law. Ethics may in turn be influenced by personal, communal, cultural and religious factors.

Approaches to medical ethics

There are a number of generic approaches to ethical decision making, each with its own inherent advantages and disadvantages.
- Virtue-based ethics: Ethical decisions are focused on the decision maker's intentions. To be 'virtuous' one needs to intend to do the best for the patient, based on gathering knowledge and experience
- Outcome based or consequentialist ethics: Ethical decisions focused on optimising the moral outcome of a situation, of which utilitarianism is perhaps best known. 'What would constitute the best outcome in this situation, and how can I bring that about'?
- Duty based or deontological ethics: Ethical decisions focused on the idea of duties and rules. For example 'never lying' regardless of outcome. 'What am I morally obliged to do (or not to do) in this situation?'

Discussing medical ethics

The 'four-principle approach' is an accessible method of identifying and framing medical ethical dilemmas. No one principle is necessarily pre-eminent amongst the rest and conflicts between principles are common.
- Respect for autonomy: Acknowledgement of, and action to promote, a person's right to make choices free from both controlling interference and from limitations that prevent meaningful decision making
- Nonmaleficence: 'Above all do no harm'. This includes taking proactive steps to avoid/minimise the risk of harm
- Beneficence: The obligation to use medical knowledge and skills constructively in order to seek patient-centred benefits
- Justice: The fair and equitable provision of medical care amongst patients, in the light of what is due or owed to them

Guidance and consensus

As a basis for discussion, this section makes reference to English and Welsh law. Legislation varies significantly according to the legal system of each country: readers should check national law and guidelines. **Figure 7** provides a pragmatic scheme for approaching and resolving ethical dilemmas as they arise in the workplace. The emphasis in all cases is on information gathering. The patient and their best interests should remain at the heart of the process.

Consent

The responsibility for ensuring valid consent prior to any intervention lies with the clinician providing the intervention. In obtaining consent in medical practice, there are legal, ethical and practical imperatives.
- Ethical: The moral obligation, as mentioned above, to promote the rights and views of the individual patient
- Practical: Patients are more likely to comply/cooperate with treatments that have a purpose they understand and value
- Legal: Doctors who fail to obtain consent from competent patients risk criminal conviction or civil liability for assault or battery. 'Assault' is, by words or actions, causing an individual to believe they are at immediate risk of personal violence, whilst 'battery' is the unlawful (including

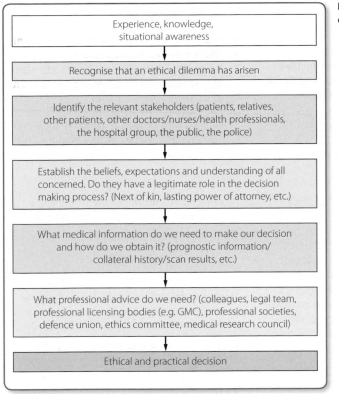

Figure 7 A stepwise approach to ethical decision making.

nonconsensual) application of force upon an individual. Touching constitutes sufficient force for a charge of battery. In addition, doctors may be found liable for clinical negligence in civil court actions where they fail to disclose important/ relevant information about medical interventions during the consent process

Valid consent

- Arises during a process of ongoing doctor–patient consultation
- Is given by the patient or by an authorised proxy decision maker where the patient lacks capacity
- Is given voluntarily for a specific intervention
- Is given by a patient/decision maker who is well informed about the possible and likely consequences of the intervention in terms of the risks and benefits
- Remains valid indefinitely unless it is actively withdrawn, or material facts emerge which compromise the premise upon which the consent was given in the first place
- Consent can be written, oral or implied (as when a patient holds out their arm to give blood)

Capacity

There are important specific issues pertaining to 'consent' and 'refusal of treatment' in relation to those deemed to lack capacity. Legislation relating to these issues varies from country to country. Here we will use he legislation of England and Wales as the framework for discussing the principles.

The Mental Capacity Act (MCA) 2005 (England and Wales)

The Mental Capacity Act (MCA) 2005 for England and Wales is discussed to demonstrate the key issues. For the purposes of this Act, all patients are presumed to have capacity unless proven otherwise. Patients lack capacity to give valid consent when they are unable to:

- Understand the relevant information, even where every practical means has been utilised in order to help them to do so (i.e. using written information for the deaf, using interpreters, allowing time for sedation to wear off)
- Retain the information long enough to make the decision
- Use or weigh the information as part of the decision-making process
- Communicate the decision effectively, by any means available (including where the only route possible is, e.g. through blinking or muscle twitching)

Prior to deciding a patient lacks capacity, all reasonable attempts must be made to help a patient regain capacity. In cases where patients lack capacity, it remains the responsibility of the clinician to act only in accordance with the patient's best interests, and in the least restrictive manner available to achieve what is necessary in the pursuit of those interests.

'Proxy' decision makers

Where a patient lacks capacity, appropriate decision makers may include parents/responsible guardians, those authorised to do so under a health welfare lasting power of attorney, or a court-appointed deputy following formal hearings. All decisions should be made in the patient's best interests. In some cases, the existence of an advance decision (formerly referred to as an advanced directive) may avoid the need for a proxy decision maker.

Advance decisions (advance directive)

These now form statutory law under the MCA 2005. A valid advance decision:

- Is made by an adult over the age of 18 years

- Is made by someone who has the capacity to make such a decision
- Is clear as to which treatments are being refused
- If including a decision to forgo life-sustaining treatment, must be signed and witnessed in written format and state clearly that the signatory wishes the directive to remain valid even where they will put their life at risk as a result

Minors

Where capacity is concerned, minors (age <18 years) represent a vulnerable and diverse patient group. In essence, the mental capacity of an individual minor should be assessed using the four elements set out in the 2005 MCA indicated above, as for adults. Minors with capacity (sometimes referred to as 'Fraser competent' following a test case in the English courts) may provide valid consent, with or without the knowledge of parents/guardians. Minors may also be able to refuse to undergo treatment, although the position in law on these cases is less clear and legal advice should be obtained.

Emergencies

It is good practice to anticipate clinical emergencies, and to establish patients' views on medical interventions at a stage in their illness where they have the time and capacity to make informed decisions (i.e. about the use of invasive ventilation in chronic obstructive pulmonary disease). However, some emergencies arise where immediate and necessary care (e.g. to preserve life or limb) is required, which precludes the possibility of obtaining formal consent. Where this is the case, good reasons for acting without consent need to be well documented, and the issues should be discussed with the patient or their next of kin at the earliest opportunity.

Further Reading

General Medical Council (GMC). Consent: patients and doctors making decisions together. London; GMC, 2008.

Department of Health. Reference guide to consent for examination or treatment, 2nd edn. London; Department of Health, 2009.

Mental Capacity Act, chapter 9. http://www.legislation.gov.uk/ukpga/2005/9/contents.

Related topics of interest

- Emergency anaesthesia (p. 70)
- Organ donation (p. 171)

Gas embolism

Key points

- Gas embolism outcome depends on the gas volume, rate of entrainment and patient health
- There are a number of methods that can be used to help detect gas embolism
- A high index of suspicion and rapid treatment is essential in this medical emergency
- Treatment is principally based on an ABC approach and measures to prevent further entrainment

Gas embolism is a potential complication of many operations and is usually due to a combination of an open vein above the level of the right atrium, a low central venous pressure (CVP) and poor surgical technique. The outcome depends on the volume and rate of air entrainment, the cardiorespiratory health of the patient, the use of N_2O and the presence of a patent foramen ovale (PFO).

A large bolus of air tends to obstruct right ventricular ejection due to its compressible nature. More insidious gas entrainment is more likely to obstruct the pulmonary vascular tree with resultant pulmonary hypertension and right ventricular failure. An inflammatory response to bubbles within the pulmonary vasculature leads to pulmonary oedema. Gas in the arterial tree (paradoxical air embolism) may arrive by transpulmonary shunting or a PFO, the latter being present in up to 27% adults. A right to left shunt may be precipitated by the use of positive end-expiratory pressure (PEEP) through an increase in right atrial pressure. Gas in the coronary or cerebral arterial circulation is particularly poorly tolerated leading to hypoxic tissue damage. Children are more likely to develop gas embolism and to suffer more profound hypotension.

Predisposing factors

- Neurosurgical and spinal surgery. Incidence of up to 76%, detected by transoesophageal echo for sitting procedures. Operating on the skull and dura (the beginning and end of the operation) places the patient at most risk, as this is when small veins are open
- Orthopaedic, especially hip and knee replacement and arthrograms
- Obstetric related. Termination of pregnancy, manual removal of placenta and whilst the uterus is open during caesarean section
- Abdominal, especially with laparoscopy or uterine insufflation
- ENT, including thyroid and head and neck surgery. A head-up position will reduce venous pressure
- Cardiac surgery. Surgical error or bypass pump failure following direct arterial cannulation
- Others, e.g. endoscopic surgery, epidurals, bronchoscopy, jet ventilation and central line placement

Prevention

Particular care should be taken when performing high-risk procedures in patients with PFO. Preoperative screening has been suggested. General preventative measures include maintenance of venous pressure with intravenous fluids or high PEEP (although not advised for sitting neurosurgical procedures) and reduction in the height of the operating site relative to the right atrium. Suitable patient positioning and attention to detail during central line placement as well as meticulous surgical haemostasis also play essential roles. Placement of central venous access to aid air aspiration prior to high-risk surgery may have a theoretical benefit and has been suggested.

Diagnosis

In the conscious patient, coughing, dyspnoea, chest pain and dizziness progressing to loss of consciousness may occur. In the unconscious patient, diagnosis is based on the signs of developing hypotension, tachycardia, jugular venous distension and decreased pulmonary compliance during an 'at-risk' operation.

It may also be made using the specific monitoring aids listed below.

Monitoring

- Basic senses. Hissing may be heard or bubbles seen being sucked into open veins
- Heart sounds. The classical 'millwheel' murmur may be heard using an oesophageal or precordial stethoscope. It is insensitive (1.5–4.0 mL air/kg) and may be preceded by cardiovascular collapse
- ECG may show development of right ventricular strain and arrhythmias, and ST segment depression
- CVP. Obstruction of right heart filling by the embolism will cause a rise in CVP
- Capnography. As emboli are trapped in the lung, perfusion falls causing an increase in physiological dead space. This results in a marked fall in the peak end expired CO_2 concentration. Capnography allows the detection of an air embolism before cardiovascular compromise occurs (1.5 mL air/kg)
- Expired gas analysis. Once alveolar denitrogenation has been completed, the detection of further nitrogen in expired gas signifies the occurrence of an air embolism
- Pulmonary artery pressure. Raised PAP occurs with air embolism. Return to 'pre-embolism' levels can be used as an indication of successful treatment and the timing of the recommencement of surgery
- Precordial or oesophageal Doppler. Ultrasonic detection of air embolism is very accurate, permitting the detection of 0.5 mL of air. A change from the usual swishing noise to a roaring sound is heard. Limitations include diathermy interference, maintenance of good patient contact and recognition of a changing noise pattern. Distinction between inconsequential gas embolism and major embolism is difficult
- Transoesophageal echocardiography can provide a two-dimensional four-chamber view in skilled hands. Although more sensitive than Doppler, it is also not specific and is unable to differentiate between air, fat and blood microemboli.

It is able to localise intracardiac air to a specific chamber, therefore detecting paradoxical air embolism

Treatment

- Initial management should follow an ABC approach. Massive embolism may require cardiopulmonary resuscitation, which should not be delayed
- Surgical. Once air embolism is detected the surgeon should flood the wound with saline or cover with wet gauze. The surgical site should be lowered below the right atrium if possible. A careful search for open veins is then made. Laparoscopy-related embolism should trigger immediate cavity desufflation
- Venous pressure may be raised by intravenous volume loading, use of PEEP or Valsalva manoeuvre and manual jugular venous compression. Neck pressure obstructs venous drainage preventing further air entry during head and neck and neurosurgery. It also increases local venous pressure, filling potentially open veins with blood
- Nitrous oxide should be discontinued and 100% O_2 given. Being 35 times more water-soluble than N_2, N_2O is rapidly transported to intravascular air increasing the bubble size. Hyperbaric oxygen will enhance bubble elimination but is only suitable for stable patients
- A multiorifice central venous catheter with the tip at the caval–atrial junction may be useful for aspiration of the air embolus. However, placement should not delay other measures and practical benefit is doubtful due to the low likelihood of successful tip placement within the airlock
- Drugs are given as indicated to support the cardiovascular system
- Position. The left lateral head down position and the Trendelenburg position may prevent a large air embolus from entering the pulmonary artery by 'trapping' it in the right ventricle
- If available, emergency cardiopulmonary bypass can effectively maintain circulatory perfusion whilst the gas is removed

Further reading

Mirski MA, Lele AV, Fitzsimmons L, et al. Diagnosis and treatment of vascular air embolism. Anaesthesiology 2007; 106:164–177.
Webber S, Andrzejowski J, Francis G. Gas embolism in anaesthesia. Br J Anaesth: Contin Educ Profess Develop Rev 2002; 2:53–57.

Wenham TN, Graham D. Venous gas embolism: an unusual complication of laparoscopic cholecystectomy. J Minim Access Surg 2009; 5:35–36.

Related topics of interest

- Airway – the shared airway (p. 10)
- Neuroanaesthesia – tumours (p. 134)
- Orthopaedics – elective (p. 174)
- Positioning for surgery (p. 220)
- Substance abuse (p. 287)
- Thyroid and parathyroid surgery (p. 300)
- Vascular access (p. 311)

Gynaecology

Key points

- Gynaecological surgery is varied in its range and patients and an increasing number of procedures are performed by minimally invasive techniques, the ramifications of which must be kept in mind
- Anxiety is common for many reasons and these patients must be treated with particular sensitivity
- The approach to most minor procedures should reference good day case anaesthesia technique

Gynaecological surgery covers a very wide range of surgical procedures, from the quick and minor cases, which are often carried out as day cases, to prolonged and complex major pelvic surgery. Equally, women presenting for gynaecological procedures are a diverse group from the young and healthy to the elderly with multiple comorbidities.

Problems

- Many women are very apprehensive preoperatively, even those scheduled for relatively minor surgery
- Those undergoing gynaecological surgery may be at higher risk of postoperative nausea and vomiting (PONV)
- Vagal stimulation is common. Good communication with the surgical team is essential. Have antimuscarinic drugs such as atropine or glycopyrrolate to hand
- Careful positioning of patients is key for this surgical discipline. Patients are commonly in the lithotomy or steep head-down position. This can result in peripheral nerve injury, aspiration of gastric contents, high airway pressures and displacement of airway devices
- Those undergoing pelvic surgery are at high risk of postoperative deep vein thrombosis
- Obesity is a risk factor for gynaecological malignancy. Many patients presenting for surgery will have a raised BMI

- Some gynaecological procedures, especially those for malignancy, can be prolonged with significant blood loss. These cases present all the normal challenges faced during major complex surgery
- An increasing number of procedures are being carried out laparoscopically. In some centres, major oncology surgery is being performed as robot-assisted laparoscopic surgery. Carefully consider the ramifications of these modes of surgery, particularly in combination with steeply tilted positions

Anaesthetic management – minor procedures

Common procedures include:
- Hysteroscopy
- Evacuation of retained products of conception (ERPC)
- Surgical termination of pregnancy (STOP)
- Thermoablation of the endometrium
- Cervical biopsy and large loop excision of the transformation zone (LLETZ)
- Laparoscopic sterilisation

Preoperative

Patients for these procedures are usually young and fit but they are commonly very anxious. Longer time should be allowed for the preoperative visit and the induction of anaesthesia. The vast majority can be done as day case procedures.

Patients should receive preoperative paracetamol and a nonsteroidal anti-inflammatory drug (NSAID) (in the absence of contraindications). Alternatively, the NSAID can be given as a rectal suppository intraoperatively (such as diclofenac 100 mg) but specific consent must be obtained for this.

Intraoperative

Those who are in their second or third trimester of pregnancy are at high risk of aspiration so should have a rapid sequence induction of anaesthesia and be intubated. Otherwise a laryngeal mask and spontaneous ventilating technique is frequently used.

Cervical dilatation can result in marked vagal stimulation. Surgical stimulation can produce laryngospasm, particularly in those who are very anxious. There is a risk of uterine perforation for all intrauterine procedures. If the surgeon suspects this, they may proceed to a diagnostic laparoscopy.

Consider the use of prophylactic antiemetics. Those undergoing ERPC and STOP may require oxytocin (5 units intravenously) to help the uterus to contract. This can result in hypotension and tachycardia, even if given as a slow bolus. Its use in the first trimester is very limited as uterine expression of oxytocin receptors is minimal at this gestation.

Postoperative

Simple oral analgesia is normally sufficient. The main postoperative complications include PONV, excess pain and bleeding.

Anaesthetic management – moderate/major procedures

Common procedures include:
- Vaginal hysterectomy
- Anterior/posterior repair for vaginal prolapse
- Total abdominal hysterectomy (+/− bilateral oophorectomy)
- Vulvectomy
- Removal of ectopic pregnancy

Preoperative

Those presenting for major gynaecological surgery tend to be older and therefore have more comorbidities. Time should be spent investigating these preoperatively. There is the potential for blood loss; therefore, all patients should have a valid blood group and save sample as a minimum.

These procedures require more postoperative analgesia than the minor procedures; options include epidural anaesthesia, caudal, spinal, patient-controlled analgesia (PCA), rectus sheath catheters or a combination of the above. Discuss the options with the patient and surgeon preoperatively.

Those presenting with a suspected ectopic pregnancy may show signs of hypovolaemic shock. They should be seen quickly and ensure they have good intravenous access and have blood available. Young patients have a large physiological reserve so compensate well for significant blood loss. Have a high index of suspicion for significant underlying hypovolaemia.

Intraoperative

Take care with positioning, especially those patients who are in the lithotomy position for prolonged periods of time. During some procedures (such as a vaginal hysterectomy) the surgeons will infiltrate local anaesthetic with adrenaline for its vasoconstrictor properties. This has the added advantage of providing postoperative analgesia. Ensure maximum recommended doses of local anaesthetic are not exceeded.

Prepare for oncological surgery to be prolonged with the potential for significant blood loss. These patients should be intubated and there should be consideration of the need for invasive monitoring such as an arterial line. Monitor the temperature intraoperatively and use active warming devices.

Postoperative

All patients should receive regular paracetamol and NSAIDs (if no contraindications). Those who have undergone abdominal hysterectomy will normally require PCA (which can be combined with rectus sheath catheters) or epidural analgesia.

Consider HDU care postoperatively for those with significant comorbidities or for those who have had significant intraoperative blood loss.

Further reading

Morosan M, Popham P. Anaesthesia for gynaecological oncological surgery. Br J Anaesth: Contin Educ Anaesth, Crit Care Pain 2014; 14:63-68.

Viira D, Myles PS. The use of the laryngeal mask in gynaecological laparoscopy. Anaesth Intensive Care 2004; 32:560–563.

Related topics of interest

Human factors in patient safety

Key points

- Human-error represents the underlying cause in the majority of adverse incidents with a significant human and financial cost
- 'Human factors' training is an approach to understanding and minimising the threat to safety posed by the human element of any system

It has become apparent in the last 15–20 years that healthcare is no different to other high-risk industries (airlines, deep-sea oil drilling, nuclear power); failures are costly in both financial and human terms and more often than not are caused by human factors. A US study found error to be the eighth highest cause of in-hospital death, costing $29 billion.

The airline industry led the way with a conference of airline captains and instructors in 1979. This was in response to a series of high-profile disasters caused by 'pilot error'. The aim was to identify the traits and practices of the best pilots which delivered a safe flight deck and then work out how to describe and teach these to all pilots. The result was CRM – Crew Resource Management. The UK Civil Aviation Authority defines this as 'a management system which makes optimum use of all available resources – equipment, procedures and people – to promote safety and enhance efficiency of flight deck operations'. All involved in commercial aviation – e.g. pilots, cabin crew, helicopter emergency medical services (HEMS) paramedics – must undergo specific CRM training annually to maintain their clearance to fly. This illustrates how this is not simply the realm of the pilot but all members of the team. Similarly, as other industries have developed their own nontechnical skills frameworks, team working has been central to all.

Anaesthesia nontechnical skills (ANTS) are central to modern practice. Appreciation of the role of human factors in safe practice takes other forms as well – checklists (e.g. the WHO Safe Surgery Checklist, AAGBI Anaesthesia Machine Check, blood administration checking and ICS

(UK) Transfer Checklists) and structured handovers to name a few. Any strategy to defeat the fallibility of the human element can potentially improve patient safety. It is also important to note that whilst some measures are designed to manage a crisis [e.g. DAS (UK) failed intubation guidance], the principal ethos is to improve routine management and avoid a crisis in the first place.

Specific examples

ANTS

The ANTS framework is the most well-established human factors management structure in anaesthesia and probably all of healthcare. This is composed of 4 categories with 14 elements (**Table 14**). Each element is then described by a number of behavioural markers which illustrate good and poor performance. Communication is conspicuous by its absence from the 4 categories but this is a deliberate reflection of how integral it is to all aspects of ANTS. Situational awareness is the ability to know what is happening around you – audible monitoring of the patient, subtle cues that the surgeons are encountering difficulty, knowledge that a junior colleague may be

Table 14	Anaesthesia non-technical skills (ANTS) system
Category	**Elements**
Team working	• Coordinating activities with team • Exchanging information • Using authority and assertiveness • Assessing capabilities • Supporting others
Situational awareness	• Gathering information • Recognising and understanding • Anticipating
Task management	• Planning and preparing • Prioritising • Providing and maintaining standards • Identifying and utilising resources
Decision making	• Identifying options • Balancing risks and selecting options • Re-evaluating

Reproduced with kind permission from Prof. R Flin, University of Aberdeen

out of their depth in an adjacent theatre. Failure to perceive or correctly interpret these cues is the first step to a potential critical incident. Experienced clinicians can recognise patterns in the cues ('mental models' or 'schemas') and use this to anticipate the next step – being 'ahead of the curve'. The wrong mental model or different models within the team or incorrect implementation of the appropriate script of actions can still lead to an adverse outcome. Integral to this is the next category – decision making. This consists of initial assessment of what the problem is and then making and enacting a suitable plan, assessing the effectiveness of the plan as it proceeds. There are a number of different models describing how decisions are made, often dictated by the stress and time pressure of the situation; a highly stressed situation favours recognition-primed decisions, the implementation of experience of what has worked before in the same situation. Others include rule-based or choice-based decisions, whilst others may call for creative decisions with improvisation and lateral thinking.

These two categories are inextricably linked to the other two – team working and task management. ANTS delineate the performance of an individual as a team member rather than directly assessing the whole team. Team-working skills are as relevant to leadership as they are to 'followership'. This focus has led to the flattening of hierarchies within teams with the express aim of enabling any team member to challenge a leadership decision in the pursuit of enhancing safety and ensuring the right outcome. Most teams, although not all, require a leader of some kind. Task management essentially describes some of the core skills of leadership. As well as reading the situation, it has been noted that the best leaders have a range of leadership styles (directive, consultative, facilitative, delegative etc.) and are able to adapt to the situation, deploying the most appropriate style.

Checklists and care bundles

Checklists and bundles have a significant role to play in standardising care and procedures related to care (e.g. checking the anaesthetic machine). They aim to reduce the chance of overlooking the seemingly mundane in a multitude of tasks to deliver safe care. By combining an array of marginal safety gains, both additively and synergistically, a significant improvement is made with comparatively little effort. Similarly in the emergency situation, where stress and multiple problems reduce mental capacity, a checklist reduces the workload on an individual. Checklists are conceived in advance so they can be comprehensively considered, streamlined and optimally sequenced to deliver the best safety gain when an emergency arises. The WHO Surgical Safety Checklist has been demonstrated to significantly reduce adverse incidents and 30-day hospital mortality.

Simulation

Simulation has a key role to play in all aspects of human factors management. This includes paper-based exercises, part-task trainers, low-fidelity and high-fidelity manikin simulators and in situ simulation. Debrief from scenario-based training, particularly with video replay, is without doubt the most valuable aspect of the training for both participants and observers. Research and training is now focussing on optimising debriefing rather than the approach to running a scenario itself.

Error reporting

An open, no-blame error reporting system is crucial to appreciate the impact of human factors in healthcare. The importance of this is illustrated by James Reason's 'Swiss Cheese' model which explains how latent flaws in several system safety features (the holes in the cheese slices) may occur simultaneously – 'lining up the holes in the Swiss Cheese' – resulting in a system failure. By reducing the number of 'holes' or increasing the number of 'layers of cheese', errors become less likely. Error reporting identifies these latent flaws or lack of checks within a system providing a focus for change and a means to evaluate the success or failure of such changes.

Further reading

Flin R, O'Connor P, Crichton M. Safety at the sharp end: a guide to non-technical skills. Farnham: Ashgate publishing, 2008.

Flin R, Patey R, Glavin R, et al. Anaesthetists' non-technical skills. Br J Anaesth 2010; 105:38–44.

Su Mallory S, Weller J, Bloch M, et al. The individual, the system, and medical error. Br J Anaesth: Contin Educ Profess Develop Rev 2003; 3:179–182.

University of Aberdeen Industrial Psychology Research Centre. ANTS; A behavioural marker system for rating anaesthetists' non-technical skills. [Online] Available from: www.abdn.ac.uk/iprc/ants [Accessed April 2014].

Related topics of interest

Hypertensive disease

Key points

- Hypertension becomes increasingly common with advancing age. Treatment is aimed at reducing long-term risk
- Evidence suggests that there is little increase in perioperative risk in patients with grade 1 or 2 hypertension
- Acute perioperative hypertensive events carry a high risk of morbidity and should be managed aggressively

Hypertension is the most frequent indication for chronic, lifelong treatment in the Western world. The vascular tree becomes less compliant with age and most hypertension is idiopathic; however, 10% may be renal, endocrine or pregnancy related.

Hypertension is directly related to cardiovascular disease, contributing to 500,000 strokes and 1,000,000 myocardial infarctions each year in the United States. Risk increases with rising arterial pressure. NICE guidelines categorise hypertension into three stages according to clinic and ambulatory/home blood pressure monitoring (**Table 15**).

Treatment is offered to patients with stage 1 disease under age 80 if they have evidence of organ damage and all patients with stage 2/severe hypertension. End-organ damage includes renal impairment, left ventricular hypertrophy (LVH), atheromatous disease and retinal artery disease. Hypertension is often undertreated with only 25% of patients being well controlled. Isolated systolic hypertension increases with age. It has become clear in recent years that systolic pressure correlates well with cardiac risk, particularly in the elderly. Raised blood pressure represents a continuum of risk; hence, the stratified management protocols set out by NICE. Thus, even high pressures considered 'within the normal range' carry an increased long-term risk of coronary/cerebrovascular death. Cardiac risk assessment calculators (e.g. JBS III cardiovascular risk assessor – see further reading below) are now commonly used when deciding how best to treat hypertension.

Problems

- Hypertensive patients may have associated medical problems, e.g. LVH (20–60% of hypertensives referred for hospital care), accelerated atherosclerosis, reduced ventricular compliance, altered autoregulation, cardiac arrhythmia)
- Untreated hypertensives show a greater fall in blood pressure following induction of anaesthesia and more episodes of perioperative myocardial ischaemia
- An exaggerated hypertensive stress response to laryngoscopy, extubation and surgical excision is common
- Patients are prone to increased postoperative hypertensive responses to pain, bladder distension etc.
- Patients with hypertensive disease have increased perioperative cardiovascular risks
- Cerebral autoregulation is shifted up in chronic hypertensive patients such that critical ischaemia is possible if the pressure is rapidly brought within normal physiological range

Causes of perioperative hypertension

- Primary or essential hypertension
- Secondary (accounts for only 10% of hypertensives)

Table 15 Stages of hypertension		
	Clinic blood pressure	Ambulatory/home pressure
Stage 1	140/90	135/85
Stage 2	160/100	150/95
Severe	Systolic >180 or diastolic >110	

- Renal, e.g. chronic pyelonephritis, chronic glomerulonephritis, renal artery stenosis, polycystic disease
- Endocrine, e.g. phaeochromocytoma, Cushing's syndrome, Conn's syndrome, acromegaly
- Pregnancy (pre-eclampsia, eclampsia) and the contraceptive pill
- Coarctation of the aorta
- Related to anaesthesia
  - Hypoxia
  - Hypercarbia
  - Light anaesthesia/inadequate analgesia
  - Fluid overload
  - Drug interactions, e.g. monoamine oxidase inhibitors
  - Surgical effects, e.g. aortic cross clamping
  - Hypothermia
  - Malignant hyperpyrexia
  - Raised intracranial pressure
  - Measurement errors, e.g. blood pressure cuff too small, an underdamped arterial trace or malpositioned transducer

Hypertension and perioperative risk

- Although it would seem intuitive, many studies have failed to demonstrate an increase in mortality in patients with a raised admission blood pressure (stage 1 or 2). There is evidence of an increase in perioperative silent myocardial ischaemia which, in turn, is associated with increased morbidity and mortality. Thus overall, there is only a weak association between perioperative cardiac morbidity and preoperative stage 1 or 2 systemic hypertension
- Isolated systolic hypertension on admission has been shown to carry a small increased risk of perioperative morbidity
- Elevated blood pressure in a nonhypertensive individual immediately prior to surgery does not appear to be associated with increased perioperative risk
- Severe hypertension carries a greater likelihood of perioperative cardiovascular instability, and although there is little clinical evidence in this population, it

is likely that perioperative morbidity is increased

Perioperative management

A complete assessment of the patient will establish whether there is evidence of end-organ damage due to hypertension and whether hypertension is idiopathic or secondary. All patients on antihypertensive treatment should remain on their therapy throughout the perioperative period, including ACE inhibitor therapy.

Investigations should include ECG and urea and electrolytes (to determine renal damage and potassium, if treated). A new finding of hypertension on admission should prompt advice to see the GP, thus allowing for further investigation and possible antihypertensive therapy with a view to longer-term risk reduction.

It seems reasonable, in the absence of strong evidence, to defer elective surgery for patients who, on admission, have severe hypertension, or stage 2 hypertension with evidence of end-organ damage. Professor Foex suggested this approach in 2004. Patients should probably be rebooked for surgery after several weeks of controlled blood pressure, although, once again, evidence is lacking.

For emergency surgery, blood pressure should be reduced by careful use of beta-blockers through the perioperative period. Invasive arterial monitoring, appropriate fluid loading and cautious use of anaesthetic agents provide a pragmatic approach to this problem.

The exaggerated haemodynamic responses to anaesthesia and surgery can increase myocardial work, predisposing to ischaemia, especially in the presence of ventricular hypertrophy and coronary artery disease. Short-acting antihypertensive agents and high-dose opioids have been used successfully to blunt the intubation hypertensive response.

All general anaesthetic agents and high sensory blockade resulting from neuraxial anaesthesia can cause myocardial depression, hypotension and alteration in heart rate. Anticipation of these effects will permit a choice of anaesthetic technique to minimise their occurrence. In particular, attention to intravascular volume status is important. Hypertensive patients often have a high resting vascular tone and a fluid-deplete circulation. Volume loading around the time of induction can significantly reduce perioperative hypotensive episodes. The combination of hypotension and tachycardia is most detrimental to the heart.

Perioperative hypertensive events, if sustained, carry a high morbidity, and treatment of the cause is essential.

Specific useful hypotensive agents include phentolamine (α-antagonist), glyceryl trinitrate (venodilator and anti-ischaemia agent), sodium nitroprusside (arteriolar dilator), labetalol (alpha- and beta-blocker) and esmolol (short-acting beta-blocker). Sublingual nifedipine is difficult to control with a variable rate/amount of absorption.

Postoperative rebound hypertension is not uncommon amongst hypertensive patients and close monitoring should continue in the early postoperative period.

Further reading

Foex P. Hypertension: pathophysiology and treatment. Br J Anaesth: Contin Educ Anaesth Crit Care Pain Med 2004; 4:71–75.

Foex P. The surgical hypertensive patient. Br J Anaesth: Contin Educ Anaesth Crit Care Pain Med 2004; 4:139–143.

Howell SJ, Sear JW, Foex P. Hypertension, hypertensive heart disease and perioperative cardiac risk. Br J Anaesth 2004; 92:570–583.

Joint British Societies for the prevention of cardiovascular disease. JBS3 Risk Calculator (2014). http://www.jbs3risk.com/.

National Institute of Clinical Excellence (NICE). Clinical Guideline 127. Hypertension: clinical management of primary hypertension in adults. London; NICE, 2011.

Related topics of interest

Infection prevention and control

Key points

- Healthcare-acquired infections (HCAIs) affect 1 in 5 surgical patients with a significant human and financial cost
- Hospitals and healthcare workers have a professional and statutory responsibility to prevent such infections
- Basic measures such as hand hygiene, appropriate antibiotic use, temperature control and aseptic techniques are crucial

Up to 20% of surgical patients suffer post-operative infections and 10% of all patients suffer a HCAI of some form. A UK National Audit Office report (2009) found that HCAIs can add £10,000 per patient to the cost of care and 3–10 days to hospital length of stay. Many of the factors predisposing to infection are modifiable and the anaesthetist has a crucial role to play.

Some particular HCAIs, e.g. methicillin-resistant *Staphylococcus aureus* (MRSA) and *Clostridium difficile* (*C. difficile*) are a particular problem of modern health care. These are largely preventable with proper care and attention to detail of basic hygiene and other simple measures such as antibiotic stewardship.

Additionally, infection control matters have implications for nonsurgical patients who may be encountered on the medical wards or critical care. Of particular importance here are catheter-related bloodstream infections (CRBSI), urinary catheter-related infection, hospital or ventilator-associated pneumonias. Proper prevention of these infections is a statutory responsibility for NHS Trusts in the UK under the Health and Social Care Act, 2008 and compliance with these laws is subject to inspection by the Care Quality Commission (CQC).

Main aspects

A successful infection prevention and control (IPC) program comprises elements which are the responsibility of the organisation and those which are the responsibility of individuals.

Organisational

- Nominated clinician director for IPC (DIPC) with an expert medical/nursing IPC team
- Adequate staff training in IPC measures and an occupational health service
- Suitable audit of key IPC policies with quarterly reports to hospital boards
- Development of a detailed antibiotic policy in conjunction with microbiologists
- Ensure that the hospital environment is kept clean
- Monitoring of specific infection rates including *C. difficile* and MRSA
- Have strategies and isolation facilities for managing outbreaks of infection
- Ensure proper disposal of waste and decontamination of infected equipment following patient care

Individual

- Adherence to all IPC policies
- Adoption of standard precautions
- Correct hand hygiene (see below)
- Adherence with infection nursing protocols (see below)
- Correct antibiotic prescribing
- Consideration to contamination of fomites (pens, stethoscopes, ultrasound and ECG machines)
- Appropriate disposal of infected material and single use equipment
- Adherence to occupational health requirements for vaccinations
- Prompt removal of old or infected vascular access devices

In addition, anaesthetists have specific responsibilities in the perioperative phase:
- Per-policy antibiotic prophylaxis within 30 minutes of incision
- External warming where anaesthetised time is >30 minutes
- Appropriate aseptic technique for vascular access, regional and neuraxial anaesthesia

including suitable skin preparation, hand washing and draping

- Appropriate theatre attire (self, team members and particularly visitors)
- Limit unnecessary numbers of individuals in theatre
- Ensure glycaemic control (blood glucose 6–10 mmol/L)
- Ensure good tissue oxygenation and perfusion: facilitates neutrophil oxygen radical generation following phagocytosis thus promoting immunity and wound healing
- Limit immunosuppressive agents, e.g. allogenic blood transfusion and steroids. Also consider immunosuppressive effects of opioids in at-risk individuals

Specific items

Antibiotics and prophylaxis

Surgery can be categorised as clean, clean-contaminated, contaminated or dirty (see **Table 16**). NICE (UK) recommends prophylaxis for all these except clean surgery not involving implantation of prosthetic materials. Prophylaxis is best given within the 30 minutes before incision. This is enshrined in the WHO Safer Surgery Checklist; risk of postoperative infection doubles if antibiotics are given after incision or >60 minutes before.

Prescription according to local policy is crucial in managing local resistance. Inadequate dosing, incomplete courses and failure to de-escalate from broad-spectrum cover once the specific sensitivity of an infecting pathogen is identified all contribute to antibiotic resistance. The four key mechanisms of resistance transmission are plasmids (which move between bacteria as separate loops of DNA), naked DNA (briefly available to be taken up after death of another bacterium), bacteriophages (viral insertion of DNA into a bacterium) and transposons (DNA fragments which also encode motility so enhancing transmission). These DNA segments engender several means of defeating antimicrobial agents. These include:

- Enzymatic inhibition, e.g. they encode an enzyme such as β-lactamase
- Modification of the antibiotic target, e.g. ribosomal changes against aminoglycosides
- Facilitate extracellular pumping of the antibiotic, e.g. tetracyclines
- Reduced cell wall or porin permeability, e.g. gram-negative bacteria or imipenem-resistant Pseudomonas
- Metabolic pathway changes, e.g. change in peptidoglycan synthesis in MRSA

Hand hygiene

The importance of this was first noted by Ignaz Semmelweis in 1847 who reduced maternal death from puerperal sepsis to <1% (from up to 35% at the time). It is now encapsulated in the WHO guidelines on hand hygiene in health care. This recommends hand hygiene procedures:

- Before touching the patient
- After touching the patient
- After touching the patient's surroundings
- Before clean/aseptic procedures
- After exposure to body fluids

Hands may be cleaned with 70% isopropyl alcohol if not visibly soiled. If visibly soiled, washing with soap and water is required. The same is true if caring for a patient infected with *C. difficile* as alcohol does not kill the spores of this organism. In addition

Table 16 Categorisation of surgical site sterility	
Clean	No breaching of GI, urinary or respiratory mucosal surfaces and full aseptic technique
Clean -contaminated	Minor breach in asepsis or oropharyngeal, biliary, GI, urinary or respiratory tract surgery with no infection present
Contaminated	In presence of acute inflammation, infected urine, gross faecal contamination or biliary pus
Dirty	Established infection but antibiotic usage is therapeutic rather than prophylaxis and choice is based on known microbial isolates
Adapted from Berard F, Gandon J. Ann Surg 1964; 160 1-192.	

guidelines state that staff should remove all jewellery except for a plain wedding band and adopt a 'bare below the elbows' dress code when in clinical areas.

Infection nursing protocols

These are vital for the protection of vulnerable patients and to prevent cross infection:

- Barrier-nursing: use of personal protective equipment (PPE) to reduce risk of transfer of pathogens from a patient or their surroundings onto staff and their clothing with risk of onward transfer
- Reverse barrier nursing: PPE to protect vulnerable patients from environmental or staff-transferred pathogens. May be combined with isolation nursing in a room with positive-pressure room ventilation
- Cohort nursing: grouping patients with a common infection in the same semi-restricted space, e.g. a ward bay with a dedicated nursing team. Less staff required than to manage all patients in separate isolation and may be less psychologically isolating to patients
- Isolation nursing: individual patient nursed in a single-patient area with appropriate PPE and positive or negative pressure room ventilation as required

Consider moving patients to the start or end of the operating list if they require the above measures to reduce the risks posed to and by other patients in the theatre suite.

Further reading

Department of Health. The Health and Social Care Act 2008 Code of Practice on the prevention and control of infections. London; DH, 2008.

Gifford C, Christelis N, Cheng A. Preventing postoperative infection: the anaesthetist's role. B J Anaesth: Contin Educ Anaesth Crit Care Pain 2011; 11:151–156.

Varley AJ, Williams H, Fletcher S. Antibiotic resistance in the intensive care unit. Br J Anaesth: Contin Educ Anaesth Crit Care Pain 2009; 9:114–118.

Related topics of interest

- Infectious diseases (p. 95)

Infectious diseases

Key points

- There are several severe infections which have the potential to be transmitted to health care workers and other patients
- The key to avoiding infection is preventative measures, using WHO Standard Precautions

Occupational exposure to infectious diseases represents a significant hazard for anaesthetists. Conditions of particular concern include tuberculosis (TB), viral hepatitis, influenza, human papilloma virus (HPV) and, of course, human immunodeficiency virus (HIV). Others, whilst less serious, can be debilitating and threaten health care infrastructure through staff illness, e.g. norovirus.

By adhering to Standard Precautions, the risks posed to health care workers by these disorders are significantly reduced. There remains a significant problem with ensuring staff take such precautions routinely, particularly with the wearing of gloves for example. Some of these diseases are untreatable and have no vaccine available, thus prevention remains the best option.

Problems

- To the health care worker and patient
  - Infection – personal illness, limiting of life, exposure of close family
  - Cost, inconvenience and side effects of postexposure treatments
  - Side effects of long-term treatments
  - Loss of earnings with subsequent problems for dependents and personal lifestyle
  - Anxiety, depression
- To the health care system
  - Potential for litigation from staff infected due to organisational failure
  - Loss of workforce
  - Cost of sick pay
  - Managing the risk of staff-to-patient transmission

Specific disorders

HIV

Lentivirus with two predominant sub-types – HIV-1 and HIV-2 (latter mainly in Africa)

- Retrovirus able to insert its genome into host-cell DNA via reverse transcriptase
- Predominant effect on CD4+ T-helper cells leading to susceptibility to malignancy and opportunistic infections
- First noted in USA homosexual population as *Pneumocystis jirovecii* (previously *carinii*) pneumonia, mucosal candidiasis and Kaposi's sarcoma. Heterosexual transmission accounts for majority now
- Treatments interfere with reverse transcriptase function (nucleotide and non-nucleotide reverse transcriptase inhibitors) or subsequent viral protein processing (protease inhibitors)
- Testing is by enzyme-linked immunosorbent assay or Western blot for anti-HIV IgG antibodies but these may take 12 weeks to form (the seroconversion period)
- Percutaneous, mucocutaneous and cutaneous exposures have 0.3%, 0.03% and 0.0% risk of infection respectively
- Gloves reduce inoculum volume of a percutaneous exposure by 10 to 100-fold
- Postexposure prophylaxis (PEP) is most effective when started within 1–2 hours of exposure but may benefit for 1–2 weeks postinjury

TB

- Caused by *Mycobacterium tuberculosis* and transmitted in respiratory droplets of 0.5–5 μm diameter
- Increasing incidence globally with around a third of the global population infected; mostly due to rising HIV infection rates
- Economic and medical poverty and overcrowded living conditions (e.g. prisons) remain key risk factors. Others include occupational lung disease (30x), smoking (2x), alcoholism and diabetes (3x)

- Drug resistance is a rapidly increasing problem with the emergence of multiple, extended and totally drug-resistant strains (MDT-TB, XDR-TB and TDR-TB)
- Manifestations are pulmonary and, in 10–15%, extrapulmonary (e.g. bone, CNS, lymph, urinary)
- Vaccination by BCG protects against disseminated disease in children but offers less certain protection against pulmonary TB, particularly outside this age group
- Screening is by tuberculin testing – induration at site of injection of purified protein derivative seen in patients with prior exposure to TB
- Specialised, close-fitting masks and negative-pressure isolation facilities are recommended in the management of those with active TB

Hepatitis B and C

Hepatitis B (a hepadnavirus) has 40% infectivity after inoculation and leads to acute viral hepatitis with a risk of fulminant liver failure and death. Ninety-five per cent of adults clear the virus within months. The remainder have chronic hepatitis, remain infective and at risk of cirrhosis and hepatocellular carcinoma. Three inoculations of surface antigen (HBsAg) should produce a positive titre of anti-HBsAg antigens. A further 5-year booster provides lifetime immunity.

Hepatitis C (a hepacivirus) has 2% infectivity but 85% progress to a chronic state of whom 20% develop cirrhosis and 3% hepatocellular carcinoma. Hepatitis C cirrhosis is the leading prompt for liver transplant. There is no vaccine but 48 weeks of pegylated interferon-α and ribavirin eliminates the virus in 70–85%. Immune serum globulin may have a role as PEP.

Others

Methicillin-resistant *Staphylococcus aureus* (MRSA) and *Clostridium difficile* (*C. difficile*) may be transmitted from patient to patient by staff but rarely cause symptoms in the carrier. MRSA may have profound career implications if staff who are found to be carriers fail to respond to eradication therapy. Norovirus is a significant cause of seasonal diarrhoea and vomiting. Staff are easily infected but long-term consequences are rare. Health care

infrastructure can be dramatically affected by widespread staff absence however. Viable HPV DNA has been detected in laser smoke from airway surgery for treating papillomas – suitable filter masks should be worn by staff.

Management to reduce transmission

There are three phases to this:

Pre-exposure: This requires adherence to immunisation recommendations of the occupational health service. Routinely this involves hepatitis B immunisation and confirmation of TB, mumps, herpes zoster and rubella immunity or prior exposure.

Periexposure: Historically this involved the application of 'Universal precautions' but this term is no longer used. They were introduced following the HIV/AIDS epidemic of the 1980s but staff were found to be indirectly discriminating against patients by not applying them universally, except to those about whom they had made a negative judgement. The WHO, Centers for Disease Control and Prevention and NHS Professionals all now have guidance on the successor, 'Standard Precautions'. Rather than a subjective judgement, these rely on objective risk assessments to determine the level of precautions required. They are equally designed to protect both patients and health care workers. The key elements that anaesthetists are directly involved in are as follows:

1. Hand hygiene
2. Gloves
3. Facial protection (eyes, nose and mouth)
4. Gown
5. Prevention of needlestick and injuries from other sharp instruments
6. Respiratory hygiene and cough etiquette
7. Environmental cleaning
8. Linens
9. Waste disposal
10. Patient care equipment

Postexposure: This refers to management of a case of suspected transmission of infection to a health care worker. For inoculation ('needlestick') injuries, the wound should be encouraged to bleed and copiously washed.

Local policy will dictate the procedure for accessing PEP and appropriate hepatitis B follow-up within 1 hour of the injury. A risk assessment of the infectivity of the source patient should be made with consideration given to obtaining consent for viral screening.

Generally, this should be undertaken by another health care professional. Those who may have been exposed to TB should similarly contact occupational health for consideration of tuberculin testing and PEP (6–12 months therapy).

Further reading

Association of Anaesthetists of Great Britain & Ireland. Safety guideline: Infection control in anaesthesia 2. London: AAGBI, 2008.
Thomas I, Carter JA. Occupational hazards of anaesthesia. Br J Anaesth: Contin Educ Anaesth Crit Care Pain 2006; 6:182–187.

World Health Organisation. Standard precautions in healthcare. Geneva; WHO, 2007.

Related topics of interest

- Infection prevention and control (p. 92)
- Lasers in surgery (p. 98)
- Liver disease and anaesthesia (p. 101)

Lasers in surgery

Key points

- LASER stands for **L**ight **A**mplification by **S**timulated **E**mission of **R**adiation
- Lasers are used for their precise tissue damage and excellent haemostasis
- Laser use is associated with dangers to staff and patients
- Airway fires are a particular hazard with disastrous consequences

Lasers are used in many branches of surgery including thoracic, urology, gynaecology, ophthalmology and, of particular importance to the anaesthetist, ENT and airway procedures. The light energy they produce is monochromatic (single wavelength), coherent (light particles are in phase) and collimated (energy minimally diverges from the origin and so are considered as being parallel). They work by causing tissue damage, cutting and haemostasis with the advantage that they can do so at various tissue depths, depending on the wavelength of light which in turn depends on the construction of the laser (**Table 17 and 20**).

Lasers can be hazardous and therefore staff must be well trained and follow established safety guidelines. The principal dangers are of damage to the eye, skin burns and ignition. There must be a designated laser protection supervisor to oversee the process. There are specific dangers associated with the use of lasers near the airway of an anaesthetised patient. It is essential that the anaesthetist minimises the risk of an airway fire and also makes preparations to rapidly treat this event should it occur to prevent further injury to the patient.

Problems

- Inadvertent thermal transfer. Lasers deliver a high-power density resulting in rapid heating. This may result in ignition of flammable materials, or burns if accidentally applied to the wrong area of a patient, or to a member of staff. Eyes are particularly susceptible to damage, in particular the cornea, retina and optic nerve. Because the beam is nondivergent, distance does little to reduce the energy deposited.

- Airway issues. Accidental heating of the endotracheal tube cuff may puncture it, resulting in loss of positive pressure ventilation and airway protection. Endotracheal tubes are combustible and generally carry an oxygen-rich mixture of flammable vapours. They may contain nitrous oxide which also supports combustion. If accidentally ignited by a laser, a fierce 'blow torch' fire directed into the trachea may result.

- Smoke. Like electrocautery, lasers produce smoke during vaporisation of tissue. Although difficult to quantify, it is likely that this forms an environmental hazard to those working with lasers.

Anaesthetic management

- During any laser surgery, staff must comply with the general laser safety considerations (**Table 18**)
- During airway surgery the anaesthetic technique must be tailored to the individual case (**Table 19**). This will involve discussion

Table 17 Components of a LASER	
Energy source	Provides energy for atoms in the laser medium to become excited, releasing photons of energy Usually electricity or light Application of energy is called 'pumping'
Laser medium	Contains the atoms which can be excited during pumping May be solid, liquid or gas Determines the properties of the laser beam (wavelength and therefore depth of tissue damage)
Reflectors	Reflect photons back into the lasing medium such that 'stimulated emission' can occur Ensures the exiting energy beam is parallel (i.e. non-divergent)

Table 18 Laser safety – general considerations

Laser protection supervisor must be employed to oversee laser safety

Signposts outside theatre that indicate a laser is in use

Theatre doors should be locked and windows blinded

Staff should wear eye protection specific to the laser being used

Surgical instruments should be nonreflective

Patient's eyes should be taped shut and covered with moist gauze

Flammable materials close to the operative field should be moistened

Smoke evacuation should be considered

Table 19 Laser safety – airway considerations

Reduce probability of airway fire

Low oxygen concentration gas mixture

Avoid nitrous oxide

Consider laser-safe endotracheal tube

Consider nasal intubation and moistened throat pack

Consider jet ventilation to avoid use of endotracheal tube

Reduce impact of cuff rupture

Double cuff endotracheal tube

Cuffs filled with saline to offer some airway protection in the event of puncture

Table 20 Types of lasers used in medical practice

Laser medium	Type	Wavelength	Clinical applications
CO_2	Gas	10,600 nm	Cutting, coagulation, laser scalpel, skin resurfacing
Ho:YAG	Solid	2100 nm	Tissue ablation, lithotripsy, dentistry
Nd:YAG	Solid	1064 nm	Cutting, coagulation, GI bleeding, ocular surgery, tattoo removal
Ruby	Solid	694 nm	Hair removal, tattoo removal, holography
Argon	Gas	500 nm	Retinal surgery, AV malformations, port-wine birthmarks
Excimer (Ar:F)	Gas	193 nm	Corneal vision correction

with the surgical team regarding access to the airway, airway protection and the risk of endotracheal tube ignition

- The anaesthetic gas mixture should be as low in oxygen concentration as is safely possible to reduce the risk of an airway fire. Below 30% is considered acceptable by many. Nitrous oxide should not be used
- Nasal intubation should be considered for procedures in the oropharynx. A moist throat pack in the posterior pharynx offers some protection of the endotracheal tube and cuff
- Specific endotracheal tubes have been designed to be safer when using lasers in a shared airway. These are coated in a laser diffusing layer, e.g. copper foil, to prevent reflection of the laser beam. There is also an absorbent layer which must be moistened before use and which further prevents the risk of ignition
- Laser-specific endotracheal tubes may also have two cuffs, which can be filled with

saline rather than air. In the event of the laser puncturing the first cuff, the spilled saline should both alert the operator and reduce the chance of an airway fire. The distal cuff maintains airway protection and allows continued positive pressure ventilation

- Jet ventilation, either via a ventilating bronchoscope or a tracheal catheter, may be the most practical solution. This has the advantage of giving improved surgical access but has the disadvantage of providing little airway protection. Oxygen concentrations should be kept below 30%

Further reading

Kitching AJ, Edge CJ. Lasers and surgery. Br J Anaesth: Contin Educ Profess Develop Rev 2003; 3:143.

Medicines and Healthcare Product Regulation Agency (MHRA). Device Bulletin: Guidance on the safe use of lasers, intense light source systems and LEDs in medical, surgical, dental and aesthetic practices. London; Medicines and Healthcare Product Regulation Agency, 2008.

Simpson E. The basic principles of laser technology, uses and safety measures in anaesthesia. anaesthesia tutorial of the week; 255, 2012. www.atotw.anaesthesiologists.org

Related topics of interest

- Airway – the shared airway (p. 10)
- Ophthalmology (p. 168)

Liver disease and anaesthesia

Key points

- Liver disease represents a wide spectrum of disorders and severities
- Perioperative mortality and morbidity are significantly increased in severe disease
- Drug handling and response are often unpredictable

In under a decade, death rates due to liver disease have risen 25% and it is now the fifth most frequent cause of death in the UK. Worldwide the most common cause is viral infection, but in the UK it is alcohol. There are a number of disease processes which can affect the liver and in turn increase the risk of postoperative morbidity, particularly in those with alcoholic liver disease.

Problems

Cardiovascular

Arteriovenous connections develop between the splanchnic and systemic circulation in cirrhosis and portal hypertension. This and increased levels of endogenous vasodilators lead to a high cardiac output state, with reduced systemic vascular resistance and systolic BP. In addition, the splanchnic circulation no longer acts as a volume reservoir and there is a reduction in plasma oncotic pressure resulting in reduced effective blood volume with impaired compensation for hypovolaemia. The response to endogenous and exogenous vasoconstrictors is also reduced due to a combination of the changes to the splanchnic circulation and excess of endogenous vasodilators. Cardiac failure may also be present.

Respiratory

In advanced liver disease, intrapulmonary shunts are common and hypoxic pulmonary vasoconstriction is impaired due to endogenous vasodilators. Atelectasis, V/Q mismatch and a reduced FRC can result from ascites or pleural effusions. Pulmonary hypertension may develop alongside portal hypertension.

Renal

There is activation of the renin–aldosterone–angiotensin system due to the circulatory changes caused by portal hypertension and reduced renal perfusion. This leads to sodium and water retention causing dilution hyponatraemia and worsening oedema and ascites. Renal failure and hepatorenal syndrome may develop.

Haematology

Production of most clotting factors (excluding factors III, IV, VIII) is liver dependant and there is a reduction in Vitamin K levels due to disruption of the biliary circulation. Thrombocytopaenia may occur due to hypersplenism and platelet function can be impaired. There is also a right-shift of the oxygen dissociation curve due to low levels of 2,3-diphosphoglycerate. Megaloblastic anaemia is common due to dietary folate deficiency and alcohol-induced inhibition of folate metabolism.

Neurology

Encephalopathy occurs when the liver fails to breakdown nitrogenous waste products, toxins and drugs due to hepatocellular damage and portosystemic shunting (**Table 21**).

Pharmacology

Pharmacokinetics are altered due to decreased total protein binding capacity, increased volumes of distribution and changes in hepatic blood flow and metabolism. Drug metabolism is unpredictable; it may be decreased due

Table 21 Grades of encephalopathy	
Grade I	Slowed mental function but alert
Grade II	Inappropriate behaviour or confusion
Grade III	Permanent somnolence
Grade IV	Coma
Adapted from the West-Haven grading.	

to hepatocellular damage or increased in alcoholic patients due to enzyme induction.

Ascites

A combination of hypoalbuminaemia, sodium and water retention and increased splanchnic capillary pressure (due to increased resistance through the liver) leading to net outflow of lymphatic fluid causes the accumulation of ascites.

Metabolic

Patients are usually malnourished and hypoglycaemia is common, particularly in those with alcoholic liver disease. Vitamin deficiency is common and thiamine should be supplemented (before glucose administration to minimise the risk of precipitating Wernicke's encephalopathy).

Anaesthetic management

Preoperative assessment

Liver disease is often asymptomatic or presents with only mild or nonspecific symptoms. Perioperative risk depends on the severity of hepatic disease, type of surgery and general status. Patients should be assessed and their nutrition, coagulation, electrolyte balance optimised and ascites/encephalopathy treated. Involve a hepatologist. Surgery should be carried out only if the benefits outweigh the risks; in patients with acute liver disease, postpone surgery until the acute episode has resolved. The most commonly used tool for risk stratification is the Child–Turcotte–Pugh (CTP) classification (**Table 22**). After abdominal surgery, patients with CTP class

A disease have a predicted mortality rate of 10%, class B 30–31% and class C 76–82%.

Baseline investigations include full blood count, coagulation, biochemistry, liver function and ECG. An echocardiogram should be performed if cardiac dysfunction is suspected and a chest ultrasound or chest X-ray if there are pleural effusions suitable for drainage. Lung function tests are indicated if there is evidence of restrictive disease or other pathology. Sedative premedication should be avoided.

Intraoperative

The risk of preoperative complications is high and worsening of hepatic function is common. Key goals are to maintain hepatic blood flow, optimise fluid status and ameliorate the risk of encephalopathy. In addition to standard monitoring, an arterial line and monitoring of urine output are usually necessary. Central venous and cardiac output monitoring may be required depending on the complexity of surgery and patient's condition. Neuromuscular block and depth-of-anaesthesia monitoring should be used. Regional anaesthesia and analgesia should be used where possible as it reduces the risk of encephalopathy associated with opioids/anaesthetic agents and reductions in hepatic blood flow. However, it may be contraindicated if coagulopathy or thrombocytopaenia are present.

If GA is necessary, short-acting agents with nonhepatic metabolism, nonhepatotoxic metabolites and minimal effects on hepatic blood flow should be used. Due to the unpredictable nature of changes in pharmacokinetics, reduced doses should be

Table 22 Assessment of liver dysfunction			
Criterion	1 Point	2 Points	3 Points
Ascites	None	Controlled with diuretics	Poorly controlled
Encephalopathy	None	Grade I–II	Grade III–IV
Total bilirubin (µmol/L)	<34	34–50	>50
Albumin (g/L)	>35	25–35	<25
Coagulation (based on INR)	<1.7	1.7–2.2	>2.2
Adapted from Child-Turcotte-Pugh assessment. A=5–6 points; B=7–9 points; C=10–15 points.			

used and titrated to effect. The clearance of propofol is not significantly affected by liver disease and is commonly used for induction and maintenance of anaesthesia. There is increased sensitivity to the sedative and cardiorespiratory depressant effects. Due to reduction in protein binding, the unbound concentration of thiopentone and hence its effect will be increased. Desflurane is the ideal volatile agent for maintenance as it is minimally metabolised, has a rapid onset and offset and has the least effect of all volatiles on hepatic blood flow. Remifentanil is useful to reduce the amount of intravenous/inhalational agent required. The action of suxamethonium and mivacurium may be prolonged in severe liver disease due to a reduction in plasma cholinesterase levels. Atracurium or cisatracurium are the most suitable nondepolarising neuromuscular blocking agents as they undergo minimal hepatic metabolism. If longer-acting opioids are required in patients with severe liver dysfunction, fentanyl should be used rather than morphine; the latter has delayed elimination in severe disease and active metabolites.

Postoperative care

Critical care support should be considered in patients with significant liver disease. Alcohol withdrawal should be anticipated and treated appropriately. Nutritional support may be required and vitamin supplements, in particular thiamine, administered. Constipation should be aggressively treated as it may precipitate encephalopathy. NSAIDs should be avoided due to the risk of renal injury and gastrointestinal haemorrhage. Paracetamol can be used for short periods, but the dose should be reduced (2–3 g/day).

Further reading

Jackson P, Gleeson D. Alcoholic liver disease. Br J Anaesth: Contin Educ Anaesth Crit Care Pain 2010; 10:66–71.

Marschall KE. Diseases of the liver and biliary tract. In: Hines RL, Marschall KE (eds), Stoelting's anaesthesia and co-existing disease, 5th edn. Philadelphia: Elsevier Saunders, 2012:259–278.

Vaja R, McNicol L, Sisley I. Anaesthesia for patients with liver disease. Br J Anaesth: Contin Educ Anaesth Crit Care Pain 2010; 10:15–19.

Related topics of interest

Liver resection surgery

Key points

- Preoperative liver dysfunction should raise concern about cirrhosis, a relative contraindication to resection
- Major bleeding is rare due to advances in surgical technique, but can still occur
- Point-of-care coagulation and blood-gas monitoring have a particular role to play

The liver is the largest solid organ in the body weighing around 1.5 kg in an adult. It has numerous functions (**Table 23**). It receives 20% of cardiac output: the portal vein provides 75% of the blood flow, but only 50% of the oxygen. The hepatic artery provides the remaining 50% of the oxygen supply. Venous drainage is via the hepatic veins, which emerge from the posterior surface of the liver and drain directly into the inferior vena cava (IVC).

Macroscopically, there are two major lobes, a larger right and smaller left, separated superficially by the falciform ligament, with two minor lobes, the caudate and quadrate, in between (**Figure 8**). The lobes can also be divided into functional–anatomical segments which can be devascularised by isolating the blood supply and drainage. This allows relatively bloodless resection of each segment. It is unusual for a patient to lose > 500 mL of blood during liver resection; however, when haemorrhage does occur it can be significant.

Generally, around 75% of the liver tissue can be resected without significant impact on function, provided this was normal preoperatively. The organ will regenerate over a number of months following surgery. Acute liver failure is a risk if more than 75% is removed.

The commonest indication for liver resection is to remove metastatic deposits from colorectal cancer. When resectable, the expected 5-year survival rate after surgery

Table 23 Key functions of the liver
Glucose, lactate, fat and protein metabolism
Bile synthesis
Clotting factor synthesis
Inactivation of hormones and drugs/toxins
Bacterial filter of intestinal bacteria in portal venous blood

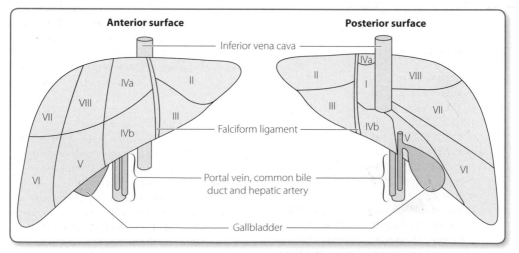

Figure 8 Gross anatomy of liver, showing Couinaud segmental division (I – caudate, II and III – left, IV – quadrate; V–VIII – right).

is around 40%. Further indications include resection of secondaries from carcinoid syndrome, melanoma and other primaries. Liver resection may also be performed for symptomatic benign liver cysts, liver trauma, cholangiocarcinoma and live donor transplants. In all of these cases, the underlying hepatic function is usually normal. Occasionally, surgical resection is performed for primary hepatocellular cancer. Such tumours usually arise in cirrhotic livers with an associated substantial risk of postoperative liver failure.

Problems

- Comorbidities due to lifestyle (smoking, diet and alcohol) and advancing age
- Many have had preoperative (neoadjuvant) chemotherapy with detrimental effects on aerobic fitness, nutrition, immune function and hepatic reserve
- Risk of major intraoperative haemorrhage due to direct trauma to vessels (including IVC) and coagulopathy
- Intraoperative haemodynamic instability due to surgical obstruction to venous return
- Postoperative biliary leak
- Acute liver failure can occur if the function of the liver remnant is inadequate
- Prolonged surgery – in the region of 3–12 hours

Conduct of surgery

There are characteristically three phases:
- Dissection to access the liver
- Resection: Systematic devascularisation of the liver, during which significant blood loss can occur. Techniques to minimise haemorrhage include:
  - Intraoperative ultrasound to characterise anatomy and exclude new metastases
  - Cavitron ultrasonic aspirator ('CUSA') for resection: Very high frequency ultrasound dislodges hepatocytes, which are then washed out with saline, leaving 'tougher' capillaries intact

  - Argon diathermy: High-energy, localised current which coagulates the cut hepatic surface and capillaries exposed by CUSA
  - Fibrin glue for oozing areas
  - Vascular inflow occlusion: Nonselective (Pringle's manoeuvre – a soft clamp across the porta hepatis) or selective (Makuuchi's manoeuvre). These may cause liver ischaemia followed by reperfusion injury
- Repair: biliary reconstruction (if required) and closure

Anaesthetic management

Preoperative

Preoperative assessment is as for any other major case, but with a focus on cardiorespiratory and hepatic reserve. Cardiopulmonary exercise testing is often used to facilitate informed discussion with patients about perioperative risk. Thirty-day mortality is around 4% for liver resection but higher in patients with poor cardiorespiratory fitness.

If preoperative liver function is abnormal, cirrhosis must be excluded; review of CT imaging and, where necessary, diagnostic laparoscopy should be considered before embarking on open resection. Staging imaging (CT or MRI) within 4 weeks preceding surgery is also important for resection planning, as well as to confirm that the cancer remains surgically resectable. Blood group and save to facilitate 'electronic issue' of blood products is required. If this is not possible, blood should be cross-matched (4 units).

Intraoperative

Standard AAGBI-recommended monitoring plus central venous pressure (CVP), urine output and temperature monitoring are required. Arterial lines are routinely used as regular lactate level checks are needed. Arterial blood gases and near-patient tests of coagulation (e.g. thromboelastography) are performed at baseline and postresection.

There is a risk of significant blood loss. Extended right-sided resections, hilar cholangiocarcinomas and patients who have had previous liver surgery or have abnormal hepatic function are at particular risk. Large-bore intravenous access is mandatory and consideration should be given to placement of an 8-French rapid infusion device (in either a central or large peripheral vein) to allow high-flow, warmed fluid resuscitation with a high-pressure infusor.

There is no specific evidence to favour any particular induction technique. Intubation and ventilation with oxygen enriched air and volatile to maintain normocapnia is required. Desflurane has minimal hepatic metabolism (0.002%) and has a quick offset time, making it the agent of choice in open liver surgery.

An atracurium infusion can minimise the risk of the patient coughing and incurring a diaphragmatic injury from fixed retractors. Vasopressor infusions are frequently employed to counteract the vasodilator effects of the anaesthetic, epidural and inflammatory response. Broad-spectrum antibiotic prophylaxis (such as co-amoxiclav) is normally administered.

The dissection and resection phases are facilitated by 'low CVP anaesthesia'. This aims to avoid raised IVC pressure and so limit back-bleeding through the valveless hepatic veins. Intravenous fluids are administered sparingly (around 2–3 L of isotonic crystalloid until resection is complete) to keep a 'low-adequate' preload. An α-1 selective vasopressor infusion is often used to maintain mean arterial pressure. Theoretically, a low venous pressure will increase the risk of venous air embolism, but in practice this is very rare. Serial lactate measurement is useful to guide fluid therapy: lactate can be expected to rise eventually due to reduced liver function, but an early rise is probably due to occult hypovolaemia.

If bleeding occurs it is often venous: difficult for the surgeon to access and control. In the case of major bleeding employ the standard protocols to maintain oxygen delivery. Tranexamic acid (1 g over 20 minutes then 1 g/12 hours) can also be used. Thromboelastography guides rational use of blood products.

Once the resection is complete and primary haemostasis is achieved, the surgeon may allow a 'haemostatic' pause. This is a good opportunity to restore intravascular volume. There is no specific evidence that minimally invasive cardiac output monitors are of benefit; however, some centres use these for stroke volume optimisation during this fluid replacement phase.

Analgesia

NSAIDs are avoided on account of the risk of bleeding and perioperative kidney injury. Paracetamol dosing is dependent on preoperative liver function, magnitude of liver resection, lactate and clotting function. Dosing is 1 g/6 hours, unless there are concerns about liver function, in which case 500 mg/8 hours can be given.

Open surgery

The incision is usually a 'roof top' subcostal or an inverted 'L', such that a midthoracic epidural may have benefits on postoperative cardiac, respiratory and gastrointestinal function in addition to analgesic efficacy. Timing of removal of epidural catheter requires careful consideration of clotting function and intervals between doses of thromboprophylaxis. Shoulder tip pain, referred from diaphragmatic irritation, is not always predictable or well controlled by epidural.

Laparoscopically assisted procedures

If hand ports and any larger incisions are lateralised to a single side, local anaesthesia (transversus abdominis plane (TAP) or intrapleural block) plus regular paracetamol and patient controlled analgesia (PCA) opioid should suffice. Intrathecal local anaesthesia with diamorphine can be opiate-sparing postoperatively but requires monitoring for respiratory depression.

Postoperative care

Unless there are significant complications, patients should be extubated to reduce the risk of lower respiratory tract infection. Planned high dependency care is usual. Normal liver function should be anticipated.

Postresection lactate is usually <4 mmol/L; higher suggests hepatic damage and is associated with a higher incidence of postoperative complications.

Acid–base status, lactate levels and clotting should be closely monitored. Postoperative fluid management should aim to maintain an adequate oxygen delivery. A vasopressor infusion may be required. Postoperative bleeding is unusual. A high index of suspicion needs to be maintained and early surgical review is advised. Rising lactate should prompt Doppler flow ultrasound to exclude venous thrombosis.

Perioperative mechanical thromboprophylaxis is usual. As long as there is no contraindication or coagulopathy, then pharmacological thromboprophylaxis can be administered on the first postoperative day (i.e. >24 hours postoperative). Enhanced recovery programmes are emerging for liver resection patients.

Further reading

Jones C, Kelliher L, Dickinson M, et al. Randomized clinical trial on enhanced recovery versus standard care following open liver resection. Br J Surg 2013; 100:1015–1024.

Stümpfle R, Riga A, Deshpande R, et al. Anaesthesia for metastatic liver resection surgery. Curr Anaesth Crit Care 2009; 20:3–7.

Wiggans MG, StarkieT, Shahtahmassebi G, et al. Serum arterial lactate concentration predicts mortality and organ dysfunction following liver resection. Periop Med 2013; 2:21 doi:10.1186/2047-0525-2-21.

Related topics of interest

Major abdominal surgery

Key points

- Major abdominal surgery is a risk factor for morbidity and mortality
- Enhanced recovery programmes utilise a multidisciplinary approach with the aim to allow early discharge from hospital

It is well established that major abdominal surgery is associated with increased morbidity and mortality especially in the high-risk patient. Anaesthetists are uniquely placed to enhance the outcome of these patients.

Problems

Major abdominal surgery covers a multitude of procedures on several different organs; upper and lower GI tracts, pancreas, spleen, liver and abdominal vasculature. Many factors collude to make these patients high risk, and therein are the potential avenues for optimisation.

- Presenting disease process
  - The underlying disorder often plays a major role in determining perioperative risk. The operative mortality for obstructed sigmoid volvulus, for example has been estimated in some studies to be as high as 57%, whereas resection for colon cancer is 5–10%
- Comorbidities
  - Many studies have shown that concurrent disease processes are risk factors for increased operative morbidity and mortality, regardless of surgical speciality
- Surgical procedure
  - Major abdominal procedures can be technically complex, of long duration and physiologically disruptive
  - Potential complications include large blood loss, significant postoperative pain, thromboembolism and fluid/electrolyte and nutritional disturbances. The advent and popularisation of minimally invasive alternatives may go some way to reducing this as a factor

- Urgency of procedure – elective or emergency
- Surgical stress response
  - Major abdominal surgery and the associated tissue trauma is a profound stimulus for the surgical stress response (a neuroendocrine/inflammatory response which may last up to weeks)
- Nutritional and fluid status
  - Poor nutrition is a major risk factor for morbidity and mortality. It is commonly associated with abdominal pathology and there is a growing awareness of the need for preoperative assessment
- Fluid status
  - Hypovolaemia has been implicated as a risk factor for adverse outcomes after major abdominal surgery and much work is being done into perioperative fluid management
- Postoperative pain and respiratory function
  - Vertical incisions are more frequently associated with postoperative pain, when compared with transverse incision. Postoperative pain is associated with reduced respiratory function and increased likelihood of respiratory tract infections

Anaesthetic management

Preoperative assessment

There is increasing evidence that preoperative optimisation can improve postoperative outcomes and this is where anaesthetists have an increasing role as perioperative physicians. A thorough assessment of functional capacity and comorbidities with appropriate investigation and referral is essential. This allows for perioperative goal setting and planning for postoperative management.

Intraoperative management

- Positioning
  - Major abdominal surgery may involve prolonged procedures and it is important to remember to manage

pressure points adequately to reduce the risk of pressure sores or peripheral neuropathies
- Monitoring
  - In addition to the AAGBI minimum standard, some patients may benefit from additional monitoring
  - Invasive arterial, central venous and cardiac-output monitoring all may be appropriate. A 2011 NCEPOD (UK) report suggested that these are still being underutilised in the high-risk patient and that inadequate monitoring was associated with a threefold increase in mortality
- Temperature management
  - Inadvertent perioperative hypothermia is a common complication of abdominal surgery and is associated with negative outcomes such as surgical wound infection, myocardial ischaemia and increased recovery stay
  - Care should be taken to monitor and maintain temperature above 36°C perioperatively. This may be achieved by the use of forced air warmers, warmed fluid and warming mattresses
- Fluid management
  - The reasons for preoperative hypovolaemia are numerous; vomiting, diarrhoea or use of bowel preparation, '3rd space losses' and bleeding, e.g. GI bleeding, aneurysmal rupture
  - Debate continues as to which fluid type (crystalloid or colloid) is most appropriate for perioperative use and whilst fluid prescription varies widely there is growing evidence that inadequate or excessive intraoperative fluid therapy adversely affects postoperative outcome
  - Cardiac output monitors may provide a way of guiding fluid therapy
- Analgesia
  - Postoperative pain can be significant and a comprehensive, multimodal analgesic plan is required. Central neuraxial (spinal or epidural anaesthesia) and regional techniques (e.g. rectus sheath or transversus abdominis plane blocks) are both

options for postoperative pain relief. Epidurals have the added benefit of reducing postoperative ileus and improving intestinal blood flow
  - Systemic opioids are an alternative option, either as intermittent boluses or PCA. However, their major limitation is their effects on bowel motility, which may prolong recovery

Postoperative care

Respiratory and cardiovascular complications are common and result in poor patient outcomes and greater utilisation of hospital resources. Therefore, close monitoring in the immediate postoperative period is important and consideration must be given to HDU/ICU admission

Patients with intra-abdominal pathology often have a degree of malnutrition. It is well known that inadequate nutrition is associated with increased morbidity and mortality in the form of increased muscle weakness, reduced immunity and wound healing and potential translocation of gut flora. Consequently, assessment and management of nutritional status perioperatively is important and may involve enteral or parenteral supplementation

Enhanced recovery programmes

Such programmes were initially used in colorectal and orthopaedic surgery and are being increasingly used in many centres across surgical specialities to improve patient flow and outcomes. They use a multimodal approach across the whole perioperative period and recommendations include:
- Preoperative
  - Increased preoperative assessment and patient education
  - Discharge planning being completed before surgery
  - Day of surgery admission
  - Avoiding prolonged fasting
  - Preoperative carbohydrate loading
  - Avoidance of bowel preparation
- Intraoperative
  - Avoidance of hypothermia
  - Surgical technique including laparoscopy, use of short and transverse

incisions and avoiding use of surgical drains or nasogastric tubes
- Anaesthetic technique including use of short-acting anaesthetic agents, regional or epidural anaesthesia and goal-directed fluid therapy
- Thromboprophylaxis
- Postoperative
  - Multimodal analgesic strategy (aiming to be opioid sparing)
- Early resumption of normal diet and discontinuation of intravenous fluids
- Early and structured mobilisation
- Early treatment of PONV
- Early removal of drains or urinary catheters
- Adequate community support and follow-up
- Regular audit

Further reading

Department of Health. Delivering enhanced recovery: helping patients get better sooner after surgery. London: DH, 2010.

McConachie I (Ed.). Anaesthesia for the high risk patient. 2nd edn. Cambridge: Cambridge University Press, 2009.

National Confidential Enquiry into Patient Outcome and Death. Perioperative care: knowing the risk. London: NCEPOD, 2011.

Related topics of interest

- Emergency anaesthesia (p. 70)
- Liver resection surgery (p. 104)
- Obesity – surgery for weight reduction (p. 150)
- Perioperative fluid management (p. 208)

Malignant hyperpyrexia

Key points

- Malignant hyperpyrexia (MH) is a rare life-threatening disorder of the ryanodine receptor
- The AAGBI has published clear guidelines for the treatment of MH
- All trigger agents should be avoided in patients thought to be susceptible to MH

This is a rare pharmacogenetic syndrome with an incidence between 1:10,000 and 1:20,000. It shows autosomal dominant inheritance with variable penetrance. The associated gene is on the long arm of chromosome 19 and is responsible for coding of the ryanodine receptor (RYR1). Multiple genetic mutations across a large site produce a similar phenotype and are found in 50–70% of affected patients. Other gene sites have been proposed and there may be considerable genetic heterogeneity.

Mortality rates have dropped from 70%–80% to around 2%, mostly due to increased awareness of the condition and its trigger agents, better patient monitoring and better treatment algorithms (especially utilising dantrolene). MH presents either during or immediately following general anaesthesia with a syndrome indicative of greatly increased muscle metabolism due to abnormal calcium ion flux from the sarcoplasmic reticulum (SR) in skeletal muscle.

Physiology

In normal physiology, the RYR1 receptor, positioned on the SR, interacts with the T-tubule voltage sensing dihydropyridine receptor, a process fundamental to excitation–contraction coupling.

The RYR1 receptor opens in response to a small rise in intracellular calcium from the opening of L-type calcium channels. This usually allows for a sudden calcium efflux from the SR through the RYR1 pore, which is utilised in muscle contraction. The RYR1 receptor is inhibited by magnesium ions and it is likely that MH trigger agents overcome the inhibitory effect of magnesium.

In MH, this dysfunction of the RYR1 receptor results in a lower activation and higher deactivation threshold. There is uncontrolled release of more ionised calcium from the SR into the cytoplasm causing myofibrillar contraction which depletes high-energy muscle phosphate stores (as ATP), increases metabolic rate, causes hypercapnia and heat production, increases oxygen consumption and produces metabolic acidosis.

Trigger agents

The clinical effects of MH are caused by exposure to trigger agents. There is little doubt that all the volatile inhalational anaesthetic agents can act as trigger agents. However, there are few recorded cases of suxamethonium triggering MH and there is some doubt regarding it's significance as a trigger agent. Despite this, it is clear that suxamethonium will provide a more marked clinical course in inhalational-agent-induced MH with far greater muscle damage and a worse clinical course. It is for this reason that suxamethonium is also best avoided. All other drugs in clinical use, including induction agents, nitrous oxide, nondepolarising neuromuscular blockers, local anaesthetics and cardiovascular drugs, are safe for use in MH patients.

Associated conditions

There are two associated conditions, Central Core Disease (CCD) and the King-Denborough syndrome. CCD is an autosomal dominant, nonprogressive congenital myopathy with abnormalities of the SR and T-tubules. MH and CCD both involve abnormalities in the genetic coding of the RYR1 receptor on chromosome 19 and there may be overlap (but not always). Patients with CCD should be tested for MH susceptibility. King-Denborough syndrome is a rare progressive myopathy with associated physical features.

Certain other neuromuscular conditions are associated with mild pyrexia, acidosis, hyperkalaemia, raised creatine kinase and acute rhabdomyolysis. Although these signs and findings are all similar to the presentation of MH, there is no increased susceptibility to MH on formal testing. These include muscular dystrophy (Becker's and Duchenne's), spinal muscular atrophy, myotonias, periodic paralysis, neuroleptic malignant syndrome, McArdle's syndrome and carnitine palmitoyl transferase deficiency.

Presentation

Masseter spasm following suxamethonium is frequently observed lasting several minutes. Signs of MH usually occur some time after the masseter spasm or not at all. Twenty-five per cent of patients with masseter spasm will be MH susceptible.

Management

Once recognised, the key principles for management of MH are:
Early management
- Declare the emergency and get help
- Remove trigger agents
- Hyperventilate with 100% oxygen using a volatile-free breathing system
- Expedite/abandon surgery

Ongoing management
- Dantrolene:
  - 2.5mg/kg IV bolus immediately
  - 1mg/kg repeated boluses up to max 10mg/kg
- Active cooling: e.g. icepacks, cool IV fluids
- Observe and treat hyperkalaemia, arrhythmia, acidosis, myoglobinaemia, coagulation derangements (DIC).
- Check arterial blood gases, coagulation, urea and electrolytes and plasma CK.

Following initial resuscitation, patients should be transferred to critical care. Patients should be monitored closely for renal failure (due to myoglobinaemia) and compartment syndrome.

Dantrolene acts by inhibiting excitation–contraction coupling within the skeletal muscle cell, reducing intracellular calcium release from the SR. Consequently, side effects include muscle weakness and prolongation of neuromuscular blocking agents.

Investigation

There are two forms of screening either by muscle biopsy or genetic screening.

Investigation is undertaken after the immediate crisis has resolved. It involves a quadriceps muscle biopsy from the vastus medialis, which includes the muscle point. Histologically this is normal but the specimen is connected to a force transducer and exposed to caffeine (2 mmol/L) or halothane (2%). If a contracture occurs, generating a force in excess of 0.2 g, the test is positive. If both tests are positive the patient is deemed susceptible (MHS), if only one test is positive the patient is equivocal (MHE) and if both are negative the patient is nonsusceptible (MHN).

The immediate relatives of the susceptible patient should also be tested. A positive biopsy test will lead to genetic screening for mutation in coding of the ryanodine receptor. A known genetic abnormality can be used to screen relatives (although, they may still require muscle biopsy if there is a negative genetic test). MH testing in the UK is co-ordinated by the MH Investigation Unit at St James Hospital, Leeds, which holds a register of all investigated patients.

Management of patients with known/suspected MH

The key principle is avoidance of trigger agents. A flushed anaesthetic machine should be used (10 L/min for 30 minutes) with vaporizers removed. Regional anaesthesia or a total intravenous anaesthesia-based technique with nondepolarising neuromuscular blockers should be used. Rapid sequence induction should incorporate rocuronium with sugammadex available. There is no place for prophylactic dantrolene.

Further reading

Glahn KP, Ellis FR, Halsall PJ, et al. Recognising and managing a malignant hyperthermia crisis: guidelines from the European Malignant Hyperthermia Group. Br J Anaesth 2010; 105:417–420.

Hopkins PM. Malignant hyperthermia: pharmacology of triggering. Br J Anaesth 2011; 107:48–56.

Malignant Hyperthermia Crisis. AAGBI safety guideline. Association of Anaesthetists of Great Britain and Ireland. London; AAGBI, 2011.

Related topics of interest

Minimally invasive surgery

Key points

- Minimally invasive surgery encompasses a wide variety of operations
- Recovery is generally faster than with conventional procedures
- Requires careful patient selection

The term 'minimally invasive surgery' evades definition whilst it spans almost all surgical disciplines and catalogues a wide variety of procedures (**Table 24**). Thomas Crozier perhaps puts it best by pointing out that it is not a matter of 'large incisions and extensive tissue destruction' but 'the invasiveness compared with that of the conventional procedure'.

Problems

The advent of the endoscope, lasers and interventional radiology has revolutionised the invasiveness of all surgical specialities. For the purposes of this topic, we will focus on endoscopic surgery, which has many potential benefits over conventional approaches, including:

- Reduced tissue trauma and incision size resulting in less postoperative pain and improved cosmetic results
- Lessened surgical stress response and morbidity
- Faster recovery and shorter hospital stay

Equipment

The endoscope is a device used to view inside a hollow organ or bodily cavity. Philipp Bozzini in Mainz described the first use of such a device (a 'Lichtleiter' or 'light conductor') in 1806. Typically they consist of:

- A rigid or flexible tube
- Light source
- Fibreoptics or lens system
- Eyepiece or monitor system
- Other channel for additional devices

Trocars are sharply pointed devices which are used to introduce ports or cannulae into cavities/hollow organs. Depending on the cavity or organ to be examined, insufflation of an inert gas (typically CO_2 to allow use of diathermy without combustion) may be required; in these instances insufflation devices are required. Two commonly used devices are the Veress needle and an insufflating trocar.

- The Veress needle is a bevelled needle (with a spring-loaded, blunt-tipped stylet within) (**Figure 9**). Once the cavity is entered, the spring extends the stylet, so structures within are not traumatised by the sharp point of the needle. Once the abdomen is inflated, the Veress needle is removed and replaced with a trocar
- Insufflating trocars (**Figure 10**) are primary trocars through which gas can be insufflated

Table 24 Types of minimally invasive surgery	
Surgical speciality	**Example of minimally invasive surgery**
Cardiac	Transcatheter aortic valve implantation
Thoracic	Video-assisted thoracoscopic surgery)
Neurosurgical	Trans-sphenoidal hypophysectomy
Vascular	Endovascular aneurysm repair
Orthopaedic	Arthroscopy
General, liver, endocrine	Laparoscopic anterior resection
Urological	Laparoscopic nephrectomy
Gynaecological	Laparoscopic hysterectomy
ENT and maxillofacial	Functional endoscopic sinus surgery
Ophthalmic	Endoscopic cyclophotocoagulation

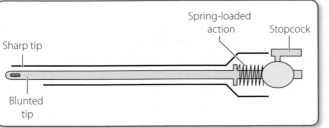

Figure 9 Veress needle.

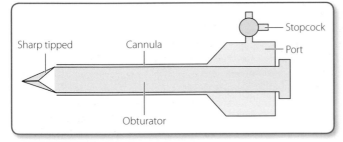

Figure 10 Insufflating trocar.

Insertion of both of these devices has the risk of tissue damage/organ puncture. An alternative is open laparoscopy, in which there is surgical dissection into the cavity before the port is inserted over a blunt-tipped trochar.

Physiological changes and other considerations

The physiological changes seen during endoscopic surgery largely depend on the cavity or organ that is being examined. We will focus on laparoscopy. The three major processes associated with physiological changes are pneumoperitoneum, positioning and gas insufflation (other changes associated with forms of endoscopic surgery are covered in **Table 25**).

Pneumoperitoneum

- Airway/respiratory
  - Increased intra-abdominal pressure (IAP) results in reduced diaphragmatic compliance, pulmonary compliance and lung volumes (e.g. functional residual capacity) whilst increasing airway resistance and pressure
  - Other effects include increased risk

of barotrauma, V/Q mismatch and possible migration of endotracheal tube tip into a main bronchus
- Cardiovascular
  - Changes are dependent on IAP
  - Heart rate – stretching of the peritoneum results in a vagally mediated bradycardia and other dysrhythmias
  - Venous return – increases with IAPs under 10 mmHg due to autotransfusion from splanchnic circulation however, with increasing IAP venous return steadily decreases as the vena cava is compressed
  - Systemic vascular resistance increases with IAP
  - Cardiac output falls with IAPs >10 mmHg
  - Regional blood flow within organs may also be affected
- Gastrointestinal (GI)
  - Increased risk of regurgitation
- Neurological
  - Raised IAP may raise intracranial pressure with an associated fall in cerebral perfusion pressure. This is compounded by absorption of CO_2 and effects of increased $Paco_2$

Table 25 Complications of minimally invasive surgery		
Speciality	**Type of endoscopy**	**Potential surgery-specific complications**
Cardiothoracic	Mediastinoscopy Thoracoscopy Bronchoscopy	Phrenic or recurrent laryngeal nerve palsy Laryngospasm Vocal cord, tracheobronchial, oesophageal or thoracic duct injury Stroke Pneumonia Chronic pain at wound site
Neurosurgery	Ventriculoscopy	Bradycardia and asystole Cranial nerve palsy Seizures Ventriculitis/meningitis Intracerebral haemorrhage/subdural haematoma Cerebrospinal fluid (CSF) leak
Orthopaedic	Arthroscopy (complications depend on joint)	DVT or PE Fluid extravasation Chrondolysis Synovitis Cartilage/ligamentous injury
Gastrointestinal	Endoscopy (upper and lower tract)	Arrhythmias Deep vein thrombosis or pulmonary embolism Regurgitation and aspiration Perforation Pancreatitis Infection, e.g. cholangitis
Urological	Cystoscopy Ureteroscopy Nephroscopy	Hyponatraemia/hypo-osmolality Haematuria/dysuria Urinary tract infection Bladder/urethral injury or perforation
Gynaecological/obstetric	Hysteroscopy Amnioscopy Fetoscopy	Bradycardia and asystole Hyponatraemia/hypo-osmolality Infection Haematuria Adenomyosis Uterine perforation Rupture of membranes
ENT and maxillofacial	Bronchoscopy Rhinoscopy Laryngoscopy Oesophagoscopy	Laryngospasm Vocal cord injury Diplopia, blindness or brain injury CSF leak Epistaxis

- Renal
  - Raised IAP results in increased renal vascular resistance and decreased glomerular filtration rate
- Endocrine/metabolic
  - Increased circulating catecholamines, adrenocorticotropic hormone, cortisol and antidiuretic hormone
  - Whilst the inflammatory aspect of the surgical stress response is reduced, the endocrine aspect is still induced with laparoscopic surgery
  - Fall in body temperature is a common complication, as a result of gas and irrigation fluid flowing through the abdominal cavity

Positioning

The three common positions associated with endoscopic surgery are Trendelenburg (head-down), reverse Trendelenburg (head-up) and lateral. General issues include:
- Intravenous access must be reliable as it may be inaccessible intraoperatively

- Need for a secure airway
- Protection of the eyes from excess pressure or corneal abrasions
- Protection of pressure points, e.g. brachial plexus

Trendelenburg (head-down)
- Respiratory – reduced lung volumes, increased V/Q mismatch and potential endotracheal tube migration and upper airway oedema (may result in stridor postoperatively)
- Cardiovascular – increased venous return and cardiac output
- Neurological – risk of cerebral oedema

Reverse Trendelenburg (head-up)
- Cardiovascular – reduced venous return, blood pressure and cardiac output (effects are most marked in the hypovolaemic patient)

Lateral position
- Respiratory – compliance and V/Q relationship depends on lung position. The nondependent lung will have increased compliance and ventilation, whereas the dependent lung will have reduced compliance and increased perfusion
- Cardiovascular – increased systemic vascular resistance and decreased venous return result in reduced cardiac output

Gas insufflation

There are many benefits of using CO_2 to insufflate the abdomen; it is nontoxic, nonflammable and its high solubility reduces the risk posed by gas embolism. However, whilst the insufflator maintains gas flow, some CO_2 will be absorbed from the peritoneum resulting in an increase in $Paco_2$ and its subsequent effects. Other effects are the result of cavity expansion and inadvertent insufflation into other tissues/organs.

Complications

Laparoscopic surgery is not totally benign and has specific complications that the anaesthetist needs to be aware of, which are classified into pneumoperitoneum, positioning or gas insufflation issues.
- Pneumoperitoneum – haemorrhage and/or tissue/organ injury from Veress needle/trocar insertion, occult bleeding due to restricted visualisation of surgical site and dysrhythmias from stretching of the peritoneum
- Positioning – peripheral compression neuropathy
- Gas insufflation – venous gas embolism, subcutaneous emphysema and pneumothorax or pneumomediastinum

Further reading

Bozzini, P. Light conductor, an invention for examing internal parts and diseases, together with illustrations. J Pract Med Surg 1806; 24:107–124.

Crozier, TA. Anaesthesia for minimally invasvie surgery. Cambridge: Cambridge University Press, 2004.

Related topics of interest

Muscular diseases

Key points

- Regional anaesthesia is usually the preferred option in muscular disease with respiratory involvement
- Muscular dystrophies are usually progressive in nature. Respiratory and cardiac involvement should be investigated prior to anaesthesia
- In general, nondepolarising neuromuscular blockers are used in reduced doses and suxamethonium should be avoided in muscular disease
- Surgery duration should be minimised where possible and there should be a low threshold for postoperative recovery in the high dependency unit

Dystrophies

The most frequent dystrophies are Duchenne and Becker's muscular dystrophy. Both are associated with X-linked defects in the gene coding for dystrophin, a cytoskeletal protein which bonds muscle cells to the extracellular matrix. Absence of dystrophin leads to chronic muscle fibre necrosis and fibrosis (observed as pseudohypertrophy).

Duchenne muscular dystrophy (DMD) has an incidence of 1:3500. One third are spontaneous mutations. There is a progressive muscle weakness (classically starting in the lower limbs) as the child ages and serum creatine kinase (CK) is raised, even in asymptomatic neonates and female carriers. Kyphoscoliosis develops and most patients are nonambulatory by teenage years. Cardiac muscle undergoes degenerative change and fibrosis affecting the conduction system and chambers. Most patients die in their 20s from respiratory or cardiac failure. Becker muscular dystrophy is a milder form with a later onset with survival usually into the 30s–40s.

Problems

- Respiratory weakness, obstructive sleep apnoea and kyphoscoliosis (reduced total lung capacity and vital capacity)
- Rhabdomyolysis and hyperkalaemia with suxamethonium and possibly inhalational agents. This may mimic malignant hyperpyrexia (MH), but appears to be pathophysiologically distinct
- Airway may be difficult due to obesity, tongue hypertrophy and limited neck movement
- Myocardial fibrosis, cardiomyopathy and dysrhythmia

Anaesthetic management

Assessment and premedication

Particular emphasis should be given to assessment of respiratory reserve and cardiac muscle involvement. Lung function tests and peak flow can be helpful in older patients and an ECG and echocardiogram are essential, although may not reveal the extent of disease. Cardiac MRI can be used to determine the degree of myocardial fibrosis, which corresponds to the severity of cardiomyopathy. The likelihood of a difficult airway should be assessed.

Conduct of anaesthesia

Regional anaesthesia should be considered where possible. For general anaesthesia, invasive cardiac monitoring should be considered and induction should be smooth, titrating small doses of induction agent.

Historically, a link between DMD and MH was accepted; however, recent evidence suggests that the incidence of MH is no greater in these patients. Suxamethonium should be avoided due to rhabdomyolysis and many specialists still advocate avoidance of volatile agents. Given the controversy, it would seem sensible to use a 'volatile-free' anaesthetic machine and employ a total intravenous anaesthesia technique. This has the added benefit of titratability and rapid elimination. If gas induction is essential, volatiles should be discontinued as soon as possible.

Nondepolarising neuromuscular blockers may be used in small doses but have a delayed and often prolonged effect. It is often possible to avoid these drugs through careful use of propofol and short-acting opiates. As with suxamethonium, anticholinesterases may cause life-threatening hyperkalaemia. Cardiac dysfunction may be unmasked by cardiac depressant drugs (including anaesthetic agents), large fluid shifts (especially haemorrhage), prone positioning and high ventilation pressures. Hypovolaemia is poorly tolerated. Coagulation may be impaired due to platelet dysfunction and vascular smooth muscle involvement.

Patient temperature should be monitored and normothermia maintained. Any evidence of rhabdomyolysis (e.g. metabolic acidosis, hyperkalaemia, raised CK, myoglobinuria) should be treated aggressively with intravenous fluids, sodium bicarbonate (to alkalinise the urine thus improving myoglobin solubility) and ICU support.

Postoperative care

Patients should be managed in the ICU with ongoing cardiovascular monitoring. Noninvasive ventilation is a useful step-down. Opioids should be carefully titrated to effect. Swallowing is often impaired and gastric emptying delayed. Asymptomatic aspiration is common and care should be taken to ensure return of bulbar function prior to feeding.

Myotonias

This group of hereditary diseases are characterised by delayed muscle relaxation following contraction. Myotonia congenita has little systemic involvement, a normal life expectancy and is very rare. Myotonic dystrophy is more common (prevalence 4 per 100 000). It exhibits autosomal dominant inheritance with anticipation (i.e. increasing severity with successive generations). A mutation in chromosome 19 is found in 99% of affected families with males and females equally affected. The pathophysiological mechanism of myotonia is abnormal closure of sodium and chloride channels in the muscle membrane following depolarisation, leading to repetitive discharge and contraction.

Clinical features include characteristic facies with frontal balding, a smooth forehead, ptosis, cataracts and a 'lateral smile'. There is muscle wasting of the neck (especially of the sternomastoids), shoulders and quadriceps. Muscle tone and reflexes are reduced once wasting has developed and foot drop is common. The disease is associated with a low IQ in 40%, gonadal atrophy, diabetes mellitus, dysphagia, constipation, respiratory muscle failure, cardiac conduction defects and cardiomyopathy. Patients usually present aged 20–40 years and die in their sixth decade from cardiac disease or bulbar muscle involvement. There is a progressive worsening of cardiac conduction with an increasing risk of tachyarrhythmia and sudden death. Myotonia is precipitated by cold, exercise, shivering, hyperkalaemia, suxamethonium and neostigmine.

Problems

- Increased sensitivity to anaesthetic drugs, e.g. propofol and thiopentone
- Drug precipitation of myotonia, e.g. suxamethonium and neostigmine
- Respiratory and cardiac involvement

Anaesthetic management

Assessment and premedication

The clinical diagnosis is confirmed by EMG, indicating spontaneous myotonic discharges. Genetic testing is used to screen affected families. Preoperative investigation should include ECG and possibly a 24-hour tape, lung function tests (reduced maximum breathing capacity and expiratory reserve volume) and blood potassium. Cardiac pacing may be necessary. Patients are sensitive to all depressant drugs and anxiolytic premedicants should be avoided. Quinine, procainamide or phenytoin may be used as symptomatic treatments for myotonia.

Conduct of anaesthesia

In addition to standard AAGBI monitoring, invasive pressure and cardiac output monitoring may be indicated. Body temperature and neuromuscular blockade should also be monitored.

Regional anaesthesia is safe and avoids the use of known precipitating agents.

However, the myotonic reflex is not blocked as this is due to the intrinsic muscle disorder. If a general anaesthetic is given, suxamethonium and neostigmine should be avoided. Nondepolarising neuromuscular blockers exhibit an increased sensitivity and should be titrated in very small doses (10–20% usual dose). Options include small doses of atracurium with spontaneous return of neuromuscular function, mivacurium (hydrolysed rapidly by plasma cholinesterase) or rocuronium followed by sugammadex.

Patients are sensitive to opioids, barbiturates and volatile agents. The use of propofol in low doses has been reported as safe in myotonic dystrophy. Potassium worsens myotonia and should be avoided in intravenous fluids. Patients must be kept warm. Myotonic contractures (e.g. masseter spasm) are not responsive to neuromuscular blocking agents or local anaesthetics and can be managed by normalising physiology and correcting the precipitating factor. Principle treatment is with antiarrhythmic agents (e.g. mexiletine).

Postoperative care

Patients may require admission to ICU if they have cardiovascular instability or have been slow to regain consciousness or normal neuromuscular function. As with the dystrophies, noninvasive ventilation can be useful and opioids should be used cautiously. Return of bulbar function should again be assured prior to feeding.

Mitochondrial and metabolic myopathies

There are over a hundred distinct rare myopathies associated with mitochondrial disorders. There may be associated metabolic derangements, such as increased serum lactate or pyruvate. Patients tolerate stresses such as fasting and systemic illness poorly and show exaggerated metabolic responses. Preoperative treatment with metabolic substrates and avoidance of prolonged fasting is paramount. Particular features that may affect anaesthesia include:

- Cardiac involvement, either cardiomyopathy or conduction defects necessitating pacing
- Encephalopathy and seizures
- Respiratory weakness
- Bulbar weakness with associated aspiration
- Other organ dysfunction, such as eye, liver, kidney and endocrine system

Preoperative assessment should focus on these issues and include a detailed cardiorespiratory evaluation. Due to the scarcity of evidence (predominantly case reports), the anaesthetic management of most of these myopathies is based on the general principles outlined for other muscular disorders outlined above. Blood glucose monitoring is essential and tight glycaemic control is required to prevent lactic acidosis. Management of the particular condition will be tailored to the individual pathology identified in the history.

Further reading

Boyle R. Antenatal and preoperative genetic and clinical assessment in myotonic dystrophy. Anaesth Intensive Care 1999; 27:301–306.

Marsh S, Pittard A. Neuromuscular disorders and anaesthesia. Part 2: Specific neuromuscular disorders. Br J Anaesth: Contin Educ Anaesth Crit Care Pain Med 2011; 11:119–123.

Marsh S, Ross N, Pittard A. Neuromuscular disorders and anaesthesia. Part 1: generic anaesthetic management. Br J Anaesth: Contin Educ Anaesth Crit Care Pain Med 2011; 11:115–118.

Related topics of interest

Myasthenia gravis

Key points

- Diagnosis is usually by antiacetylcholine (anti-Ach) receptor antibodies or edrophonium test
- Thymectomy is largely successful and is the treatment of choice for younger myaesthenic patients
- Regional anaesthesia is preferred. Patients usually require mechanical ventilation if undergoing general anaesthesia
- The principal critical events are myaesthenic crisis and cholinergic crisis. The later is due to overtreatment

Myaesthenia gravis (MG) is an autoimmune disease. Around 90% of patients have antibodies to the nicotinic ACh receptors in the postsynaptic membrane of the neuromuscular junction. The correlation between absolute antibody levels and disease severity is weak. Muscarinic ACh receptors, and thus the autonomic nervous system, are spared. Thymus disease is associated with MG; 75% of patients have histological evidence of an abnormality (e.g. germinal centre hyperplasia), whilst 10% have a benign thymoma. Other autoimmune disorders and certain HLA subgroups are associated with MG (e.g. thyroid disease, pernicious anaemia). The prevalence of MG is around 5:100 000 with young women being affected most commonly (peak onset 20–30 years of age). Men over the age of 50 are the next most commonly affected (including most patients with MG-associated thymoma).

Neonatal myaesthenia is rare and is seen in infants of myaesthenic mothers. It presents at birth and results from the passage of anti-ACh receptor antibodies across the placenta. Congenital myaesthenia is very rare and is not associated with antibodies to the ACh receptor. Anaesthetists may be asked to care for myaesthenics during surgery, especially for thymectomy, or in critical care when the patient is in crisis (myaesthenic or cholinergic) or has developed respiratory failure.

Problems

- Muscle weakness especially of the bulbar (aspiration risk) and respiratory muscles
- Abnormal response to muscle relaxants, both depolarising and nondepolarising
- Complications of drug therapy; difficulty interpreting response to muscle relaxants, immunosuppression and drug-induced exacerbation

Clinical features

The muscle weakness of MG is typically made worse by exertion and is improved by rest. The characteristic distribution of affected muscles, in descending order, is extraocular, bulbar, cervical, proximal limb, distal limb and trunk. Thus patients frequently complain of ptosis and diplopia, and dysphagia. Severe bulbar weakness leaves them at risk of frequent pulmonary aspiration.

The Eaton-Lambert syndrome, by contrast, is characterised by muscle weakness which improves on exertion and spares the ocular and bulbar muscles. It is a condition associated with small-cell carcinoma of the bronchus and, like myasthetics, sufferers are equisitely sensitive to nondepolarising muscle relaxants.

Investigations

- Anti-ACh receptor antibodies. Detected in the serum of 80–90% patients, these are pathognomonic. It is much less sensitive in ocular myaesthenia
- Edrophonium test. The diagnosis of MG is established by administering an intravenous dose of the short-acting anticholinesterase edrophonium. Anticholinesterases increase the amount of ACh available at the neuromuscular junction. An improvement in muscle function following edrophonium thus supports the diagnosis (although other conditions such as amyotrophic lateral sclerosis will also give a positive result).

The principal side effect is severe bradycardia. Patients with weakness due to cholinergic crisis will worsen and may become apnoeic after edrophonium

- A test dose of 2 mg of edrophonium is administered intravenously, followed (in the absence of adverse effects) by 8 mg 1 minute later. The absence of clinical improvement would suggest cholinergic crisis or an alternative cause of weakness
- Electromyography. A decremental response in the size of the compound motor action potential after repeated electrical stimulation of a motor nerve can support the diagnosis. This is true even in the majority of those with only ocular symptoms

Treatment

- Anticholinesterases. Pyridostigmine bromide 60 mg is given four times a day and increased until an optimal response is achieved. It may not be possible to abolish all weakness and increasing the dose in an attempt to do so may precipitate a cholinergic crisis
- Anticholinergics. May be required to control side effects of anticholinesterase administration such as salivation, colic, and diarrhoea. They are not used as a matter of routine in all patients
- Immunosuppression. Corticosteroids are the most frequently used immunosuppressive agents. They may benefit patients with pure ocular symptoms and those whose response to anticholinesterases is suboptimal. Administration may be associated with an initial deterioration and improvement may take several weeks. Plasma potassium levels should be monitored to ensure that steroid-induced hypokalaemia (enhanced renal potassium loss) is not adding to muscle weakness. Azathioprine and ciclosporin are used in those with severe myaesthenia unresponsive to other measures and are thought to act predominantly on the T cell but can take months to work
- Plasmapheresis. Some patients show a short lived but dramatic improvement in weakness following plasma exchange through the reduction in circulating antibodies. Maximum response is usually seen about a week after a series of five or so daily exchanges. Improvement lasts for around a month. It may be a useful technique for those is severe myaesthenic crisis or to allow weaning from ventilation.
- Intravenous Immunoglobulin. The mechanism of action is poorly understood, but indications and effects are similar to plasmapheresis
- Thymectomy. Usually results in clinical improvement in around 80% of all myaesthenics although the mechanism has not been fully elucidated. This is the treatment of choice in adults with MG up to the age of 60 and produces a more rapid onset of remission with a lower mortality than medical therapy alone. Patients due to undergo thymectomy should have their respiratory function optimised preoperatively. Plasma exchange and steroids may help. Thymectomy often leaves patients more sensitive to the effects of anticholinesterases and cholinergic crisis may ensue after surgery. It is for this reason that the dose of pyridostigmine should be reduced preop as much as possible without compromising respiratory function. In addition, the intraoperative management of neuromuscular blockade is easier in the presence of a mildly myaesthenic patient

Anaesthetic management

Regional anaesthesia should be used where possible. Assessment of muscle function (e.g. ability to sustain a head-lift off the pillow or generate a negative inspiratory pressure >25 cmH$_2$O) and arterial blood gas analysis is essential. Predictors of poor postoperative respiratory function include MG for >6 years, coexisting respiratory disease, reduced forced vital capacity (FVC) and major surgery.

Almost all procedures will require tracheal intubation and assisted ventilation. An anaesthetic technique is usually chosen that will either reduce the dose of neuromuscular relaxants given or avoid their use altogether. Suxamethonium gives an unpredictable response and nondepolarising agents such as atracurium should be used in 10–25% of the normal dose. Responses should be monitored. Neuromuscular function should be allowed to return spontaneously as the administration of reversal agents may cause confusion in the presence of continued weakness.

Myaesthenic crisis

This is a severe life-threatening exacerbation of MG. It can progress rapidly to respiratory failure necessitating urgent tracheal intubation and respiratory support. Myaesthenic crises can be precipitated by infection, pyrexia, surgical or emotional stress and certain drugs. These drugs include aminoglycoside (e.g. gentamicin) and macrolide antibiotics, membrane stabilising antiarrythmics (e.g. quinidine, procainamide, lignocaine), anticonvulsants (e.g. phenytoin) and antidepressants (e.g. lithium).

If the patient's FVC falls below 10–15 mL/kg or they are unable to adequately expectorate secretions, they require intubation and respiratory support. Many then withdraw all anticholinesterase therapy and rest the patient, believing that the sensitivity of the motor end plate to ACh will increase under such circumstances. Plasma exchange or immunosuppressive therapy may be required to wean the patient from mechanical ventilation. Subcutaneous heparin should be given for prophylaxis against thromboembolism.

Cholinergic crisis

A cholinergic crisis is caused by an excess of ACh available at the neuromuscular junction and usually follows excessive administration of anticholinesterase. It too may present with respiratory failure, bulbar palsy and virtually complete paralysis. It may be difficult to distinguish from a myaesthenic crisis but often includes an excess of secretions, which may worsen the respiratory failure. Other symptoms more likely during a cholinergic crisis include abdominal pain, diarrhoea and blurred vision. The differential may be made be administering a small dose of intravenous edrophonium. Patients in myaesthenic crisis should improve, whereas those with a cholinergic crisis will get worse.

Further reading

Blichfeldt-Lauridsen, Hansen BD. Anaesthesia and myasthenia gravis. Acta Anaesthesiol Scand 2011; 56:17–22.

Related topics of interest

- Muscular diseases (p. 118)
- Neurological disease – demyelinating and neurodegenerative diseases (p. 137)
- Thoracic surgery (p. 297)

National audit

Key points

- National audit projects are funded by government, arm's length bodies or charities
- The GMC recognises the importance of involvement in audit for clinicians
- The anaesthetic NAP audits, and NCEPOD, focus on particular areas of clinical practice in each cycle

Clinical audit is a quality improvement tool, systematically evaluating the procedures used in patient care and allowing examination of how associated resources are used with a view to improvement in patient outcome. The safety and quality domain of 'Good Medical Practice', published by the GMC, makes it clear that all doctors are expected to contribute to local and national audit where appropriate.

This discussion will be limited to national audit projects in the UK. Many other countries have their own national audit programmes.

NCEPOD

The National Confidential Enquiry into Patient Outcome and Death (NCEPOD) audit programme started in 1982 and has published over 30 reports since then. As a charitable independent organisation, their remit now includes both deaths and 'near misses' in all specialties, not just surgery. They are funded through the Healthcare Quality Improvement Partnership. Key reports (and recommendations) pertinent to anaesthesia are discussed below.

Knowing the risk: a review of the perioperative care of surgical patients (2011)

'High-risk' patients do worse in the United Kingdom than other countries. Recommendations include clear identification of this group to allow improved preoperative preparation, perioperative monitoring and postoperative critical care.

Elective and emergency surgery in the elderly: an age old problem (2010)

Recommends greater involvement of elderly care physicians. Note that delay in surgery in the elderly has a worse outcome. Acute kidney injury and perioperative hypotension should be avoidable.

Trauma: who cares? (2007)

Sixty per cent of trauma patients received suboptimal care. A lack of seniority and recognition of illness severity contributed. Recommended regional planning for trauma services include trauma centres.

Abdominal aortic aneurysm: a service in need of surgery? (2005)

Consideration for abdominal aortic aneurysm repair to be done in tertiary centres only and by fewer anaesthetists. Emergency patients transferred to tertiary centres do no worse than those admitted direct.

An acute problem (2005)

A review of pre-ICU care of critically ill patients. Recommended that a consultant physician see patients within 24 hours and ICU admissions seen by a consultant within 12 hours. All hospitals should have a track-and-trigger system to rapidly detect deterioration.

Who operates when? I (1997) and II (2003)

Following the 1997 report, which described complex surgery occurring out-of-hours by trainees with inadequate supervision, the 2003 report indicated a reduction in out-of-hours operating. Out-of-hours work is still carried out mostly by trainees. Over 50% elective surgery is day case, performed by career grade anaesthetists.

Recommendations included consultant involvement in complex cases, consultant supervision of trainees and appropriately specialised and trained surgical and anaesthetic teams for the patient's condition. Improved critical care facilities and more rapid surgery for emergency patients are required. They also recommend regular audits of operative results, with joint meetings with surgeons, with morbidity and mortality discussed.

CMACE

The Centre for Maternal and Child Enquiries (CMACE) report (2011) supersedes the CEMACH and CEMD reports and covers the periods 2006–2008. The audit started in 1952 and produces a report every 3 years.

The most frequent causes of direct maternal death were sepsis (26), pre-eclampsia (19), thromboembolism (16), amniotic fluid embolism (13) and haemorrhage (9). There were 7 direct deaths caused by anaesthesia. Anaesthesia-related factors included failure to ventilate, failure to consult with critical care/senior, obesity, suboptimal management of pre-eclampsia, sepsis and haemorrhage.

Key recommendations: Improved preparation of high-risk patients, including prepregnancy counselling, interpreters, preoperative assessment, multidisciplinary care and better communication. Systolic hypertension (>160 mmHg) and genital tract infection should be treated early. There should be regular clinical skills training and incident reporting.

National audit projects

The Royal College of Anaesthetists has undertaken a number of national audit projects (NAPs) since 2003. In 2011, the administration of NAP was taken over by the Health Services Research Centre, a subsidiary of the National Institute of Academic Anaesthesia. Projects are discussed below.

NAP1: Supervisory role of consultant anaesthetists 2003

Most trainees are satisfied with their level of supervision, although often consultants are not immediately available to assist.

NAP2: Place of mortality and morbidity review meetings 2003

Three quarters of anaesthetic departments have systems in place to review mortality and morbidity. Meetings are well attended and valued. Recommendations included multidisciplinary meetings and a focus on constructive criticism within a no-blame culture.

NAP3: Major complications of central neuraxial block in the United Kingdom (2009)

Reported 84 major complications out of 700,000 procedures performed. Permanent injury had an incidence of 1:24-54,000 procedures. Paraplegia/death had an incidence of 1:50,000-140,000. The distribution of 'permanent harm' was epidural (60%), spinal (23%) and CSE (13%).

NAP4: Major complications of airway management in the United Kingdom (2011)

Fifty-six per cent of general anaesthetics involve a supraglottic device, 38% have an ETT and 5% facemask. Particular areas of concern include failure to assess and anticipate the difficult airway, failure to plan adequately and failure to use fibreoptic intubation equipment. Other findings of note were a 60% failure rate with needle cricothyroidotomy and that a third of events occurred at emergence. Aspiration was noted as the leading cause of airway-related death.

NAP5: Accidental awareness during general anaesthesia in the United Kingdom (2013)

Baseline incidence of awareness is 1:15,000, much lower than previously thought. Around half of the cases occurred around induction of anaesthesia. Depth of anaesthesia monitors were used in <2% of centres.

NAP6: Anaphylaxis

Data collection window anticipated 2015–2016.

ICNARC

The Intensive Care National Audit and Research Centre (ICNARC) reports annually on outcomes and activity of participating intensive care and high dependency units in the United Kingdom. It is a sister organisation of the Intensive Care Society. The two principal audits are the National Cardiac Arrest Audit (relating to in-hospital cardiac arrest) and the Case Mix Programme Database, concerning patient outcomes from critical care units. The latter is a voluntary database collecting information from around 95% of UK ICUs. Data collected includes age, acute severity, comorbidity, surgical status, reason for admission and outcome of admissions. Data is validated, analysed and risk adjusted using the APACHE II and ICNARC (2011) models to predict mortality and now contains validated data on over a million admissions to participating critical care units.

Quarterly comparative data analysis reports are generated for each unit concerning case mix, activity and outcome.

The Critical Care Minimal Dataset (CCMDS) can be extracted by participating units and used for payment-by-results submissions to the Department of Health. In addition, the reports form part of the resource used by governing bodies, commissioners and providers to aid the organisation of critical care.

TARN

The Trauma Audit and Research Network (TARN) is Europe's largest trauma database with over 200,000 cases taken from over 50% of trauma-receiving hospitals in England and Wales as well as centres in other parts of Europe. Data has been collected electronically since 2005. Akin to ICNARC, data collected can be used for research or to provide comparison of trauma care at the local or national level. It also produces evidence upon which commissioners and governing bodies can plan trauma care in the United Kingdom. Reports are produced monthly, quarterly or ad hoc.

Further reading

McWilliam A, Smith A. National UK audit projects in anaesthesia. Br J Anaesth: Contin Educ Anaesth Crit Care Pain Med 2008; 8:172–175.

National Confidential Enquiry into Patient Outcome and Death (NCEPOD). Trauma: who cares? London; NCEPOD, 2007.

Royal College of Anaesthetists National Audit Projects. http://www.rcoa.ac.uk/clinical-standards-safety-and-quality/national-audit-projects

Saving Mothers' Lives: Reviewing maternal deaths to make motherhood safer: 2006–2008. Executive Summary. BJOG: An International Journal of Obstetrics and Gynaecology 2011; 118:e12–21.

Related topics of interest

- Airway – the emergency airway (p. 7)
- Emergency anaesthesia (p. 70)
- Obstetrics – emergencies (p. 160)

Neuroanaesthesia – subarachnoid haemorrhage

Key points

- Anaesthesia for cerebral vascular surgery requires an understanding of the effects of subarachnoid blood on the brain and other organ systems and awareness of potential immediate complications and their management, including delayed cerebral ischaemia (DCI) and rebleeding
- Anaesthesia should aim to minimise risk of rebleeding, provide good conditions for surgery and allow rapid wakening and assessment

Incidence of subarachnoid hemorrhage (SAH) is about 8/100,000 population per year. Approximately 80% of all patients with SAH will have bleeding from an aneurysm. The other 20% result from trauma, stroke or a variety of rarer causes.

Problems

Both therapeutic options are high-risk interventions with significant mortality and morbidity.

Endovascular platinum coiling

- Induces thrombosis of aneurysm sac
- Takes place in radiology suite
- Problems associated with anaesthesia in a remote location:
  - Different processes for preassessment, consenting and WHO checklist
  - Lack of recovery unit
  - Location/distance to help
- Availability of emergency equipment
- Require heparinisation

Surgical clipping of aneurysm neck

- Long surgery
- Relatively uncommon now
- Clinical grading of subarachnoid haemorrhage
- Risk of air embolus
- Risk of significant bleeding; may require induced hypotension, management of major haemorrhage

Clinical features

Patients can present with no symptoms (incidental finding), sudden severe headache, neurological signs, collapse and death. Prognosis is related to grading which depends on symptoms or CT findings (**Tables 26 and 27**). About 10% patients die before arrival in hospital and another 12% within the first 24 hours. Up to 40% of patients with poor grade (IV or V) and 10% of good grade (I or II) SAH die. Incidence of aneurysms increases with age and has a genetic component. Modifiable risk factors include smoking, hypertension and alcohol intake.

Major complications after SAH include rebleeding, DCI, hydrocephalus, seizures and cardiopulmonary dysfunction. Rebleeding risk is highest in the few hours after the initial bleed but has a cumulative incidence thereafter of 1.5% per day. It is associated with significantly increased morbidity and mortality, thus early intervention is recommended.

Patients with SAH, especially of poorer grade, may have systemic effects including hypovolaemia, hyponatraemia (probably due to cerebral salt wasting), pulmonary oedema and cardiac dysfunction (ECG changes, raised troponin and echocardiographic evidence of reduced ventricular function and wall motion abnormalities). Cardiac compromise tends to be reversible and the prognosis is good, although it may require supportive treatment with inotropes.

Table 26 Clinical grading of subarachnoid haemorrhage		
Grade	Motor deficit	Glasgow Coma Score
I	Absent	15
II	Absent	13–14
III	Present	13–14
IV	Present/absent	7–12
V	Present/absent	3–6
Adapted from World Federation of Neurological Surgeons' grading		

Table 27 Radiological grading of subarachnoid haemorrhage	
Grade	CT findings
1	No blood detected
2	Diffuse thin layer of subarachnoid blood (vertical layer <1 mm thick)
3	Localised clot or thick layer of subarachnoid blood (vertical layer >1 mm thick)
4	Intracerebral or intraventricular blood (with or without diffuse subarachnoid blood)
Adapted from Fisher grading of subarachnoid haemorrahge on CT scan	

DCI may occur in up to 30% of patients with SAH. Incidence and severity may correlate with the amount of blood seen at CT. It is associated with significant increases in morbidity and mortality and risk peaks at about 7 days post-bleed. Symptoms include focal neurology and decreased conscious level: it may be associated with vasoconstriction seen at CT. Historically 'vasospasm' was thought to be the cause of this deterioration, but DCI is now thought to be a distinct entity with other predisposing and causative factors. Nimodipine is the only therapy that has been shown to reduce incidence and should be given prophylactically to all patients with SAH.

Investigations

CT brain and CT angiography will likely have been performed already to grade the SAH. Full preoperative assessment should be undertaken. Pupillary signs and Glasgow Coma Score should be checked and documented prior to induction of anaesthesia. Patients should have appropriate investigations to allow rapid access to cross-matched blood. Cerebral vascular lesions can bleed significantly and quickly. Abnormalities may be seen preoperatively on ECG.

Treatment

The decision to coil or clip is made on the basis of grade of aneurysm, clinical status of patient and imaging review between the neuroradiologist and neurosurgeon. For low-grade bleeds from anterior aneurysms, the evidence now favours coiling with a 7% reduction in mortality and a number needed

to treat (NNT) of 14. Some aneurysms are inappropriate for coiling; they may be difficult to access radiologically, have other vessels arising close to their neck or be wide necked. Evidence regarding posterior circulation aneurysms is less clear.

Anaesthetic management
Preoperative

Opiate premedication should be avoided; it may mask changes in neurological state and cause respiratory depression with hypercapnia or hypoxia which affects intracranial pressure (ICP).

Intraoperative

Invasive arterial monitoring allows accurate measurement of blood pressure which facilitates therapeutic hypertension or hypotension in the event of complications. Other haemodynamic monitoring may be warranted depending on patient status. Ensure appropriate intravenous access.

A number of factors must be considered when inducing anaesthesia. Patients may may have raised ICP secondary to intracranial bleeding or oedema. Areas of ischaemia/ tissue damage often have disrupted autoregulation. Finally, the risk of further bleeding from the aneurysm is related to the pressure difference across the wall of the aneurysm (transmural pressure). Induction should therefore be smooth, avoiding coughing or straining and maintaining systemic blood pressure without peaks or troughs so the transmural pressure is stable. Most centres now use short acting opiate infusions (remifentanil 0.25–0.5 µg/kg/ min) plus either propofol infusion or volatile anaesthetic gases (desflurane and sevoflurane probably have least effect on cerebral blood flow). Blood pressure should be maintained using an infusion of an appropriate vasopressor. RSI may be indicated in which case suxamethonium may be used. Rocuronium is an alternative as long as there is access to sugammadex. Neuromuscular function should be monitored using a peripheral nerve stimulator; intermittent boluses may be required.

Coiling

Anticoagulation with heparin will be requested by the radiologist. Aim for an activated clotting time (ACT) of 2 x baseline, usually by point of care testing. Ongoing ACT assessment is required during the procedure. Protamine should be available for rapid reversal should the aneurysm rupture; this may be visible on the screen or be signalled by cardiovascular instability (hypo- or hypertension and ECG changes). Good communication with the neuroradiology team is vital. In such an event, reverse any continuing anticoagulation, induce hypotension (bearing in mind the requirement to maintain cerebral blood flow to other areas of the brain) and be prepared to relocate to theatre urgently if bleeding cannot be controlled. The responsible neurosurgeon should be involved in decision making at an early stage as the outcome is likely to be poor. In this situation the patient is likely to remain intubated and may require further imaging or intervention e.g. external ventricular drain (EVD).

Clipping

The same principles regarding likelihood of further rupture relating to transmural pressure apply. Bleeding may be very significant. Procedures for managing major haemorrhage may be required. Even a small amount of bleeding can make it impossible for the surgeon to control the source. In this case the anaesthetist may need to induce profound hypotension to allow placing of haemostatic clamps. This can be achieved by beta-blockade, bolus doses of anaesthetic (remifentanil and propofol boluses) and may also require boluses of adenosine to temporarily arrest the circulation and allow visualisation of the bleeding point for the surgeon. Cerebral 'protection' should be used in this situation with either a thiopentone (EEG burst suppression or 'sleep dose') or propofol bolus.

In some cases surgeons will opt to use temporary clips to allow safer dissection around the aneurysm prior to the permanent clip. Distal blood flow relies on collateral circulation and there is a risk of brain ischaemia and infarction, which is time sensitive. Surgeons may request cerebral protection at this point.

Postoperative care

It may be appropriate to wake the patient immediately after surgery depending on preoperative status and intraoperative course. Haemodynamic stability is desirable. Analgesia can be managed with paracetamol and short acting opiates (fentanyl and fentanyl patient-controlled analgesia). Postoperative care should be in a Level 2 area or higher after cerebral vascular surgery. Patients who are slow to wake may require a CT scan in case of hydrocephalus, oedema, bleeding or vasospasm and may require further operative procedures (evacuation of haematoma, EVD insertion or ICP monitor).

Further reading

Diringer MN, Bleck TP, Hemphill JC, et al. Critical care management of patients following aneurysmal subarachnoid hemorrhage: recommendations from the Neurocritical Care Society's Multidisciplinary Consensus Conference. Neurocrit Care 2011; 15:211–240.

Molyneux AJ, Kerr RS, Yu LM, et al. International subarachnoid aneurysm trial (ISAT) of neurosurgical clipping versus endovascular coiling in 2143 patients with ruptured intracranial aneurysms: a randomised comparison of effects on survival, dependency, seizures, rebleeding, subgroups, and aneurysm occlusion. The Lancet 2005; 366:809–817.

Rowland MJ, Hadjipavlou G, Kelly M, et al. Delayed cerebral ischaemia after subarachnoid haemorrhage: looking beyond vasospasm. Br J Anaesth 2012; 109:315–329.

Related topics of interest

- Blood transfusion and salvage (p. 22)
- Gas embolism (p. 80)
- Neuroanaesthesia – traumatic brain injury (p. 131)
- Radiology – interventional radiology (p. 250)
- Total intravenous anaesthesia and target-controlled infusions (p. 303)

Neuroanaesthesia – traumatic brain injury

Key points

- Management aims to prevent secondary brain injury
- Management is time critical
- Attention to detail greatly improves outcomes

Traumatic brain injury (TBI) remains a major cause of death and disability in trauma. Primary brain injury occurs at the moment of impact, resulting in immediate damage to structures in the brain. Secondary brain injury follows as indirect mechanisms cause further damage to brain structure and function. It has been shown that prompt, specialist care can reduce the effect of secondary brain injury and improve outcomes.

The Monroe-Kelly doctrine describes the cranium as a fixed container, containing brain tissue, blood and cerebrospinal fluid (CSF). An increase in the volume of any one of these contents needs to be balanced by a decrease in the volume of another, to maintain a constant intracranial pressure (ICP). CSF, and to some extent blood, acts as a buffer for small rises in brain tissue volume. Once this buffering system is exhausted, any small increase in volume leads to a sharp rise in ICP (**Figure 11**).

Cerebral perfusion pressure (CPP) is dependent on the differential between the systemic blood pressure and the ICP:

$$CPP = MAP - ICP$$

Manipulation of these variables to maintain adequate CPP is part of the strategy for the prevention of secondary brain injury, the principal causes of which are as follows:

- Hypotension
- Hypoxia
- Hypercapnia
- Raised ICP
- Seizures
- Hyperthermia
- Hyperglycaemia

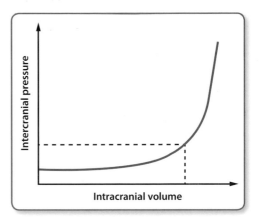

Figure 11 Intracranial compliance curve demonstrating the inflexion point where a small increase in volume produces a dramatic increase in pressure.

Treatment

Several aspects of treatment deserve particular mention.

Management of raised ICP

To facilitate venous drainage, patients should be nursed 30° head-up, the cervical collar should be loose, and tape – not ties – should be used to secure the endotracheal tube. Coughing should be avoided with adequate sedation and paralysis. Mannitol 0.25–1 g/kg bolus can be given before ICP monitoring when signs of transtentorial herniation or progressive neurological deterioration not explained by extracranial causes are seen. It is generally given on the advice of the receiving neurosurgeon. Hypertonic saline can also be used (1–2 mL/kg of 5% saline).

Management of seizures

Seizures increase the cerebral metabolic rate and may lead to a critical rise in ICP. They should be treated aggressively. The ABC sequence should be rechecked, and a bolus of benzodiazepine should be given. This can be followed by a loading dose of phenytoin (15 mg/kg). Neuromuscular blockers may mask seizure activity; check for pupil or gaze abnormalities in the presence of tachycardia and hypertension.

Reduction in cerebral metabolic requirements

If ICP remains persistently high despite the basic therapy, an infusion of thiopentone or propofol will reduce the cerebral oxygen requirement. EEG monitoring of burst suppression is recommended. Pyrexia should be avoided as it increases metabolic requirements and cerebral blood flow. Some advocate therapeutic hypothermia (<35°C) for refractory ICP, but its role in TBI is still unclear.

Anaesthetic management

Management of a head injury is time-critical. There is evidence to show that the time between initial insult and definitive care at a specialist centre is a key factor in determining outcome. Initial resuscitation of a head injury should follow the ABCDE approach and other injuries identified.

Airway

Casualties with Glasgow Coma Score (GCS) <9 should be intubated and ventilated for protection against aspiration and for optimal management of secondary brain injury. Cerebrally agitated patients with a GCS of 13–14 have a 12.5% risk of an abnormal CT head requiring neurosurgical intervention and may well need intubation at least to facilitate the CT scan.

A single episode of hypoxia (Spo$_2$<90%) is associated with worse outcomes. Maintaining a patent airway right from the initial impact is key. Traditionally, nasopharyngeal airways are avoided in head trauma due to the risk of intracranial placement in a base of skull fracture. Many experts now routinely use these airway adjuncts in head injury with no reported problems as avoidance of even short-lived hypoxia is so important.

A rapid sequence induction is performed, with cricoid pressure and in-line cervical spine stabilisation. A difficult airway should be anticipated. Routine use of a bougie can decrease the number of attempts at intubation and maintain oxygenation. Cricoid pressure may need to be removed to improve the view at laryngoscopy. A surgical airway may be required, particularly if there is severe facial trauma.

On induction, care should be taken to avoid hypotension (associated with worse outcomes) or hypertension and raised ICP. There is much debate over choice of induction agent. Etomidate is relatively cardiovascularly stable, but depresses cortisol production. Thiopentone and propofol both reduce cerebral metabolism, but cause hypotension. Ketamine has historically been linked to raised ICP although the evidence suggests this can be attenuated by adequate ventilation, and there may even be some neuroprotective benefits. The original studies demonstrating raised ICP were primarily in patients undergoing surgery for CSF drainage problems. Fentanyl at 3 μg/kg and lignocaine 1.5 mg/kg given intravenously over 1 minute, 3 minutes before induction have both been used to attenuate the response to laryngoscopy.

Once intubated, paralysis with longer acting neuromuscular blockers should be given and an orogastric tube inserted.

Breathing

Ventilation to achieve low normocapnia is the goal (Paco$_2$ 4.0–4.5 kPa). Hyperventilation to Paco$_2$(<3.5–4 kPa) causes vasoconstriction, reduced cerebral blood flow and reduced CPP. High levels of positive end-expiratory pressure should be avoided as it can impair venous drainage from the cranium and contribute to raised ICP. Ventilation should be guided by capnography and arterial blood gas sampling.

Circulation

In an isolated head injury, resuscitation should aim to achieve a CPP of 60–70 mmHg. In the absence of intracranial monitoring, an ICP of 20 mmHg is presumed, therefore a mean arterial pressure (MAP) of 80–90 mmHg is the target. Isotonic intravenous fluids (0.9% saline) are given to restore blood volume.

A vasopressor (e.g. noradrenaline) may be required to counteract the effects of ongoing sedation. Fluid overload is detrimental. An arterial line is optimal for accurate blood pressure measurements but the insertion of this should not delay transfer to CT or definitive care. In polytrauma, where permissive hypotension is initially employed, it is suggested that a systolic blood pressure of 100 mmHg is a reasonable compromise. Patients who are being treated with antiplatelet or anticoagulant therapy also present with head injury and are a group with particularly high morbidity and mortality. In patients with evidence of intracranial haemorrhage, rapid reversal of the therapy is required. Those on antiplatelet therapy can have type-specific platelet infusions (10 units), whilst those on anticoagulation can have 50 μg/kg prothrombin complex concentrate or 15 mL/kg fresh-frozen plasma, followed by 5–10 mg intravenous vitamin K.

Disability

A rapid neurological assessment, including GCS, pupillary reaction and focal signs, should be documented prior to induction. This has important prognostic significance. Blood glucose should be checked, and kept within the normal range.

Further reading

Brain Trauma Foundation. Guidelines for the management of severe traumatic brain injury, 3rd edn. J Neurotrauma 2007; 24:S1–106.

Harris T, Davenport R, Hurst T, et al. Improving outcome in severe trauma: what's new in ABC? Imaging, bleeding and brain injury. Postgrad Med J 2012; 88:595–603.

Related topics of interest

Neuroanaesthesia – tumours

Key points

- These procedures all carry a significant risk of major bleeding and gas embolism
- These are long procedures with occasionally complex positioning requirements
- Understanding of cerebral physiology and its manipulation is crucial to optimal neuroanaesthesia

Anaesthesia for craniotomy for brain tumour requires a sound understanding of cerebral anatomy and physiology and the effects of anaesthesia on this. A good relationship with the surgeon is important to plan the approach and understand the risks associated with the particular tumour. Many controversies still remain in the practice of neuroanaesthesia.

Clinical features

Brain tumours are a heterogeneous group of pathologies ranging from a primary malignancy, through metastatic deposits to meningiomas, which can be large and vascular. They can affect any anatomical area of the brain and arise from any of the structures within the skull. Brain tumours may be discovered incidentally but otherwise present with signs of raised intracranial pressure (ICP) or focal or generalised neurological signs and symptoms.

Anaesthetic management

Preoperative

Tumour type and position will affect surgical approach and access. Proximity to vascular structures, brain stem or cranial nerves and vascularity of tumour are all important. Enquire about neurological signs and symptoms looking especially for signs of raised ICP, seizures and focal neurological signs. A recent neurological examination should be documented in the notes to allow accurate assessment of neurological function postoperatively. A standard assessment should also be made of any other comorbidities.

Patients may already be taking medications including antiseizure medications and dexamethasone in addition to those for other comorbidities. Avoid sedative or opiate premedication (effects on Pa_{CO_2} and ICP) and nonsteroidal anti-inflammatory drugs (NSAIDs) (risk of bleeding). All patients should receive paracetamol unless contraindicated.

Intraoperative

Surgical requirements for a craniotomy are good positioning, controlled ICP, a still patient (avoid coughing or straining during surgery which may raise ICP, cause a catastrophic surgical mistake or lead to brain herniation) and a patient who wakes smoothly and rapidly.

At the preop briefing use the mnemonic 'DAMP' for:

- Dexamethasone – does the patient require dexamethasone at induction? If given early at induction, it has a more profound effect on brain swelling
- Antibiotics – according to hospital policies
- Mannitol – may be required to improve surgical access. Initial dose 0.25–0.5 g/kg. All patients who have mannitol will require a urinary catheter. It may cause a profound diuresis which can make accurate management of fluid balance very difficult
- Phenytoin – certain tumours are at higher risk of causing seizure activity: a loading dose of phenytoin may be required. Infuse via a central venous catheter if possible and give slowly as it may cause profound hypotension

Invasive arterial monitoring should be used for all tumour resections and be placed prior to induction in all cases where there is a suspicion of raised ICP.

Perform standard induction with propofol plus opiate (to obtund the hypertensive response to laryngoscopy and intubation). Avoid coughing or straining on intubation as it causes a rise in ICP. Total intravenous anaesthesia with propofol and remifentanil allows good control of blood pressure (BP) during induction and is the technique of choice in many units. Volatile agents can cause flow-metabolism uncoupling at high concentrations, although sevoflurane is thought to be superior to isoflurane and may be used at concentrations up to 1.5 MAC. Patients require intubation as ventilation must be controlled to maintain normoxia and normocapnia intraoperatively. It is common practice to use a flexi-metallic endotracheal tube (ETT) to reduce the risk of kinking. Maintain systolic BP at preinduction levels to optimise cerebral blood flow. This tends to be easier to achieve with a metaraminol infusion but boluses can be used.

The ETT should be taped rather than tied. The eyes can be vulnerable to contamination from skin preparation agents and pressure damage. They should be appropriately taped and covered. If there is a significant risk of bleeding, e.g. meningioma or particularly high risk of venous air embolus, then consider central venous access in addition to reliable, large-bore peripheral intravenous access. Tumours can bleed significantly and suddenly.

Positioning will depend on the anatomical position of the tumour. Patients may be supine (often with quite significant head turn – consider resulting venous congestion and its potential effect on ICP), prone (for posterior fossa surgical approaches), full lateral (park bench) or sitting. Most will involve head-up. Many patients will be positioned with Mayfield pins. The stimulating effects of this should be attenuated with an appropriate opiate bolus.

These are long procedures. Attention should be paid to positioning, pressure areas, glucose control (often deranged by steroids), temperature and mechanical thromboprophylaxis. Check access to lines and cannulae after positioning. Maintain normothermia and euvolaemia. Urine output should be measured. Avoid glucose-containing solutions as they can worsen cerebral oedema.

Postoperative care

The majority of patients should be woken immediately after surgery. In those for whom this is not appropriate (major haemorrhage, cerebral oedema) an ICP monitor may be placed to allow measurement in the sedated patient. Extubation should be managed to minimise coughing and allow rapid recovery of neurological function for early assessment.

A balanced approach to analgesia is preferred with scalp infiltration of local anaesthetic agent or scalp block. Fentanyl boluses given at the end of surgery form the mainstay of immediate postoperative analgesia. Regular paracetamol and patient-controlled analgesia (PCA) fentanyl provide good analgesia postoperatively. NSAIDs remain controversial. Prophylactic antiemetics should be given.

Failure to wake, neurological deterioration or seizures in the immediate postoperative period will require urgent CT imaging to exclude bleeding or hydrocephalus. Processes should be in place to allow urgent transfer to CT with appropriately skilled personnel should this be required. Most craniotomies are cared for in a Level 2 setting postoperatively. Some simpler cases may be suitable for an extended recovery stay prior to returning to a neurosurgical ward.

Special circumstances

Tumours at or near the brainstem may require insertion of a lumbar drain immediately preoperatively. This allows controlled drainage of cerebrospinal fluid intraoperatively which may improve surgical access. Consideration should be given to the risks of this in a patient with raised ICP.

Electrophysiological monitoring may be used to minimise damage to adjacent structures e.g. facial nerve stimulator in acoustic neuroma surgery. There are a wide range of neurophysiological monitors currently available. There is as yet little consensus on the best indications and monitors for particular circumstances.

Very vascular tumours may benefit from preoperative embolisation. This requires an interventional radiology procedure, usually under general anaesthesia. Patients require level 2 care after this procedure as embolisation inevitably causes a degree of cerebral oedema. These patients may deteriorate clinically after this procedure. Ease and accuracy of access to small and awkwardly positioned lesions has been greatly improved by the use of image-guided techniques.

Awake craniotomy, which is in routine use for epilepsy surgery, is increasing in popularity to allow maximal resection of tumour close to eloquent areas. Many techniques have been described including local anaesthesia, conscious sedation and GA with an asleep-awake-asleep technique. None is yet proven to be superior and centres tend to develop their own processes and procedures.

Further reading

Dinsmore J. Anaesthesia for elective neurosurgery. Br J Anaesth: Contin Educ Anaesth Crit Care Pain 2007; 99:68–74.

Wilson S, John R. Anaesthesia for neurosurgery. Anaesth Intensive Care Med 2013; 14:391–394.

Related topics of interest

Neurological disease – demyelinating and neurodegenerative diseases

Key points

- Autonomic instability is common in neurological disease
- Respiratory muscle function should be assessed prior to embarking on anaesthesia in neurological disease
- Management of Guillain–Barré syndrome is largely supportive. It carries a 5% mortality
- Medical management of neurological disease, particularly Parkinson's disease, should be continued through the perioperative period wherever possible

Guillain–Barré syndrome

This is a progressive (but reversible) acute demyelinating polyneuropathy, usually starting a week after a respiratory or gastrointestinal infective illness. Motor symptoms occur in the lower limbs, although it can present with upper limb or cranial nerve involvement. The flaccid lower motor neurone paralysis, with loss of reflexes progresses, can involve the respiratory muscles. Sensory symptoms are less severe, but include pain (in 50% of patients) and paraesthesia. Autonomic dysfunction affects 70% of patients, presenting as cardiovascular instability and paralytic ileus.

Diagnosis is clinical although a high cerebrospinal fluid protein is common (usually >3 g/L). Antiganglioside antibodies can assist in differentiating Guillain-Barré syndrome subgroups. Anti-GM1 (present in 25%) carries a worse prognosis. Brain CT is indicated to rule out other differential diagnoses. The Miller Fisher variant comprises ophthalmoplegia, ataxia and areflexia. Twenty-five per cent also have limb weakness.

Anaesthetic management

Patients require meticulous multidisciplinary input throughout the course of the disease. Daily vital capacity, forced expiratory volume in 1 second (FEV_1) and peak expiratory flow rate are used to assess disease progression. Critical care with ventilatory support is required in 30% and is likely if the vital capacity falls below 1 L or there is loss of airway protection. Tracheostomy may be required due to prolonged paralysis, which can last weeks. There is a 5% mortality, related most frequently to secondary infection, autonomic instability and thromboembolism.

Management is supportive with specific therapy comprising plasma exchange (plasmaphoresis) or immunoglobulin therapy. Both accelerate recovery to a similar extent. There is no evidence that steroids are effective.

Induction of anaesthesia and tracheal suction may precipitate cardiovascular instability due to autonomic disturbance. In particular, an exaggerated hypotensive response should be expected following intravenous induction. Suxamethonium should be avoided due to the potential for hyperkalaemia and associated arrhythmia. Poor prognostic indicators include age >40, rapid onset, severe weakness and association with campylobacter infection. Following the acute illness, psychological counselling is vital.

Multiple sclerosis

MS is a chronic disease with an unpredictable, fluctuating course. Classically it presents in patients aged 20–40, with a transient neurological deficit that develops over a few days and resolves over a few weeks. It is twice as common in females than males and is more frequently seen in Caucasians. Demyelination of white matter occurs in the brain and spinal cord, leading to retrobulbar neuritis, upper motor neurone and sensory deficits. Ocular, cerebellar and bladder dysfunctions are common. Severity varies from mild infrequent episodes causing little interference with life to a chronic progressive course leading to severe disability.

The aetiology is unclear, with environmental, genetic and immunological factors implicated. The incidence varies dramatically with geographical latitude (incidence increasing further from the equator). In the UK, prevalence is 1:2000. Diagnosis can be difficult and is often based on MRI demonstration of demyelination accompanied by at least two clinical episodes. Symptoms are exacerbated by stress, pyrexia, infection, trauma and exertion.

Problems

- Risk of exacerbation
- Existing neurological deficits, especially bulbar dysfunction
- Concurrent medications

Anaesthetic management

A careful assessment of the existing neurological deficit should be made. Severe disease can affect bulbar and pharyngeal muscle function necessitating rapid sequence induction. There is no evidence that general anaesthesia itself precipitates relapse. Autonomic instability should be anticipated, particularly hypotension during induction. Hyperthermia (including the use of anticholinergics, which can increase temperature) should be avoided. Suxamethonium should be avoided in severe disease. Nondepolarising neuromuscular blocking agents can be used safely in usual doses.

Regional anaesthesia does not carry an increased risk of relapse; however, there is experimental data suggesting local anaesthetic histotoxicity in plaques in the spinal cord following neuraxial blockade. Most anaesthetists avoid spinal anaesthesia on this basis unless there is a significant clinical advantage to this technique.

Motor neurone disease

It is a progressive degenerative loss of motor neurones within the CNS with variable course. Sensory and higher functions remain normal. Incidence is 1:100,000 and it is more frequently seen in males. It may present as upper, lower or mixed motor neurone lesions. The aetiology is unclear, but may include

excess excitatory neurotransmitters, free-radical damage or abnormal growth factors. Diagnosis is made clinically and on EMG studies. Treatment options are limited. Several distinct forms have been identified:

- Amyotrophic lateral sclerosis: Mixed upper and lower motor neurone disease featuring hyper-reflexia and spasticity
- Progressive Bulbar Palsy: degeneration of brainstem nuclei, presenting as lower motor neurone symptoms
- Progressive Muscular Atrophy: Lower motor neuron symptoms initially occurring in the arms

Pseudobulbar palsy may occur when upper motor neurones are affected. Although pathologically distinct, Friedreich's ataxia is an autosomal recessive progressive ataxia with muscle weakness involving the spinal cord, peripheral nerves, pancreas and causing cardiomyopathy.

Problems

- Increased sensitivity to nondepolarising neuromuscular blocking agents
- Respiratory muscle weakness
- Risk of aspiration due to brainstem involvement

Anaesthetic management

The degree of respiratory muscle and brain stem involvement must be assessed with particular attention to the risk of aspiration. Suxamethonium should be avoided due to the risk of hyperkalaemia. Other neuromuscular blocking agents may be used in reduced doses with responses titrated according to nerve stimulator response. Mechanical ventilation is often required.

Regional anaesthesia, including neuraxial techniques, are considered safe, provided they do not compromise respiratory function. Postoperative high dependency care is usually required, including ventilation.

Parkinson's disease

Parkinson's disease has a prevalence of 1% in people over 65. Although Parkinsonism may be caused by other pathology such as head trauma, metabolic conditions and atherosclerosis, Parkinson's disease itself has an unknown aetiology. Risk factors include advancing age and family history. The pathological process comprises loss of dopaminergic neurones in the substantia nigra leading to the characteristic cogwheel rigidity, tremor, bradykinesia and postural instability.

Therapeutic options include:

- Dopamine precursors: e.g. levodopa, converted into dopamine centrally
- Dopamine agonists: e.g. ropinirole, apomorphine (one of the few intravenous Parkinson's medications)
- Monoamine-oxidase-B inhibitors: e.g. selegiline: reduces CNS dopamine metabolism
- Anticholinergics: Orphenadrine
- Deep brain stimulation or surgical ablation: Surgical implantation of stimulation devices as well as ablation within the basal ganglia can significantly improve symptoms

Problems

- Autonomic instability, especially orthostatic hypotension, due to drugs or the disease itself
- Respiratory muscle weakness
- Coexisting drug therapy
- Aspiration risk due to upper airway dysfunction
- Difficult airway due to reduced neck movement and rigidity

Anaesthetic management

Medication should be continued up to surgery and recommenced as soon as possible after. Levodopa has a 1–3 hour half-life and can be given by nasogastric tube intraoperatively in prolonged procedures. Intravenous apomorphine can be used in patients with malabsorption (e.g. acute abdomen), although it can be difficult to ascertain the correct dose. Airway assessment may reveal neck flexion deformity and glycopyrrolate may be required to treat sialorrhoea. Lung function tests may reveal a restrictive defect and there is an increased likelihood of obstructive sleep apnoea.

General anaesthesia will eliminate tremor and thus often provides better surgical conditions; however, there is a greater impact on respiratory function. Autonomic dysfunction should be anticipated and requires judicious use of induction agents to prevent profound hypotension. Inhalational agents are safe. Hyperkalaemia has been reported following suxamethonium, which should probably be avoided in severe disease. Large doses of opiates are known to increase muscle rigidity.

Regional anaesthetic techniques generally have less impact on respiratory and cardiovascular systems, but tremor and rigidity can be problematic. Postoperative course may require critical care input for respiratory support and chest physiotherapy. Patients with severe disease may not be able to operate a patient-controlled analgesia device. Some antiemetics (metoclopramide, droperidol) can increase symptoms; however, ondansetron, domperidone and cyclizine are considered safe.

Further reading

Neurologic diseases. In: Fleisher LA (ed.), Anesthesia and uncommon diseases, 5th edn. Philadelphia; WB Saunders, 2006.

Nicholson G, Pereira AC, Hall GM. Parkinson's disease and anaesthesia. Br J Anaesth 2002; 89:904–916.

Richards KJC, Cohen AT. Guillain-Barre syndrome. Br J Anaesth: Contin Educ Profess Develop Rev 2003; 3:46–49.

Related topics of interest

Neurological disease – epilepsy

Key points

- Anaesthetic concerns primarily relate to perioperative seizure management and implications of antiepileptic drugs (AEDs)
- Perioperative conditions can induce seizures in predisposed patients
- Status epilepticus is a medical emergency and neurological injury can develop if it is not controlled in a timely manner

Epilepsy has a prevalence of 1:200. Surgical procedures are usually unrelated to epilepsy, but surgical options for treatment of epilepsy are becoming more frequent. Surgical excision of a seizure focus, burr hole placement of neurostimulation electrodes (often positioned under sedation) and vagal nerve stimulators are all procedures successfully used to improve seizure control.

Broadly speaking, epilepsy is an unrestrained imbalance between excitatory and inhibitory activity within the brain. Therapeutic agents act by either reducing voltage-gated ion flow (Na^+, Ca^{2+}), decreasing excitatory transmitter activity or increasing inhibitory transmitter activity (e.g. GABA).

Newer agents target alternative binding sites to achieve these aims (**Table 28**).

Sensory, motor, autonomic and higher centre function can be involved. There is usually a focal origin, but different patterns of epilepsy are seen, including grand mal, petit mal, focal, psychomotor and myoclonic epilepsy. Epilepsy may be caused by cerebral tumour or abscess, HIV infection, meningitis, cerebrovascular disease, drugs, metabolic disorder, a head injury or idiopathic.

Problems

- Risk of further seizures
- Drug therapy for epilepsy. Older agents (e.g. phenytoin, carbamazepine, barbiturates) and topiramate have liver enzyme-inducing properties with a resultant reduction in plasma concentration of hepatic-metabolised drugs. Liver enzyme inhibition (e.g. by erythromycin) can lead to carbamazepine toxicity
- Potential for anaesthetic agents to affect the EEG and predispose to seizures (**Table 29**)
- Underlying aetiology of the epilepsy

Table 28 Proposed mechanism of action for common antiepileptic drugs	
Medication	Proposed mechanism of action
Benzodiazepines, Barbituates	GABA receptor agonist
Carbamazepine	Enhance sodium channel inactivation
Gabapentin	Unclear mechanism, but may have a binding site associated with voltage gated calcium channels
Lamotrigine	Possibly reduces presynaptic glutamate release
Phenytoin	Mechanism unclear, but likely action on sodium ion channels and possibly other mechanisms for membrane stabilisation
Sodium Valproate	Unclear, but several mechanisms proposed, including sodium channel blockade, GABA transaminase inhibition and possibly GABA production
Topiramate	Likely multiple mechanisms including Glutamate antagonism and sodium channel blockade
Vigabatrin	Blockade of GABA transaminase

Table 29 Effects of anaesthetic agents on epilepsy

Inhalational agents	
Sevoflurane	Produces seizure-like activity, but probably not proconvulsant
Isoflurane	Anticonvulsant properties
Opioids	Remifentanil, fentanyl, alfentanil and morphine reported to cause generalised seizures
Induction agents	
Thiopentone	All appear to produce excitatory activity at low doses, but are all generally considered
Propofol	anticonvulsive in higher doses and used for refractory status epilepticus. Ketamine may
Etomidate	be useful in status epilepticus refractory to other agents. Etomidate may increase seizure
Ketamine	duration during electroconvulsive therapy
Benzodiazepines	All are anticonvulsant
Local anaesthetics	High systemic doses increase seizure likelihood. Intravenous lidocaine has been used experimentally to successfully treat status epilepticus
Neuromuscular blockers	No effect on seizure activity
Anticholinergics	Atropine can produce the central cholinergic syndrome with associated seizures unlike glycopyrrolate which does not cross the blood–brain barrier

Anaesthetic management

Assessment and premedication

The pattern of epilepsy and the frequency of seizures are ascertained. Any underlying cause should be determined and the current drug therapy with any associated side effects noted. Anticonvulsants should not be omitted preoperatively. Only sodium valproate, phenytoin and levetiracetam are available in injectable form, so patients with poor oral absorption may require therapeutic conversion to one of these drugs. Advice should be sought from a neurologist. Premedication with a benzodiazepine is appropriate. Presence of a vagal nerve stimulator should not affect anaesthesia per se; however, diathermy can damage the device and MRI is contraindicated.

Conduct of anaesthesia

Any anaesthetic must avoid the precipitating causes of seizures (see below). Drugs that induce, precipitate or exacerbate seizures should be avoided. Both propofol and thiopentone may be used for induction, whilst maintenance with isoflurane probably carries the lowest risk of seizure provocation. Regional anaesthesia can reduce the requirement for opioids and should be considered where possible.

Postoperative care

Provided no seizures have occurred, no special postoperative care is required and the normal anticonvulsant regimen should be recommenced as soon as possible. Emergence myoclonus and shivering is common and can mimic epileptic seizure.

Seizures during anaesthesia

Patients who suffer seizures during an anaesthetic are usually known epileptics. Children are more predisposed than adults. Good anaesthetic technique will avoid most of the preventable precipitating factors. If a seizure occurs *de novo*, without a clear cause, then investigations should be performed to determine the aetiology.

Causes

- Anaesthetic, including hypoxia, hypercarbia, hypocarbia and 'light anaesthesia'
- CNS disease or old head injury
- Acute intracranial event
- Metabolic. A low blood sugar, sodium, magnesium or calcium and uraemia lower the threshold for convulsions
- Hyperpyrexia
- Drugs, e.g. local anaesthetic toxicity
- Eclampsia

Management

If a seizure occurs during anaesthesia the airway should immediately be protected and 100% O_2 given by controlled ventilation. Midazolam or thiopentone are usually the most available anticonvulsants and may be given to control the seizure. Lorazepam, clonazepam or diazepam are alternatives. The above list of causes will direct investigation and further management (**Figure 12**).

The use of prophylactic anticonvulsants to prevent seizures in the postoperative period should be considered. Immediate head CT may be required postoperatively to determine intracranial pathology.

Status epilepticus

Status epilepticus (seizure activity >30 minutes with failure to regain consciousness) is a medical emergency. Most seizures lasting over 5 minutes will not terminate spontaneously and need treatment, as prolonged activity beyond 20–30 minutes will result in cerebral damage. Cerebral metabolic rate is significantly raised such that oxygen and glucose demand outstrip supply and eventually autoregulation is impaired. Systemic catecholamine release leads to hypertension, tachycardia and increases in cardiac output.

Uncontrolled epilepsy may necessitate intensive care with ventilatory support whilst therapeutic control is obtained. First line medication is a benzodiazepine, followed by phenytoin/fosphenytoin (**Figure 12**). Benzodiazepine responsiveness reduces

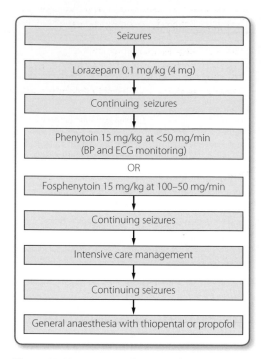

Figure 12 Management of status epilepticus.

with time. General anaesthesia and muscle relaxants may be required to prevent acidosis from the severe muscle activity associated with seizures. Subclinical seizure activity may continue and EEG monitoring is mandatory when general anaesthesia and muscle relaxation are used. Cerebral protective strategies similar to those used in head injury should be employed to ensure optimal oxygen delivery and cerebral perfusion.

Further reading

Control of the epilepsies. British National Formulary 2013; 4.8.1: Control of the Epilepsies. Joint Formula Committee. British National Formulary (67). London; BMJ group and Pharmaceutical Press, 2014.

Gratrix AP, Enright SM. Epilepsy in anaesthesia and intensive care. Br J Anaesth: Contin Educ Anaesth Crit Care Pain Med 2005; 5:118–121.

Perks A, Cheema S, Mohanraj R. Anaesthesia and epilepsy. Br J Anaesth 2012; 108:562–571.

Related topics of interest

- Electroconvulsive therapy (p. 67)
- Neuroanaesthesia – subarachnoid haemorrhage (p. 127)
- Neuroanaesthesia – traumatic brain injury (p. 131)
- Neuroanaesthesia – tumours (p. 134)
- Neurological disease – demyelinating and neurodegenerative diseases (p. 137)

Nutrition

Key points

- Avoidance of malnutrition remains important to prevent poor surgical outcomes
- Enhanced Recovery After Surgery (ERAS) nutritional guidelines aim to minimise insulin resistance by providing preoperative carbohydrate loading, and subsequent release of insulin perioperatively
- Immunonutrients such as arginine, omega-3 fatty acids, RNA or nucleotides, which may influence the immunological response to surgery, may be beneficial and are included in European guidelines

Nutritional status of patients is crucially important to perioperative outcomes. Low body mass index (BMI, <17 kg/m^2) increases risk of complications, especially after emergency surgery. Malnutrition remains poorly recognised in many patients, and is potentially amenable to treatment. Modern ERAS guidelines have emphasised the importance of avoiding prolonged starvation before elective surgery and minimising insulin resistance. Certain 'immunonutrients' may be beneficial in certain disease states.

Malnutrition

Malnutrition is still present in 50% of hospitalised patients and has been shown to worsen after admission to hospital in some cases. The most reliable identifier of malnutrition is a history of weight loss before admission. Weight loss of >10–15% may indicate severe malnutrition. Other methods of identifying malnutrition such as anthropometric measurements (e.g. triceps skin fold), serum markers (e.g. albumin levels) or immunological markers are not reliable alone. Patients at highest risk mirror those at increased risk of postoperative complications, i.e. the very young, the elderly, the obese and patients with diabetes mellitus.

Patients who are severely malnourished may require nutritional therapy if surgery can safely be delayed. Beneficial outcomes are only seen from preoperative parenteral nutrition in severely malnourished patients receiving 5–7 days of parenteral nutrition before surgery. This limited treatment does not reverse all the effects of chronic malnourishment and is only used in a minority of patients presenting for elective surgery. Enteral nutrition remains more effective, more convenient and safer than parenteral treatment. Average normal adult daily nutritional requirements are shown in **Table 30**. Requirements after surgery may vary markedly, depending on nature of the procedure and time to normal intestinal function.

Metabolic response to surgery and insulin resistance

Major surgery induces catabolic hormones such as cortisol, catecholamines and glucagon to boost energy substrate mobilisation. The action of insulin (the main anabolic hormone) is reduced. Since repair and recovery occur when the body is in an anabolic state, it follows that measures to reduce catabolism and promote anabolism will give better outcomes.

Table 30 Average normal daily nutritional requirements	
Water	30–40 mL/kg
Nitrogen	0.2 g/kg
Energy	30–40 kCal/kg
Sodium	1 mmol/kg
Potassium	1 mmol/kg
Chloride	1.5 mmol/kg
Phosphate	0.2–0.5 mmol/kg
Calcium	0.1–0.2 mmol/kg
Magnesium	0.1–0.2 mmol/kg
Iron	0.2 mg/kg
Zinc	0.2 mg/kg
Selenium	1 µg/kg

In the catabolic state after surgery, insulin resistance is encountered. The relative lack of insulin reduces peripheral uptake of glucose into tissues, preventing metabolically useful substrate from entering cells. Gluconeogenesis, lipolysis and proteolysis are increased causing hyperglycaemia, whilst depleting fat and protein (muscle) stores and inducing a negative nitrogen balance. The reduction in muscle function may last several weeks and significantly contributes to fatigue following major surgery. Insulin resistance is associated with increased inflammatory response, poor wound healing, longer hospital stays and increased morbidity.

Various strategies may be adopted to reduce the effect of insulin resistance after surgery. Intensive insulin therapy has been used postoperatively, but carries the risk of hypoglycaemia. It is more pragmatic to reduce the magnitude of catabolism and insulin resistance after surgery. Preoperative starvation is known to induce catabolism, hence the drive to reduce periods of starvation to minimal levels. There are also immunological consequences from even short periods of starvation (see below). American (1999) and British (2001) guidelines reduced starvation times from 12 to 6 hours for solids and 2 hours for clear fluids.

Patients with morbid obesity, or type-2 diabetes mellitus, have the same gastric emptying rate as other patients; however, patients with diabetic neuropathy may have delayed gastric emptying for solids (there is no conclusive data for fluids).

Carbohydrate loading

Most clear fluids do not provide significant nutritional intake to switch the body from a 'fasted' to a 'fed' state. Ingestion of 50 g of carbohydrate stimulates sufficient insulin production to mimic a meal, thus preoperative carbohydrate loading targets this figure. Protocols usually recommend 100g of carbohydrate drink the night before surgery and then 50g 2 hours before surgery. This regime does not seem to cause hyperglycaemia in nondiabetic patients. Specialist hypo-osmolar drinks (e.g. 12.5% maltodextrins) have been developed which promote gastric emptying, making them suitable for administration 2 hours before surgery. The role of carbohydrate loading in diabetic patients has yet to be established. It would be prudent to monitor serum glucose and treat excessive hyperglycaemia should this occur.

Carbohydrate loading has been shown to reduce perioperative hunger, thirst and anxiety, as well as reducing nitrogen and protein loss, maintain muscle strength and accelerate recovery. Enhanced Recovery After Surgery (ERAS) guidelines consist of multiple interventions which have been shown to reduce complications and hospital stay after major surgery. Initial protocols for colorectal surgery were produced, but use is increasingly common in orthopaedic, urological, gynaecological and upper gastrointestinal surgery. The nutritional component of ERAS packages include minimal starvation, carbohydrate loading, avoidance of gastric tube insertion and rapid reintroduction of oral diet after surgery. Overall, ERAS protocols have shown reduced morbidity and hospital stay and reduced health care costs.

The immunological role of the intestine

The intestine has a complex role in the immune system. The threat from bacteria within the intestine is normally attenuated by a number of mechanisms, including thick mucous secretion and immunological cell activity within the intestinal wall. Enteral nutrition maintains structural and functional integrity of the epithelium and stimulates bowel motility which may sweep pathogenic bacteria downstream, reducing the total number of bacteria in the proximal gut. Surgical stress leads to an increase in intestinal permeability, a decrease in villous height and a weaker barrier to intestinal bacteria.

Enteral nutrition also encourages gut blood flow. It has been proposed that some IgA immunocytes and T-helper 2 CD4+ lymphocytes may migrate out of the intestine into other organs such as lung, kidney or liver. These produce an anti-inflammatory effect in the systemic circulation, which may mitigate the proinflammatory effect of T-helper 1 lymphocytes, produced after a variety of insults, including major surgery.

Immunonutrition

Attempts have been made to modulate the immunological response to major surgery by providing specific nutrients to influence the immune system. The most extensively studied nutrients include arginine, omega-3 fatty acids, nucleotides and RNA. Arginine is involved in many metabolic pathways. It is a precursor of nitric oxide and hydroxyproline, a key factor in connective tissue repair and is also an essential substrate for immune cells, particularly lymphocytes.

Omega-3 fatty acids are commonly found in fish oils. They exert an anti-inflammatory effect in chronic disease states such as cardiovascular disease, rheumatoid arthritis and inflammatory bowel disease. Actions include production of anti-inflammatory cytokines (as opposed to proinflammatory cytokines produced by omega-6 fatty acids) and beneficial effects on membrane structure and function. They are precursors for novel molecules called resolvins and protectins which are produced specifically to downregulate inflammation and mediate healing processes. Omega-3 fatty acids also increase vagal stimulation and have antiarrhythmic effects, particularly after cardiac surgery.

Although there are now many trials concerning immunonutrition, meta-analyses often show wide heterogeneity between studies in both patients and diseases studied and interventions provided. Interactions between arginine, omega-3 fatty acids and other immunonutrients are not fully understood and dose-response studies are still required to identify optimal dosage. The European Society for Clinical Nutrition and Metabolism recommend that all patients undergoing major surgery for neck cancer (laryngectomy or pharyngectomy) or abdominal cancer (oesophagectomy, gastrectomy or pancreatectomy), regardless of nutritional status should receive enteral supplementation with arginine, omega-3 fatty acids and nucleotides.

Further reading

Bozzetti F. Peri-operative nutritional management. Proc Nutr Soc 2011; 70:305–310.

Braga M. Perioperative immunonutrition and gut function. Curr Opin Clin Nutr Metab Care 2012; 15:485–488

Burden S, Todd C, Hill J, Lal S. Pre-operative nutrition support in patients undergoing gastrointestinal surgery. Cochrane Database Syst Rev 2012; 11:CD008879. DOI:10.1002/14651858.CD008879.pub2

Kratzing C. Pre-operative nutrition and carbohydrate loading. Proc Nutr Soc 2011; 70:311–315.

Related topics of interest

- Major abdominal surgery (p. 108)
- Oesophagectomy (p. 165)

Obesity – incidental surgery

Key points

- Obesity is defined as a body mass index (BMI) >30 kg/m² and the UK prevalence has almost doubled in the last 20 years and now affects 1 in 4 in men
- Obesity has a multisystem impact and most issues arising have direct significance for the anaesthetist
- Pharmacology needs careful consideration in the context of the obese patient

Over the past 20 years the prevalence of obesity (BMI >30 kg/m²) in adult males has increased from 15% to 25% in the UK. Morbid obesity (BMI >40 kg/m²) rates are currently 1.5% in males and 3.5% in females, more than double the rate of 1993. BMI is an expression of the proportion of excess body mass: weight in kilograms divided by square of height in metres (kg/m²) with a normal range of 20–25. Although widely used due to its simplicity, BMI does not measure fat distribution, which may better correlate with health. Skin fold thickness and hip, waist or neck circumference may be more clinically relevant. Fat distribution is broadly divided into android and gynaecoid ('apples' and 'pears'). Higher intraperitoneal fat content seen in android obesity has a greater pathophysiological significance. Visceral fat-related comorbidities are multisystem and there is a significant proinflammatory component.

Problems

Cardiovascular

Dysregulated overexpression of hormones, such as tumour necrosis factor-alpha and angiotensinogen, secreted by intra-abdominal visceral fat directly or indirectly account for maladaptive cardiovascular changes seen in obesity. Left ventricular hypertrophy is a consequence of hypertension resulting from increased metabolic demands, sympathetic drive and activation of the hypothalamic–pituitary–adrenal axis.

Left ventricular dilatation occurs due to increased preload from blood volume expansion. When hypertrophy fails to keep pace with dilatation, this leads to obesity cardiomyopathy and congestive cardiac failure. Diastolic dysfunction may also occur due to impaired myocardial relaxation (negative lusitropy).

Arrhythmias may occur due to a range of factors including fatty infiltration of the conducting system, myocardial hypertrophy, hypoxaemia, diuretic-related hypokalaemia, coronary artery disease and increased circulating catecholamines.

Respiratory

Hypoxaemia and impaired gas exchange result from impingement of closing capacity upon tidal volume and reductions in lung compliance and functional residual capacity. This is compounded by an increased metabolic rate with higher oxygen consumption and CO_2 production. Lung hypoxaemia leads to pulmonary vasoconstriction, pulmonary hypertension and cor pulmonale with right ventricular strain and failure.

V/Q mismatch and intrapulmonary shunt occur as the closing capacity encroaches on tidal volume with obesity. This is more marked in the supine position and under anaesthesia. A reduced expiratory reserve volume further increases shunt through poorly ventilated lung bases. Obstructive sleep apnoea (OSA) increases proportionally to the weight of the patient. Identification and treatment preoperatively may significantly improve gas exchange and reduce systemic and pulmonary hypertension.

Obesity hypoventilation syndrome is caused by OSA in nearly 90% of patients and presents as impaired ventilatory drive and awake chronic hypercapnia ($Pa\text{CO}_2$ >5.3 kPa). These patients have greater hypoxaemia at rest, a tendency to rapid desaturation and an increased risk of pulmonary hypertension.

Gastrointestinal

Gastric acid secretion is increased and its pH tends to be lower. With an increased incidence of hiatus hernia and gastro-oesophageal reflux, the risk of aspiration is high.

Endocrine

Type 2 diabetes results from fatty liver disease and both hepatic and peripheral insulin resistance. Peripheral insensitivity is predominantly due to intracellular insulin signalling defects in adipocytes and skeletal muscle.

Metabolic syndrome (sometimes referred to as syndrome X; not to be confused with cardiac syndrome X – angina with angiographically normal coronary vessels) is a progressive, proinflammatory state of hyperglycaemia, dyslipidaemia and hypertension. It is a metabolic consequence of insulin resistance and central obesity. The prevalence is 34% in the United States and patients have a three times greater mortality risk from coronary artery disease. Cushing's syndrome, hypothyroidism and polycystic ovarian syndrome are endocrine causes of obesity.

Investigations

Attendance at preoperative assessment clinic is recommended in those with a BMI >40 kg/m^2 or >35kg/m^2 with significant comorbidities. Appropriate investigations include a full blood count, renal function, liver function, blood glucose and an ECG. Respiratory function tests and blood gases should be considered.

Anaesthetic management

Preoperative

Routine premedication of ranitidine or a proton-pump inhibitor and simple pre-emptive analgesia is ideal. Sedative drugs should be avoided.

Intraoperative

Appropriately trained staff and correct equipment are essential. This includes an operating table with sufficient maximal weight allowance. Attention to patient positioning and pressure points is important with suitable limb supports available. A HoverMatt air transfer system (or similar) should be considered to ease patient transfer.

Ideally anaesthesia should be induced in theatre to minimise the handling of unconscious obese patients with risks to both staff and patients. Intravenous access may be difficult although an antecubital fossa or even trunk vein can usually be cannulated for induction. Central venous access should not generally be required unless otherwise indicated.

During induction, airway conditions should be optimised using 20–30° head up positioning in the ramped position (ear level with sternal notch). Provide full preoxygenation with a good mask seal as rapid desaturation often occurs. RSI is not indicated for obesity without other risk factors for aspiration, such as delayed gastric emptying. There is evidence to demonstrate that patients begin to desaturate less rapidly during apnoea following rocuronium administration than following suxamethonium during RSI. Facemask ventilation may be difficult and the early use of airway adjuncts should be considered. Obesity is a weak predictor for difficult intubation but inappropriate airway management strategies (e.g. laryngeal mask airway use) resulted in twice the rate of airway complications in these patients compared with the general populace (see Royal College of Anaesthetists NAP 4 project). Awake fibreoptic intubation is not routinely indicated. Patients should be extubated sitting up.

Pharmacokinetics and drug dosing is complex. Generally, use ideal body weight for hydrophilic drugs and lean or total body weight for more lipophilic drugs (**Table 31**). Short-acting volatiles or total intravenous anaesthesia are acceptable maintenance with a focus on rapid wakeup for airway control and minimal respiratory depression. Minimal or short-acting opioids should be used with adequate reversal of neuromuscular relaxants.

Regional anaesthesia offers the potential to avoid the problems of a general anaesthetic but may be technically difficult. Patients may be unable to tolerate lying supine. Failure of regional anaesthesia, both peripheral and neuraxial, is more frequent in obese patients and may necessitate urgent general anaesthesia with fewer options and more

Table 31 Weight-based drug dose guidelines for morbidly obese patients	
IBW dosing	TBW dosing
Propofol (induction dose)	Midazolam
Rocuronium	Suxamethonium
Alfentanil	Atracurium
Fentanyl	
Remifentanil	Propofol maintenance – CBW dosing
Morphine	

IBW, ideal body weight; TBW, total body weight; CBW, corrected body weight according to Servin's formula = IBW + 0.4 (TBW–IBW).

Hydrophilic   *Lipophilic.*

potential risk. The dose of agent for epidural or subarachnoid block is 80% of normal on a mg/kg basis.

Postoperative

Analgesia should be multimodal including paracetamol and NSAIDs and avoiding long acting opioids. Use of patient-controlled analgesia may be the safest approach. Postoperative complications include a higher incidence of chest infection, wound infection, deep vein thrombosis and pulmonary embolism compared with normal-weight patients. Early mobilisation should be encouraged with active measures against venous thromboembolism.

Further reading

Cook TM, Woodall N, Frerk C. Fourth National Audit Project. Major complications of airway management in the UK: results of the Fourth National Audit Project of the Royal College of Anaesthetists and the Difficult Airway Society. Br J Anaesth 2011; 106:617–631.

Ervin B. Prevalence of metabolic syndrome among adults 20 years of age and over, by sex, age, race and ethnicity, and body mass index: United States, 2003–2006. National Center for Health Statistics, Center for Disease Control and Prevention, 2009.

Fox W, Harris S, Kennedy N. Prevalence of difficult intubation in a bariatric population using the beach chair position. Anaesthesia 2008; 63:1339–1342.

Public Health England. National Obesity Observatory. [Online] www.noo.org.uk/NOO_pub/Key_data [Accessed April 2014].

Related topics of interest

Obesity – surgery for weight reduction

Key points

- Patients undergoing malabsorptive or restrictive surgery have the potential to lose in excess of 50% body weight with a concurrent reversal of obesity-related comorbidity
- Careful patient selection and a cohesive, multidisciplinary approach to all phases of care are crucial to the success of these procedures as part of a comprehensive weight reduction package
- The overall anaesthetic approach should be as meticulous as that for an obese patient having nonobesity surgery under general anaesthesia

Obesity poses a significant health and economic burden on the UK. There are a number of obesity-related conditions that may benefit from weight reduction. Weight loss of 5–10% of initial body weight can improve hypertension, hyperlipidaemias and type 2 diabetes and reduce cumulative cardiorespiratory risk. Symptomatic joint disease and psychosocial factors may be improved. Bariatric surgery is part of a weight loss program and is the only current treatment proven to achieve significant and sustained weight loss in the morbidly obese (body mass index, BMI, >40 kg/m^2). Eligibility for surgery should be objectively assessed. In the UK, for example, NICE recommends a set of criteria which defines those likely to benefit most (**Table 32**).

Types of surgery

Both restrictive and malabsorptive surgeries induce weight loss by reducing the gastric volume.

Restrictive

Restrictive surgery includes adjustable gastric bands (AGBs), sleeve gastrectomy and gastric balloons. AGBs result in approximately 40–60% excess weight loss above a notional maximal ideal BMI of 25. Risks are low (0.1%) but there is a 10–20% long-term risk of reoperation over 10 years due to infection, slippage, erosion or leak.

Malabsorptive

Laparoscopic Roux-en-Y gastric bypass is the most common surgical weight loss procedure worldwide. It combines gastric restriction with a degree of malabsorption. Approximately 60–70% excess weight loss is achieved, more quickly and with improved resolution of diabetes (occurs in 70% of patients), hypercholesterolaemia and hypertension. The risk of mortality is higher (0.5–2%) and surgery is irreversible.

Investigations

Preoperative assessment should include assessment of perioperative risk. A commonly applied tool is the obesity surgery mortality risk score (OS-MRS) (**Table 33**). High-risk patients should be managed in a High Dependency Unit postoperatively.

Table 32 Criteria for bariatric surgery
Patients have a BMI 40 kg/m^2, or between 35 and 40 kg/m^2 with coexisting disease that could be improved with weight loss
All attempts at nonsurgical intervention have failed to achieve/maintain clinically beneficial weight loss after a minimum trial of 6 months
Patients are receiving or will receive intensive management in a specialist obesity service
Patients are generally fit for anaesthesia and surgery
Patients are committed to the need for long-term follow-up
Adapted from NICE CG43. BMI, body mass index.

Table 33 OS-MRS criteria
BMI $\geq$ 50 kg/m^2
Male patients
Hypertension
Defined risk of PE - prior history, presence of a vena cava filter or evidence of pulmonary hypertension
Age $\geq$ 45
1 point for each, 1 = low risk (1 in 500), 2–3 = intermediate risk (1 in 100) 4–5= high risk (1 in 50)
BMI, body mass index; PE, pulmonary embolism.

Comorbidities affecting anaesthesia are discussed in *Obesity – incidental surgery*. Symptoms and signs of cardiac failure and obstructive sleep apnoea should be actively sought. Many morbidly obese patients have limited mobility and may appear relatively asymptomatic despite significant cardiorespiratory dysfunction. Comprehensive airway assessment should be undertaken. In particular, a large neck circumference (>40 cm) and a Mallampati score of 3 have been identified as predictors of a potentially difficult intubation.

Anaesthetic management
Preoperative

A detailed preoperative assessment with investigations as above should be performed well in advance of surgery. Early engagement of surgeons, anaesthetists, endocrinologists, dieticians and bariatric nurse specialists is important to determine suitability of surgery, address comorbidities and develop a tailored perioperative plan. Patients should be advised to stop smoking at least 6 weeks prior to admission. Prophylactic antacid medication and simple analgesia are appropriate. Sedative premedication is best avoided.

Patients are encouraged to walk to theatre and position themselves on the table with 20–30° head up. At least two intravenous cannulae are inserted and the upper limbs are kept accessible. Intra-arterial access is generally not indicated and noninvasive blood pressure (NIBP) measurements can be reliably performed on the forearm. Mechanical thromboprophylaxis (e.g. foot pumps) should be employed until full postoperative mobilisation.

Intraoperative

Induction follows full preoxygenation in a ramped position with the ear level with the sternal notch (target ETo$_2$ of ≥85%). Facemask ventilation may be difficult; consider giving neuromuscular drugs early in the intubation sequence. Careful bag mask ventilation with a low threshold for adjuncts is important to avoid gastric distension. RSI is not routinely indicated.

A modified Lloyd-Davies position (reverse Trendelenburg, legs separated and raised) with right lateral tilt is used. Foot rests and leg strapping are applied to prevent slipping down the table. Attention to pressure areas is vital; distal limb nerve injury is a particular risk.

Maintenance anaesthesia includes either short-acting volatiles or total intravenous anaesthesia (TIVA). The aim is to achieve rapid offset and awakening to promote early airway control, reduce respiratory depression and allow earlier mobilisation. Modern volatile pharmacokinetics are only moderately influenced by obesity due to low blood–gas and oil–gas solubilities. Propofol and remifentanil must be used with caution as they rely on estimated population-based kinetics which are not validated in the obese population. Depth of anaesthesia monitors should be routinely used with TIVA. Remifentanil may decrease volatile and propofol requirements. Respiratory effort is also ablated but persisting muscle tone will reduce the size of the laparoscopic work space if neuromuscular blocking drugs are not also used.

For laparoscopic Roux-en-Y bypass, an orogastric bougie is inserted to assist gastroenterostomy formation. The anastomosis integrity is subsequently tested using blue dye through an orogastric tube. Patients should be warned preoperatively about staining; this can affect the face (but cleans easily with chlorhexidine) and hair (particularly blonde hair, which can be permanently dyed).

Intravenous fluid is generally restricted in line with the principles of Enhanced Recovery. This surgery poses a high risk of nausea and vomiting due to manipulation of the upper stomach and at least two antiemetics should be administered. Opiates should be used judiciously to reduce the risk of airway compromise, vomiting and respiratory depression.

Postoperative

Extubation should be performed sitting up and fully awake. An air-assisted mattress can be used to aid patient transfer. In recovery, they should be nursed at 45° with standard monitoring including pulse oximetry and NIBP. Demonstration of an adequate cough and deep breathing exercises is encouraged. Postoperative pain is often less than expected and this is partly attributed to high patient motivation. Patient-controlled analgesia and epidural anaesthesia are rarely necessary due to increased minimally invasive surgery.

Deep vein thrombosis (DVT) is the most common complication of bariatric surgery with an incidence of 2.4–4.5%. Patients should be encouraged to sit out on the same day to improve respiratory dynamics and reduce DVT risk. Low molecular weight heparin should be continued for 10 days postoperatively but may be used preoperatively in high risk patients. Most patients are discharged home after 3 days.

Further reading

Adams JP, Murphy PG. Obesity in anaesthesia and intensive care. Br J Anaesth 2000; 85:91–108.

Brodsky JB, Lemmens HJ, Brock-Utne JG, et al. Morbid obesity and tracheal intubation. Anesth Analg 2002; 94:732–736.

Demaria EJ, Portenier D, Wolfe L. Obesity surgery mortality risk score: proposal for a clinically useful score to predict mortality risk in patients undergoing gastric bypass. Surg Obes Relat Dis 2007; 3:134–134.

National Institute for Health and Care Excellence. Obesity: guidance on the prevention, identification, assessment and management of overweight and obesity in adults and children (CG43). London: NICE, 2006.

Related topics of interest

Obstetrics – anaesthesia

Key points

- Physiological changes of pregnancy impact on anaesthetic management
- Extensive neuraxial blockade is required for caesarean section
- Good communication is vital for maternal satisfaction

Anaesthesia for obstetric patients may be required at any stage of pregnancy for surgery, delivery or problems in the immediate postnatal period. Perinatal anaesthesia is the focus of this chapter. Changes in physiology produce several considerations for the anaesthetist (**Table 34**) and pathology may alter the technique chosen.

Caesarean sections should generally be stratified on an objective basis to determine urgency. For example, in the UK, the Royal College of Obsetetricians and Royal College of Anaesthetists categorise on a scale of 1 (emergency) to 4 (elective) according to risk to mother and/or foetus. NICE (UK) guidance states that categories 1 and 2 should be performed as soon as possible (category 2 within 75 minutes in most situations; Royal College of Anaesthetists recommendations in fact suggest 45 minutes). These times should be used as audit standards rather than to categorise performance.

Neuraxial blockade is now the most frequently used technique and has resulted in significant reductions in anaesthesia-related maternal deaths in the confidential enquiry reports. A block level from sacral segment 5 (S5) to thoracic segment 4 (T4) to cold and S5 to T5 for light touch is required for caesarean section due to the innervation pattern of the intraperitoneal viscera. Lower levels of blockade may be adequate for instrumental deliveries, although these may rapidly progress to caesarean section requiring blockade to T4.

Problems

Hypotension

Spinals and epidural top-ups result in a loss of sympathetic vascular tone. Intravenous fluid 'co-loading' and vasopressors such as phenylephrine or metaraminol are used to maintain normotension and the patient must be tilted to the left to avoid aortocaval compression.

Inadequate anaesthesia

This can be exceptionally distressing and should be managed aggressively. Inadequate anaesthesia before delivery of the foetus is highly likely to require general anaesthesia (GA) unless an epidural catheter is *in situ* (allowing top-up). Options for management include:

- Entonox
- Alfentanil/fentanyl
- Epidural top-up (avoid toxic dose of local anaesthetic)
- Local anaesthesia infiltration by obstetrician
- GA

Treatment options should be discussed with the woman and reassessment must be continuous. Clear, contemporaneous documentation is essential.

Anaesthetic management

Single-shot spinal

Commonly used when no epidural or a poorly functioning epidural is in situ. Produces a rapid-onset, predictable, dense block. About 2.2–2.5 mL of hyperbaric 0.5% bupivacaine is generally used although there is variation in practice. Additive agents include opioids to increase density and duration of postoperative analgesia.

The 'rapid sequence spinal' has been suggested for clinically urgent situations involving some alterations to increase speed (e.g. aseptic no-touch technique, limited attempts) whilst allowing preoxygenation should rapid recourse to GA be required.

Epidural top-up

An epidural providing good labour analgesia should be topped-up to surgical anaesthesia as soon as the decision for operative delivery is made, with continuous anaesthetic presence. Topping-up a poorly functioning epidural is rarely successful and although a fresh epidural can be inserted, it will take time to develop anaesthesia. All epidurals require careful assessment to ensure adequate block prior to incision. Commonly used solutions are:

- (Levo-) bupivacaine 0.5% up to 20 mL
- Lignocaine 2% + adrenaline 1:200 000 +/− 8.4% bicarbonate 2 mL (total volume 20 mL)
- +/− Opioid

Large volumes of local anaesthetic agents are administered in a short time with potential for a total spinal or local anaesthetic toxicity if catheter migration occurs. Every dose should be treated as a test dose.

Combined spinal epidural

Useful especially where surgery may be prolonged or cardiovascular comorbidity requires slow onset of blockade and careful titration of vasopressor to maintain stability. Techniques include 'needle-through-needle' or insertion of an epidural at one interspace and spinal a level below. An epidural test dose cannot be administered before onset of spinal block when using the 'needle-through-needle' technique; this should be remembered if the epidural catheter is subsequently utilised.

General anaesthesia

For patients unsuitable for regional techniques (refusal or contraindication), or where there is immediate risk to mother or foetus (the 'category 1 caesarean'). Focussed preinduction assessment is vital:

- Indication for caesarean
- Current/past medical history
- Obstetric history
- Last food/drink
- Allergies
- Anaesthetic history
- Airway assessment

Intrauterine resuscitation should be instituted if there is foetal compromise (see below) and monitoring should resume as

System	Physiological change	Anaesthetic consideration
Table 34 Maternal physiological changes of particular relevance to the anaesthetist		
Cardiovascular	↑Circulating volume ↑Cardiac output (by 40–50% at term) ↓ Systemicvascular resistance (30–35%)	Great cardiovascular stress especially if impaired myocardial function
	Nonautoregulated placental circulation (i.e. pressure dependent)	Maintain MAP to perfuse placenta
	Aortocaval compression (gravid uterus compresses great vessels) from 20 weeks	Tilt to the left/manually displace uterus
Respiratory	↑Minute ventilation and ↓Pa_{CO_2} ↓FRC (small airway closure may occur when supine) ↑Oxygen consumption (60%)	Vulnerable to hypoxaemia Rapid desaturation if apnoeic
	Potential oedema/congestion of upper airway and larynx	Difficult intubation 1 in 250 May require smaller endotracheal tube
Gastrointestinal	↑Risk aspiration ↓Tone lower oesophageal sphincter and ↑intra-abdominal pressure ↓Gastric emptying/gastroparesis in labour	Antacid medication in high-risk patients Sodium citrate pre-GA Orogastric tube pre-extubation
Haematological	Haemodilution – anaemia of pregnancy Procoagulant state (↑clotting factors and ↓ fibrinolysis)	Thromboprophylaxis
Neurological	↓Volume epidural space	↓ Volume spinal drugs compared with nonobstetric population
Other	Placental transfer of drugs to foetus Uterine contraction postdelivery	Minimise use of drugs which can cross placenta until after delivery Bolus doses/infusions uterotonics required

soon as the patient is in theatre to facilitate continuous assessment and decision making by obstetric and anaesthetic teams. Elements of intrauterine resuscitation of the foetus:

- **Syntocinon off**
- **Position full left lateral**
- **Oxygen** (15 L/min via non-rebreathe mask)
- **Intravenous fluid bolus** (caution in pre-eclampsia)
- **Low blood pressure** – use vasopressors, e.g. ephedrine
- **Tocolysis** (e.g. terbutaline)

Where time allows, consider premedication with ranitidine and sodium citrate to ameliorate the effects of potential gastric regurgitation and pulmonary aspiration. Positioning of the patient should be optimised for intubation just prior to induction. An RSI with preoxygenation in a left-tilted position with cricoid pressure is performed. The induction agent used has historically been thiopentone although propofol has increasing popularity in some centres. Once endotracheal tube position is confirmed, anaesthesia is maintained with volatile agent in an oxygen/nitrous oxide mixture. Typically, no opioids are administered until delivery following which morphine, antiemetics and simple analgesics should be given. Transversus abdominal plane blocks or local anaesthetic infiltration to the wound will improve analgesia postoperatively. Consider a large bore orogastric tube to empty the stomach prior to extubation, particularly if significant oral intake has occurred prior to anaesthesia. The patient should be extubated awake at the end of surgery.

Further reading

Centre for Maternal and Child Enquiries (CMACE). Saving mothers' lives: reviewing maternal deaths to make motherhood safer: 2006–08. The Eighth Report on Confidential Enquiries into Maternal Deaths in the United Kingdom. Br J Obstet Gynaecol 2011; 118:1–203.

National Institute for Health and Care Excellence (NICE). CG 132 – caesarean section. London: NICE, 2011.
Royal College of Obstetricians & Gynaecologists and Royal College of Anaesthetists. Classification of urgency of LSCS - a continuum of risk: Good Practice No.11. London: RCOG, 2010.

Related topics of interest

Obstetrics – analgesia

Key points

- For safe and effective analgesia in pregnancy, the physiology of the pregnant mother and the foetus must be taken into consideration
- Maternal wishes regarding mode of analgesia are paramount

Women require analgesia during pregnancy for:
- Pre-existing pain problems
- Pain problems related to pregnancy
- Incidental surgery in pregnancy
- For labour
- Postcaesarean section (CS)

The thalidomide catastrophe shaped current licensing arrangements for drug use in pregnancy. The British National Formulary states that 'no drug is safe beyond all doubt in early pregnancy'. Furthermore many drugs commonly used by anaesthetists are not actually licensed for use in pregnancy.

The possibility of pregnancy should be considered in any women of childbearing age presenting for surgery. If possible delay surgery until the second trimester when organogenesis is complete and teratogenicity risk is lower; miscarriage rates are high before this (e.g. 10–20% with appendicectomy). Use regional techniques to avoid systemic administration of drugs. Analgesics considered safe in pregnancy include paracetamol, codeine, Oramorph and morphine. Nonsteroidal anti-inflammatory drugs (NSAIDs) can be used unless delivery is imminent; they cross the placenta and perinatal administration can lead to failure of ductus arteriosus closure. Local anaesthetics used in UK obstetric anaesthetic practice include bupivacaine, levobupivacaine, ropivacaine and lignocaine.

Pharmacokinetics and pharmacodynamics

Absorption can be affected by vomiting.

Volume of distribution is increased in pregnant women due to elevated total body water and altered plasma protein profile. Increased cardiac output redistributes drugs more quickly. pH changes can occur in labour affecting drug ionisation. Hepatic metabolism is affected in conditions such as HELLP syndrome, pre-eclampsia and fatty liver of pregnancy. Minimum alveolar concentration and the minimal blocking concentration of local anaesthetics are reduced, probably due to increased progesterone concentrations. Glomerular filtration rate and clearance are increased. Breast milk is an additional route of elimination.

The foetus represents an additional compartment as most drugs cross the placenta. The foetus eliminates drugs less efficiently. Factors affecting placental transfer of a drug are as follows:
- Molecular weight
- Degree of ionisation
- Lipid solubility
- Protein binding

In labour

Nociceptive signals from the uterus and cervix travel via Aδ and C fibres in the thoracolumbar parasympathetic (T10-L2) and sacral sympathetic (S2-S4) pathways. First stage labour pain is referred to these dermatomes followed by lower and sacral dermatomes as labour progresses. Somatic pain may be caused by pressure on and tearing of pelvic structures.

Approximately 50% of women experience severe or very severe pain in labour. Fear, fatigue, anxiety and poor support enhance pain perception. Good antenatal education and the continuous presence of a midwife or doula reduce the amount of pain reported. First labours and those of older primiparae are more painful. Malposition, occipitoposterior presentation, and augmentation of labour with oxytocic drugs increase pain. Untreated pain causes an increase in circulating maternal catecholamines and stress hormones. Maternal pain and acidosis are associated with reduced uteroplacental blood flow and fetal acidosis.

Nonpharmacological pain relief

- Active labour. Walking, rocking, positional change, breathing techniques and warm water immersion can be used to help cope with pain
- Hypnosis. Hypnobirthing has gained popularity. Women can learn techniques to focus their mind on positive experiences and associations. The word 'pain' is not used with contractions being described as 'powerful'. Visualisation techniques can be rehearsed prior to labour. Women who succeed with this technique can appear quiet and dissociated in labour
- Transcutaneous nerve stimulation. Involves the administration of electrical current via electrodes placed on the skin to interfere with the transmission of pain signals. There is good evidence to support its use. Electrodes are usually placed on the lumbar spine. They should not be placed over the uterus
- Acupuncture. There is conflicting evidence concerning the benefits of acupuncture. A recent meta-analysis suggested that the effects of acupuncture are no better than placebo

Pharmacological pain relief

- Entonox. 50:50 mixture of N_2O and O_2 used widely as an inhaled analgesia. It has emetic side effects
- Pethidine. A synthetic phenylpiperidine derivative with anticholinergic properties, administered by midwives as an IM injection. It has a high lipid solubility and readily crosses the placenta. In the foetus, it is metabolised to an active but less lipid soluble derivative, norpethidine, which accumulates. Levels peak 4 hours after the maternal injection and can cause hallucinations and grand mal seizures. Its effects are not reversed by naloxone. Pethidine interacts with monoamine oxidase inhibitors
- Diamorphine. A diacetylated morphine derivative. It is an inactive pro-drug. Administered as an IM injection during labour, and as an analgesic adjunct in spinals and epidurals

- Remifentanil. A synthetic phenylpiperidine and pure µ-agonist. It is rapidly broken down by nonspecific plasma and tissue esterases. This results in an elimination half-life of 3–10 minutes. It can be administered via patient-controlled analgesia (PCA) during labour as a bolus dose of 20–40 µg with a 2-minute lockout. Midwife training and anaesthetic support should be available as respiratory depression can occur

Regional techniques

Epidural analgesia provides the most consistently effective form of pain relief during labour. Most UK units provide a 24-hour epidural service. The most commonly used mixture in the UK is bupivacaine 0.1–0.125% with fentanyl 2–2.5 µg/mL. Levobupivacaine is also used. Opioids reduce total dose of local anaesthetics required and the degree of motor block.

Epidural regimens include intermittent top-ups of 10–15 mL/hour, infusions of 10–12 mL/hour or by patient-controlled epidural anaesthesia (PCEA), an 8–15 mL/hour infusion with a patient-delivered 4–6 mL bolus limited by a 5–20 minute lockout. Infusions and PCEA are associated with better maternal satisfaction and lower total drug delivery. Computer-integrated PCEA regimens are in development. These combine variable background infusions and intermittent boluses in response to patient demand. They are not yet in widespread use but aim to improve analgesia and reduce total drug administration.

Consent in labour is controversial as women are often exhausted and distressed at the point of opting for an epidural. However, side effects and complications need to be discussed before verbal consent can be obtained (**Table 35**). Standard contraindications to an epidural apply but consider specifics such as pre-eclampsia (as a cause of thrombocytopaenia/coagulopathy). Maternal co-operation is essential for the safe insertion of an epidural.

Epidural analgesia can be readily topped up for instrumental or caesarian delivery.

Table 35 Risks associated with epidural in labour	
Side effect	Incidence/risk
Backache	No increased risk
Caesarean section	No increased risk
Length of first stage	No increased length
Second stage of labour	Increased on average by 15 minutes
Need for instrumental delivery	1.4 increased risk
Itching	1:10
Adjustment/additional analgesia required	1:10
Heavy legs	1:20
Difficulty passing urine	1:20
Significant hypotension	1:50
Failure	1:50
Headache	1:200 (operator dependent)
Temporary nerve palsy	1:3000
Permanent nerve palsy	1:15000
Total spinal	1:15000
Paraplegia	1:100000

Combined spinal epidural (CSE); some units employ this technique routinely, others rarely. The benefits include rapid onset of pain relief and absence of significant motor block. The epidural can also be left in situ for post-CS analgesia; however, there is additional risk of complications and increased cost.

Spinal drug regimens (via CSE) for labour analgesia vary, e.g. 5–15 µg fentanyl and 25 mg of bupivacaine made up to a 2 mL volume with saline. An alternative would be to use 3–5 mL standard epidural mix (0.1% bupivacaine and 2 µg/mL fentanyl). These prescriptions will provide 60–90 minutes analgesia. Further analgesia can be given via the epidural (bolus or infusion).

Pudendal nerve block may be used to reduce the discomfort of forceps delivery. Additional infiltration of the perineum and labia is required to block branches of the ilioinguinal and genitofemoral nerves. The block is usually performed by the obstetrician 5 minutes prior to delivery using 1% lignocaine via a transvaginal approach.

After caesarean section

Careful consideration should be given to analgesia at each phase of management. In the UK for example, NICE guidance states that, 'women who have a caesarean section should be prescribed and encouraged to take regular analgesia for postoperative pain' and recommends the following:

Perioperative

Neuraxial opiates are key to good analgesia in the first 24 hours following CS. There is strong evidence that pain scores are improved and the use of additional opioid analgesia reduced, e.g. diamorphine 0.3–0.4 mg intrathecal or 2.5–5.0 mg epidural administered intraoperatively. NSAIDs should be used unless contraindicated; rectal diclofenac 100 mg is commonly given, 20–40 mg parecoxib is an alternative.

Postoperative

NICE currently recommends regular paracetamol and ibuprofen with codeine for breakthrough pain. However, codeine has recently been contraindicated in breast-feeding women (MHRA and UKDILAS recommendations) due to its variable metabolism and the risk of respiratory arrest in the neonate.

Other drugs used and considered safe in breast-feeding women include, morphine (intravenous or PCA), Oramorph and tramadol. Further research is ongoing into the most effective way of providing good analgesia for women post-CS, including the use of transversus abdominis plane catheters to provide analgesia following caesarian under GA.

Further reading

Cho S-H, Lee H, Ernst E. Acupuncture for pain relief in labour: a systematic review and meta-analysis. Br J Obstet Gynaecol 2010; 117:907–912.
Cookhttp://bja.oxfordjournals.org/content/102/2/179 - aff-1 TM, Counsell D, Wildsmith JAW. Major complications of central neuraxial block: report on the Third National Audit Project of the Royal College of Anaesthetists. Br J Anaesth 2009; 102:179–190.

Medicines and Healthcare Regulatory Agency. Drug safety update, Volume 6, Issue 12, Issue 12, A1. London: MHRA, 2013.
National Institute of Health and Care Excellence(NICE). CG55: Intrapartum care: management and delivery of care to women in labour. London: NICE, 2007.
National Institute of Health and Care Excellence (NICE). CG132: Caesarian Section. London: NICE, 2011.

Related topics of interest

Obstetrics – emergencies

Key points

- Multidisciplinary management with senior clinician involvement is vital
- Sepsis is now the most common direct cause of maternal mortality in the UK

Obstetric emergencies are extremely stressful and can be traumatic for medical professionals, patients and their families. Guidelines exist for many situations and common factors for improvement identified by the UK Centre for Maternal and Child Health Enquiries (CMACE) report include:

- Communication
- Team-working
- Clear leadership
- Early identification and management of unwell women
- Up-to-date clinical knowledge and skills
- Involvement of senior clinicians and consultant-delivered care of high-risk cases
- Availability of additional skilled clinicians when the workload is extreme

Most obstetric patients are young with no (or minor) comorbidities and will compensate for prolonged periods prior to sudden collapse. Prevention requires rapid identification and aggressive management. Familiarity with the clinical environment is also important, e.g. where emergency blood, equipment (including defibrillators, eclampsia and anaphylaxis kits) and drugs are kept.

Major haemorrhage

It is an important cause of maternal mortality. Blood loss is often underestimated or concealed and clinical signs may be incorrectly attributed to labour. Early multidisciplinary management can be life saving. Declaration of an obstetric major haemorrhage on labour ward, in theatre and the haematology laboratory allows simultaneous rapid resuscitation and decision making.

Local guidelines should be available. Specific considerations are outlined in **Table 36**.

Pre-eclampsia and eclampsia

Untreated systolic hypertension (>180 mmHg) and eclamptic seizures (**Table 37**) are medical emergencies. Alterations to anaesthetic practice should be considered in pre-eclampsia (**Table 38**).

Local anaesthetic toxicity

Guidelines exist to manage this situation, e.g. those from the AAGBI. Key points include:

- Stop injecting local anaesthetic
- Call for help
- Supportive management of airway, breathing and circulation
- Control seizures
- Give intralipid 20% (1.5 mL/kg bolus plus 15 mL/kg infusion over 1 hour)

Failed intubation

The incidence of obstetric failed intubation is approximately 1 in 300. Contributory factors may include difficulty inserting laryngoscope blade due to large breasts or weight gain, airway oedema, distortion due to cricoid pressure and/or tilted patient and operator stress. Desaturation is also rapid due to reduced FRC and high oxygen consumption.

The overriding priority is maintenance of oxygenation NOT intubation (**Figure 13**) and experienced assistance is crucial. The clinical situation will dictate whether waking the patient or continuing with surgery is most appropriate.

Maternal sepsis

Genital tract sepsis is the commonest direct cause of maternal death in the UK (typically due to Group A β-*Haemolytic streptococcus*). Symptoms and signs of SIRS plus sore throat or respiratory infection (either the patient or her family) are important. Severe abdominal pain, 'after-pains' or diarrhoea are also significant. The approach is as for any other cause of sepsis.

Table 36 Specific measures for maternal haemorrhage	
Clinical aim	**Intervention**
Stop bleeding Tone Tissue Trauma Thrombin	Bimanual compression uterus Uterotonics Surgical intervention Remove retained products Repair trauma Uterine balloon tamponade B-lynch suture Interventional radiology Ligation uterine/iliac vessels Hysterectomy
Replacement fluid/ blood	Large-bore intravenous (IV) access High volume giving sets and warmer Blood products Declare major haemorrhage to haematology laboratory O-negative, type specific or cross-matched Cell salvage Attention to coagulation and red cell replacement
Monitoring	Consider invasive monitoring – initial priority is resuscitation Near-patient tests Haemoglobin Coagulation (e.g. TEG) Laboratory-based tests – may not reflect rapidly changing clinical situation Blood gases
Drug therapy	Uterotonics Syntocinon 5 units repeated once and infusion Ergometrine 500 µg slow IV or intramuscular (IM) Carboprost 250 µg IM every 15 minutes (8 doses max - caution in asthma) Misoprostol 1000 mg PR Antifibrinolytics (tranexamic acid 15 mg/kg) Consultant haematologist input Recombinant Factor VIIa Adequate haemoglobin, INR, platelet, fibrinogen levels and pH >7.2 required for efficacy Calcium chloride/gluconate for hypocalcaemia
Ongoing care	Consider optimal place of care

Table 37 Management of eclamptic seizure
Call for help
Minimise trauma to woman and foetus
Turn left lateral
Administer oxygen, maintain airway
Intravenous access
$MgSO_4$ – 5 g over 20 minutes and infusion 1 g/hour
Most eclamptic seizures are self-limiting – consider alternative diagnoses if seizures continue
Careful planning of ongoing management including delivery – senior involvement required

Maternal cardiac arrest

Management is according to Resuscitation Council UK guidelines. Additional factors in obstetric patients include:

- Left-lateral uterine displacement (avoids aortocaval compression and improves efficacy of chest compressions)
- Delivery by perimortem caesarean section within 5 minutes of cardiac arrest (to optimise maternal survival)

Table 38 Anaesthetic considerations in pre-eclampsia	
Potential problems	Considerations
Cardiovascular lability:	
Hypertensive response to laryngoscopy	Obtund, e.g. alfentanil 1–2 mg/fentanyl 100–2000 µg (inform paediatrician)/labetalol 10–20 mg/MgSO$_4$ 30 mg/kg
Exaggerated response to vasopressors	Vasopressors often not required after neuraxial block Reduce dose/careful titration
Caution with uterotonics	Profound hypotension after syntocinon Administer very slowly and dilute Ergometrine/syntometrine contraindicated – risk extreme hypertension
Thrombocytopenia/HELLP syndrome	No neuraxial block if platelets <80 or INR >1.5 (follow local guidelines)
Capillary leak/hypoproteinaemia	Care with intravenous fluids – may rapidly develop pulmonary oedema
Magnesium sulphate	Prolonged action of nondepolarising neuromuscular blocking agents

- Consider local anaesthetic toxicity and total spinal anaesthesia in addition to standard causes of cardiac arrest

Magnesium toxicity

Magnesium levels are not usually measured in pre-eclampsia unless renal dysfunction is present. Toxicity causes:
- Nausea, vomiting and flushing
- Widened QRS complexes (may occur within therapeutic range 2–4 mmol/L)
- Lost patellar reflex (4.2–5 mmol/L)
- Respiratory depression (>5 mmol/L)
- Muscle paralysis (6.2–7 mmol/L)
- Cardiac arrest (approximately 12.5 mmol/L)

Management is supportive: stop infusion and, for respiratory or cardiac symptoms, administer calcium gluconate 1 g (=10 mL 10%) over 20 minutes.

High regional blockade

Anaesthesia extending above the thoracic dermatomes may occur due to an unpredictable block or unexpected subarachnoid or subdural placement of an epidural catheter. Symptoms include breathlessness or a 'heavy chest' as the intercostal muscles are paralysed. Paraesthesia in upper limbs occurs as cervical dermatomes become blocked and will extend to the face if the block spreads further. A block above T1 on testing will often be associated with partial or complete diaphragmatic paralysis as the dermatome above T1 on the trunk is C5. Respiratory compromise, slurred speech, sedation, apnoea, bradycardia (due to block of the cardiac accelerator fibres T1-4), profound hypotension and loss of consciousness may follow.

For moderately high blocks simple reassurance will be adequate. Extensive blockade will require anaesthesia and respiratory support:
- Call for help
- 100% O$_2$
- Intubation with small dose induction agent (to avoid awareness)
- Fluid bolus and vasopressor – adrenaline may be necessary
- Delivery to prevent fetal hypoperfusion and relieve aortocaval compression
- Supportive management until block recedes

Tocolysis

Certain circumstances may necessitate abrupt reduction in the force of uterine contraction due to life-threatening conditions affecting mother or baby. These are unusual but include:
- Uterine inversion or rupture
- Retained but separated placenta
- Foetal entrapment, e.g. transverse lie at caesarian section

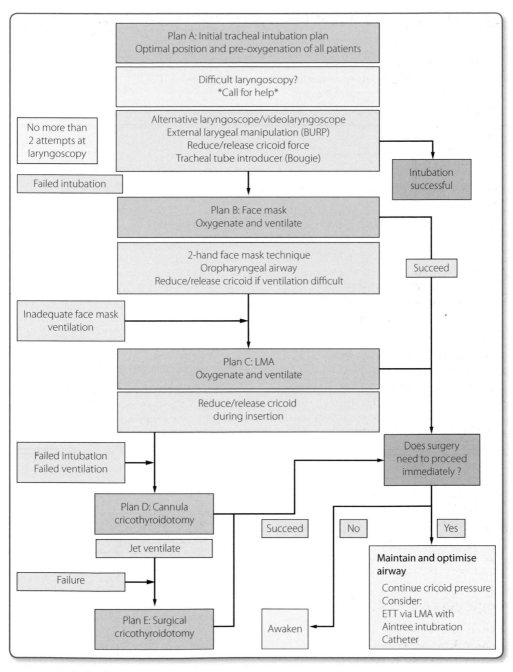

Figure 13 Failed obstetric intubation. With permission from Dr M Rucklidge and Dr C Hinton.

- External cephalic version for delivery of second twin
- Cord prolapse

Therapy will be guided by the obstetrician but in these circumstances the anaesthetist will likely be responsible for administering

treatment. Typical agents include nitrates (e.g. 100 μg intravenous glyceryl trinitrate), β-2 agonists (e.g. ritodrine, terbutaline) or calcium channel blockers (e.g. nifedipine). Tocolysis is also used to arrest pre-term labour but anaesthetists are not involved in this treatment.

Further reading

Association of Anaesthetists of Great Britain and Ireland. Management of severe local anaesthetic toxicity. London: AAGBI, 2010.

Centre for Maternal and Child Enquiries (CMACE). Saving mothers' lives: reviewing maternal deaths to make motherhood safer: 2006–08. The Eighth Report on Confidential Enquiries into Maternal Deaths in the United Kingdom. Br J Obstet Gynaecol 2011; 118:1–203.

Rucklidge M, Hinton C. Difficult and failed intubation in obstetrics. Contin Educ Anaesth Crit Care Pain 2012; 12:86–91.

Related topics of interest

Oesophagectomy

Key points

- Oesophagectomy is a major procedure carrying an appreciable morbidity and mortality risk
- Abdominal, thoracic and minimal access approaches offer specific challenges to the anaesthetist
- Careful attention to intraoperative ventilation strategy, fluid administration and postoperative analgesia is vital to minimise postoperative complications

Oesophageal cancer is the 9th commonest malignancy in the UK, accounting for 5% of cancer deaths. Seventy per cent of all cases are in those over 65 years of age, and there is a 2:1 male preponderance. Relative survival rates for oesophageal cancer remain poor, and the disease incidence is rising. Risk factors vary between the two main histological subtypes: adenocarcinoma (obesity, gastro-oesophageal reflux, Barrett's oesophagus) and squamous cell carcinoma (smoking, alcohol).

Surgical approach

Most resectable tumours are found in the distal oesophagus, and are commonly treated by a two-stage (Ivor-Lewis) gastro-oesophagectomy in which an abdominal and a thoracic approach are required. More proximal tumours may require a three-stage approach involving a cervical anastomosis.

For a two-stage oesophagectomy, surgical access can be via midline laparotomy or laparoscopy for gastric mobilisation in the abdominal stage, followed by right thoracotomy or thoracoscopy for the oesophageal resection and anastomosis. Any combination of approaches can be employed, encompassed under the term minimally invasive oesophagectomy (MIO). The insufflation of carbon dioxide into the abdomen or chest for this procedure offers some specific anaesthetic challenges.

Anaesthetic management

Preoperative management

Preoperative, neoadjuvant chemo- and radiotherapy may have been given to increase the chance of successful resection. Surgery is scheduled for the therapeutic window (typically 3–5 weeks after the final cycle) to maximise the benefits of tumour shrinkage whilst having allowed the patient to recover from treatment side effects. Many patients will be enrolled in an enhanced recovery programme, and a clear explanation of what the patient should expect in the postoperative recovery period is vital.

A thorough preoperative assessment is required, with close attention paid to risk factors such as smoking, alcohol use, obesity, reflux and cardiorespiratory disease. An assessment of functional capacity is extremely important, and traditional investigations such as echocardiography and pulmonary function tests are now being complimented by the use of cardiopulmonary exercise testing. This helps in risk stratification and informed decision making, particularly given that in-hospital mortality rates are in the range of 5–10%, and major complications occur in up to 25% of patients.

Intraoperative management

Careful intraoperative anaesthetic management not only contributes to the immediate technical success of the operation but also has significant implications for postoperative recovery. The usual concerns of attention to fluid administration, haematocrit and temperature apply, and the use of one-lung ventilation introduces some additional considerations.

Capnothorax may be a particular problem. Carbon dioxide from the creation of a capnoperitoneum can pass into the chest or mediastinum during a laparoscopic gastric mobilisation. This may cause an increase in absorbed CO_2 coupled with difficulties with ventilation, as well as a reduction in venous return and a fall in cardiac output. This may range from a mild, transient phenomenon, to a situation not unlike that of a tension pneumothorax, necessitating evacuation of gas and conversion to an open technique. Other complications such as surgical emphysema or massive gas leak with inability to maintain a suitable operating field are also possible.

A double-lumen tube is most frequently employed and the usual considerations for one-lung ventilation apply. Tidal volumes, peak inspiratory pressures and the use of positive end-expiratory pressure (PEEP) should always be adjusted so as to provide optimal oxygenation at the lowest risk of lung injury. Episodes of hypoxia can be predictive of postoperative pulmonary complications and should be corrected rapidly. Malposition of the double-lumen tube is a common complication, and flexible fibreoptic bronchoscopy should be immediately available. The use of optimum PEEP may also help the surgeon by raising the mediastinum up into the operative field.

Intraoperative fluid monitoring is attractive in theory, though associated with practical difficulties. Oesophageal Doppler probes are clearly not appropriate, and the combination of abdominal and thoracic procedures, with changes in position (+/- capnoperitoneum) make interpretation of derived cardiac output measurements problematic. In general, a restrictive fluid regimen is favoured, minimising the risk of pulmonary oedema. Oesophagectomy is frequently performed with a total blood loss of less than 500 mL, though the potential for significant haemorrhage and hence major blood transfusion should never be forgotten.

Postoperative care

Postoperative destination depends upon the stability of the patient and local practice. Early extubation is preferred, and is undertaken as long as the patient's temperature, cardiovascular status and gas exchange allow. Noninvasive ventilation is not advised postoperatively due to the high likelihood of causing gastric insufflation and an anastomotic leak. Care in a high dependency environment may be required for ongoing vasopressor support. Some units routinely care for oesophagectomy patients in a Level 1 area on the surgical ward. Local experience is a key factor to make this work safely.

Analgesic strategy may vary according to local practice. Epidural catheters offer potentially excellent analgesia; however, they can cause hypotension necessitating vasopressor support (and hence High Dependency Unit admission) or aggressive fluid administration. Paravertebral catheters (placed by the surgeon under direct vision) combined with patient-controlled analgesia can offer very good analgesia with limited sympathetic blockade. This can be particularly appropriate for MIO.

Pulmonary complications can occur following inappropriate ventilation strategies (causing lung injury), overaggressive fluid administration, or retained secretions and poor pulmonary toilet related to inadequate analgesia. Extravascular lung water is increased following one-lung ventilation, and attention to infused fluid volumes is vital.

Anastomotic leaks and mediastinitis are serious and potentially fatal complications that may be heralded by fever, dysrhythmias or increased chest drain output. Careful attention to fluid balance and perfusion pressure is paramount. Judicious use of low-dose vasopressors may maintain tissue perfusion, especially in the face of sympathetic blockade caused by epidural analgesia. Clearly a balance must be struck between the use of fluids and vasopressors to maintain perfusion; an excess of either may cause gut ischaemia and impaired healing.

Cardiac dysrhythmias are not uncommon following oesophagectomy, and frequently herald the onset of an infective complication such as a chest infection or anastomotic leak. Furthermore, the associated reduction in cardiac output further impairs anastomotic perfusion. Any dysrhythmia should be treated promptly.

Further reading

Davies RG, Myles PS, Graham JM. A comparison of the analgesic efficacy and side-effects of paravertebral vs. epidural blockade for thoracotomy – a systematic review and meta-analysis of randomized trials. Br J Anaesth 2006; 96:418–426.

Ng J-M. Update on anesthetic management for esophagectomy. Curr Opin Anesthesiol 2011; 24:37–43.

Tandon S, Batchelor A, Bullock R, et al. Perioperative risk factors for acute lung injury after elective oesophagectomy. Br J Anaesth 2001; 86:633–638.

Related topics of interest

Ophthalmology

Key points

- The majority of elective eye surgery is performed under local anaesthesia
- General anaesthesia offers a few specific advantages but is often only selected where regional techniques are contraindicated
- Those presenting for ophthalmological procedures are often either children or the older patient, each with specific considerations which must be accounted for

Elective eye surgery is generally performed on two populations with their own unique problems – children and elderly, comorbid adults. The former almost invariably require general anaesthesia. In adults, however, regional anaesthesia is regarded as the technique of choice, and more than 90% undergo cataract or glaucoma surgery without sedation or general anaesthesia. Some procedures are amenable to topical local anaesthesia. Meanwhile, a range of regional blocks exist which will briefly be discussed, although a detailed explanation of technique is beyond the scope of this book.

Problems

Patient:
- Elderly
  - Inability to lie flat
  - Confusion
  - Comorbidity; affects 75% of cataract patients – 35% ASA 3, 1% ASA 4
  - Polypharmacy including anticoagulants
- Paediatric
  - Require GA

- Oculocardiac reflex (OCR)
- Systemic conditions associated with the ophthalmic problem; may include metabolic disorders or syndromes associated with airway difficulties for example

Procedure:
- Pain
- Duration
- Requirement for ocular akinesia (varies with surgeon and procedure)

Anaesthetic technique:
- General
  - Less likely to be suited to a day case approach
  - Postoperative nausea and vomiting
  - Less cooperative during immediate postoperative period, e.g. positioning after intracameral gas injection
  - OCR remains intact
- Regional
  - Complications of the techniques (**Table 39**)
  - Intolerance of the anaesthetic procedure or subsequent surgery
  - Disinhibition or sudden waking from sedation

Investigations

A routine preassessment should proceed in case general anaesthesia becomes necessary. This should include pulse-oximetry and an assessment of the ability to lie flat. If regional techniques are planned, ultrasound-determined axial length should be noted; a myopic eye with an axial length of >26 mm is at significantly greater risk of globe perforation.

Table 39 Complications of regional techniques		
Minor	Failure Chemosis Subconjunctival haemorrhage	
Major	Scleral injury (0.1%, pain on injection, may lead to retinal detachment) Optic nerve injury (<1% but especially with retrobulbar injection if gaze is up/medial) Systemic reactions, e.g. seizures, brain stem anaesthesia (3.4 in 10,000 but 1–3 in 1000 for retrobulbar) Retrobulbar haemorrhage (up to 2%, ophthalmic emergency – threatens retinal perfusion with rapid sight loss, inform surgeon immediately Allergy (very rare, may be due to local anaesthetic agent or hyaluronidase if used) Muscle palsy (rare, due to local anaesthetic muscle toxicity or direct intramuscular injection)	

In patients who are anticoagulated or on antiplatelet agents, it is usually safe to perform regional anaesthesia as long as the international normalised ratio (INR) is within the therapeutic range for the given indication. If the indication is, however, a mechanical heart valve, this will have a much higher target INR. A joint discussion between the anaesthetist, surgeon and haematologist is recommended to consider the risks and benefits in this circumstance. In the UK, for example, The Royal College of Anaesthetists/ Royal College of Ophthalmologists joint consensus guidance states other blood tests are only necessary if they would have been required regardless of surgery occurring. The only other exception to this advice is that patients on dialysis should have their electrolytes checked. This would also be advisable for those prone to arrhythmias or who have a pacemaker implanted (this should also be checked by the pacemaker technician).

Anaesthetic management

In the case of regional anaesthesia, the minimum monitoring for topical anaesthesia is clinical observation, good communication and pulse oximetry. Any patients with cardiovascular comorbidity (however minor) and all those having more than topical anaesthesia should have blood pressure and electrocardiogram monitoring. All those having regional anaesthesia and/or sedation must have intravenous access.

Regional techniques

There remains little consensus as to whether any of these is superior, although sharp-needle blocks, particularly using needles larger than 25G and longer than 25 mm, appear to be less safe. Specific circumstances may exist where a particular type of injection may be impossible or strongly contraindicated and these are outlined in **Table 40**.

Modified retrobulbar injection deposits local anaesthesia within the fibromuscular conus behind the globe. The peribulbar technique is an injection into the extraconal space. A similar approach is used as for the modified retrobulbar injection but the needle remains anterior to the posterior limit of the globe and does not enter the conus so remaining clear of the optic nerve. Both techniques carry a risk of scleral injury in myopic eyes or those with circumferential bands. The sub-Tenon's injection is within the episcleral space. This is entered with a blunt, curved sub-Tenon's cannula following a small surgical incision and blunt dissection around the inferonasal aspect of the globe. It is safer in myopic eyes than other techniques but may be impossible following vitreoretinal procedures.

Sedation

Sedation may occasionally be required but case-selection, good analgesia, support, communication and hand-holding are proven to reduce the need. All but minimal sedation requires preoperative fasting. Beware of patients suddenly moving or becoming more disinhibited. It is not a suitable alternative to general anaesthesia in confused or demented patients.

General anaesthesia

This is generally only required where regional techniques are contraindicated. It has the advantage of offering a totally

Table 40 Contraindications to regional anaesthesia	
Absolute	**Relative**
Patient refusal Local sepsis/inflammation Allergy	Myopia Unable to lie flat or cooperate for any reason Children Marked communication difficulty, e.g. severe deafness Bleeding diatheses Previous scleral buckle/vitreoretinal surgery High intraocular pressure Single eye/single-effective eye

still eye. Intraocular pressure may also be better controlled. Measures used to control intraocular pressure are similar to those used for intracranial pressure manipulation. For many children requiring general anaesthesia, this will be the first of many procedures thus a positive, nonthreatening experience is crucial to facilitate subsequent visits. Children undergoing squint surgery are at particular risk of the OCR (severe reflex vagal bradycardia with extraocular muscle traction or globe compression sensed via the ophthalmic division of the trigeminal nerve) especially in the presence of hypercarbia. Occurrence of the OCR further elevates the associated risk of postoperative nausea and vomiting (PONV). Peribulbar block will ablate the afferent loop of the OCR but is inadvisable in children; atropine premedication is preferable. Avoid morphine due to worsening PONV and consider paracetamol, non-steroidal anti-inflammatory drugs (NSAIDs) or sub-Tenon's block at completion of surgery. Multimodal antiemetic prophylaxis is required.

For vitreoretinal surgery involving the use of intracameral gas injection (typically sulphur hexafluoride) it is vital to avoid nitrous oxide; this will increase the size of the gas bubble and disrupt the repair. In emergency eye surgery, suxamethonium is not contraindicated where rapid sequence induction is required: the airway is the priority and laryngoscopy with suboptimal paralysis provokes coughing and a much greater risk of extrusion of ocular contents. Rocuronium with sugammadex available is a suitable alternative however.

Further reading

Joint guidelines from the Royal College of Anaesthetists and the Royal College of Ophthalmologists. Local anaesthesia for ophthalmic surgery. London: RCoA/RCO, 2012.

The New York School of Regional Anaesthesia. Opthalmologic anesthesia. [Online] http://

www.nysora.com/regional-anesthesia/sub-specialties/3029-local-regional-anesthesia-for-eye-surgery.html [Accessed April 2014].

Parness G, Underhill S. Regional anaesthesia for intraocular surgery. Br J Anaesth: Contin Educ Anaesth Crit Care Pain 2005; 5:93–97.

Related topics of interest

- Day surgery (p. 51)
- Elderly patients (p. 64)
- Lasers in surgery (p. 98)
- Paediatric anaesthesia – basic concepts (p. 179)
- Paediatric anaesthesia – basic practical conduct (p. 183)
- Procedural sedation (p. 242)

Organ donation

Key points

- For every organ transplanted in the UK each year, there are currently nearly three people awaiting a transplant
- Many organs may now be successfully implanted following donation after cardiac death
- Care for the donor prior to donation after brain death involves different therapeutic targets than the neuroprotective care which preceded the diagnosis of brain stem death

The UK Organ Donation Task Force set a target in 2008 to increase organ donation by 50% in 5 years. This was achieved in 2012/13 with 3,112 organs transplanted. There has been an annual increase of 8% in donation after brain death (DBD) but donation after cardiac death (DCD) is rapidly increasing with a 16% increase in 2012/13 on the previous year. However, around 10,000 people remain on the list awaiting a transplant and the need to maximise donations on a national strategic and individual patient-clinician level is ever present.

Circumstances of donation

The process of organ donation stands on the basis that autonomy has ethical primacy. Upholding the patient's wish to be an organ donor is a final opportunity to respect an autonomous decision made in life and, in the absence of harm, this justifies the interventions of donor care and the retrieval process. Benefit to the recipients should not be a consideration and, in fact, would represent a conflict of interests if it became apparent the donation process was no longer in the donor's interests.

The family must be treated with respect and sensitivity. A specialist nurse for organ donation should be involved at a very early stage to explain the process and manage the authorisation process and retrieval team activation. The UK (except Wales) operates an opt-in system whereby donors must voluntarily join the donor register or at least make their wishes clear to their family. Whilst the family has no right in law to refuse donation when an individual is on the register, their authorisation is always sought and typically respected. To do otherwise would be insensitive and also risk the reputation of the organ donor programme. Scottish law requires family members to sign a document making it clear that they understand they are contradicting their relative's wishes in this circumstance. There are other countries, such as Spain and Austria, which operate variations of the opt-out system with correspondingly higher donor rates than elsewhere.

In the UK DBD occurs following confirmation by two clinicians (one a consultant, the other at least fully registered with the GMC for 5 years) that the patient is brain stem dead. The preconditions for brain stem death testing (**Table 41**) are as follows:

- Established irreversible brain damage
- Exclusion of possible reversible causes (including sedation, metabolic, endocrine or electrolyte disturbance or primary hypothermia)
- Exclusion of primary causes of apnoea, e.g. neuromuscular blocking drugs (high cervical cord injury is a special case)

The tests should generally only be undertaken when the diagnosis is virtually certain. The tests must be performed twice, once by each doctor. Although the second, confirmatory set of tests are often performed immediately after the first, the legal time of death is the time of completion of the first set. DCD may occur where death is certain but brain stem function is retained. Active treatment is withdrawn as with any other case of palliation and extubation, for example is at the discretion of the clinician in charge. Invasive monitoring must remain in place. Analgesia and sedation may continue. Once the systolic blood pressure falls below 50 mmHg for >2 minutes (or SpO_2<70%) the functional warm ischaemic time begins. This ends at the point of cold perfusion of the organs at retrieval. From the start of functional warm ischaemia, there is a fixed limit before the organs become nonviable (**Table 42**). If the patient

Table 41 Key elements of brain stem death testing

Test	Cranial nerves examined (afferent → efferent)
Pupillary light reflex	II → III
Corneal reflex	V → VII
Oculovestibular reflex (cold caloric test)	VIII → III, VI
Cranial response to central pain	V → VII
Gag reflex	IX,X → IX, X
Deep cough	X → (phrenic nerve)
Apnoea test	N/A

Table 42 Viability limits for functional warm ischaemic time

	Minutes of viability
Liver	20 (maximum 30, consider age and steatosis)
Pancreas	30
Lungs	60 (to inflation)
Kidneys	120 (maximum 300 in selected donors)

does not suffer a confirmed asystolic cardiac arrest within these times, organ donation cannot occur. Duration of functional warm ischaemic time, rather than time from treatment withdrawal to reach the start of this phase, appears to be the determinant of graft success.

Donor care

This is of principal relevance to the DBD situation. There are two physiological phases following brain stem death, although the first may not be apparent in all patients:

1. Hyperdynamic phase: Catecholamine surge with hypertension, tachycardia and the risk of myocardial ischaemia
2. Cardiovascular collapse: Extreme vasodilation, myocardial depression (phosphate depletion, tri-iodothyronine insufficiency, electrolyte disturbance), loss of sympathetic tone and hypovolaemia (diabetes insipidus, diuresis due to hyperglycaemia or use of mannitol)

Maintenance of optimal organ function is vital during this gradual decompensation:

Pulmonary: Neurogenic pulmonary oedema, pneumonia and aspiration pneumonitis are problems. Regular physiotherapy, 2-hourly turning, inflation breaths and aseptic tracheal toilet are required. Antibiotics may be necessary. Limit positive end-expiratory pressure to 5 cmH$_2$O and minimise inspired oxygen to achieve a Pao_2 of 10 kPa.

Cardiovascular: Echocardiography should be used to evaluate cardiac function and a pulmonary artery catheter may be required if the left ventricular ejection fraction is <40%. Fluid, inotropes and vasopressors should be used to maintain a central venous pressure of 4–10 mmHg, mean arterial pressure 60–80 mmHg, heart rate of 60–100 beats in sinus rhythm and a cardiac index of >2.1 L/min/m^2. This also aims to minimise the chance of pulmonary oedema jeopardising retrieval of the lungs.

Endocrine: Pituitary function is lost with resulting diabetes insipidus, hyperglycaemia and cardiovascular depression due to reduced thyroid function. Infusions of tri-iodothyronine, vasopressin and insulin and boluses of methylprednisolone help address this.

Renal: In this particular context, there is evidence that low-dose dopamine improves postimplantation function of renal grafts.

Temperature: Hypothermia develops due to hypothalamic dysfunction and vasodilatation. Active warming should be employed.

Haematology: Maintain haemoglobin >90 g/L and treat coagulopathy with fresh-frozen plasma and platelets; disseminated intravascular coagulopathy is common due to release of tissue thromboplastin from necrotic brain.

Do not neglect care of the family at this very distressing time. Some nursing staff may find the transition from treating to save life to treating to sustain organ function difficult and they should be fully supported.

Retrieval process

For DCD this must proceed immediately following confirmation of death. The family should be warned in advance that they will have the 5 minutes of asystolic time required for confirmation of death to pay their respects before the donor is moved swiftly to theatre. If they need further time, the retrieval should be stood down.

For DBD, most cardiothoracic retrieval teams will bring their own anaesthetist. For an abdominal-only retrieval, the local anaesthetic team will be involved. The goal is continuation of organ optimisation. Opiates and neuromuscular blocking agents will help control reflexive hypertension and muscle contraction thus aiding organ preservation and surgical progress respectively.

Anaesthetic agents are not required. Once the organs are mobilised, the surgical team leader will ask for ventilation to be stopped and the organs will be removed following aortic cross-clamping.

Further reading

Academy of Medical Royal Colleges. A code of practice for the diagnosis and confirmation of death. London: AoMRC, 2008.

Intensive Care Society. Organ and tissue donation (2005). [Online] http://www.ics.ac.uk/ics-homepage/guidelines-standards/(2013)

NHS Blood and Transplant. Donor care. [Online] http://www.organdonation.nhs.uk/about_transplants/donor_care/index.asp (2013).

Related topics of interest

*   Ethics and consent (p. 76)
*   Major abdominal surgery (p. 108)

Orthopaedics – elective

Key points

- Neuraxial anaesthesia confers an unsustained early mortality benefit compared with general anaesthesia in lower limb surgery
- Venous thromboembolism has an incidence of up to 50% in hip surgery. Prophylaxis is essential for hip and knee surgery
- Bone cement implantation syndrome (BCIS) can cause significant haemodynamic changes and can be reduced by good surgical technique
- There is an increasing trend to perform upper limb surgery under regional anaesthesia. Large doses of local anaesthetic required risk local anaesthetic toxicity

Elective orthopaedic patients tend to be at the extremes of age, they may have multisystem disease and the procedures performed can have special hazards. Patient positioning, prolonged procedures, hypothermia and postoperative pain are problems common to many orthopaedic operations.

Lower limb prosthetic surgery

Predominantly older patients with osteoarthritis or rheumatoid arthritis present for knee or hip replacement. Over 60% of total hip replacements occur in patients over 65 years old. Exercise tolerance can be difficult to ascertain due to reduced mobility. As the population ages, revision surgery is becoming more frequent. Duration of surgery, blood loss and perioperative complications are significantly increased, in comparison to primary surgery. Invasive monitoring and cell salvage are often required.

Blood loss with total hip replacement may be large and can be reduced by cell salvage and tranexamic acid. Controlled hypotension and regional anaesthesia will reduce perioperative blood loss. Neuraxial techniques appear to carry an early survival advantage over general anaesthesia; however, there is no proven long-term benefit.

Intrathecal opioids can significantly improve postoperative analgesia, whilst postoperative epidural infusions are becoming less popular. Concurrent peripheral nerve blocks, such as femoral nerve block can also, contribute to postoperative analgesia. Nerve blocks may be associated with delay in early mobilisation, thus there is a trend towards use of lower concentrations of local anaesthetic for blocks. Enhanced recovery techniques for arthroplasty are gaining popularity using local anaesthetic wound infiltration and omission of intrathecal opioid with a view to earlier mobilisation.

Bone cement implantation syndrome (BCIS) is a poorly understood condition related to the insertion of methyl methacrylate cement. Clinical features include hypotension, hypoxia, arrhythmias, increased pulmonary vascular resistance and, rarely, cardiac arrest. The aetiology is not clear. Potential mechanisms include a direct cement-mediated effect, embolic (fat, marrow or cement) phenomena and models involving histamine and complement activation. It can be minimised by use of a cement gun (rather than placement by hand), medullary lavage and by venting the medulla to avoid high pressure (which can reach 600 mmHg) within the bone. Patients should be fluid preloaded prior to cementing and vasopressors may be needed. An increase in monitoring vigilance is required at this time. A drop in Sao_2 and end-tidal CO_2 may be seen.

Patients undergoing joint replacement are at high risk of deep vein thrombosis and mechanical and chemical prophylaxis should be used.

Upper limb surgery

Elective upper limb surgery has its own issues. Patient age and comorbidity are more diverse than hip and knee replacement surgery. Regional anaesthesia, in the form of brachial plexus blockade, is particularly useful for upper limb surgery. Interscalene block is most useful for shoulder surgery, whilst supra/infraclavicular or axillary block (+/- supplemental forearm nerve blocks) is more suited to hand and forearm surgery. Tourniquet pain may still be problematic unless dense plexus block is achieved. Regional anaesthesia can provide perioperative anaesthesia in the awake patient as well as excellent postoperative analgesia.

Care should be taken not to exceed the maximum safe dose, which may be easily reached, especially in underweight patients. Brachial plexus perineural catheters may be used in to provide ongoing analgesia in the postoperative period. Regional anaesthesia alone or with light sedation is now the norm for many centres providing elective hand surgery.

The main issues relate to patient positioning (often deck-chair for shoulder surgery), proximity of the surgical field to the airway, risk of air embolism and management of postoperative pain. Significant blood loss is also a risk, especially during shoulder arthroplasty.

Limb tourniquets

Tourniquets are contraindicated in peripheral arterial disease, crush injuries and sickle cell disease. The limb is exsanguinated by compression (e.g. with an Esmarch's bandage) or elevation for 4 minutes prior to inflation to 100 mmHg above the systolic blood pressure. Maximum inflation times, which should be documented, are 1 hour for the arm and 2 hours for the leg. Even with a fully functioning regional block, considerable discomfort from the tourniquet may be seen. Problems include skin and soft tissue damage, nerve palsy, ischaemic contracture, pulmonary embolism and severe hypotension on release. Sudden reperfusion of the ischaemic and acidotic limb can result in a severe systemic acidosis and, rarely, cardiac arrest. Bilateral tourniquets should be deflated with at least a 5-minute interval between them.

Further reading

Beecroft CL, Coventry DM. Anaesthesia for shoulder surgery. Br J Anaesth: Contin Educ Anaesth Crit Care Pain Med 2008; 8:193–198.

Borghi B, Zimpfer M, Blaicher AM (editors). 2nd European Congress of Orthopaedic and Trauma Anaesthesia. Anaesthesia 1998; 53:1–80.

Donaldson AJ, Thomson HE, Harper NJ, et al. Bone cement implantation syndrome. Br J Anaesth 2009; 102:12–22.

Loach A. Orthopaedic Anaesthesia, 2nd Ed. London: Hodder Arnold, 1994.

Related topics of interest

Orthopaedics – emergency

Key points

- Fracture neck of femur carries a significant mortality. This can be reduced by minimising the time to definitive surgery. Patients commonly have multiple comorbidities
- Open fractures require urgent surgery, although delay of up to 13 hours may not increase infection risks
- Compartment syndrome has an incidence of 4% in tibial shaft fracture. Regional anaesthesia remains controversial, although evidence of harm is scant

The majority of emergency orthopaedic surgery is due to physical trauma. The patient group is diverse and includes those at the extremes of age. The AAGBI recommend provision of dedicated trauma lists to ensure that emergency patients are managed by skilled teams during daylight hours, rather than out-of-hours by junior staff.

Hip fracture surgery

Nearly 80,000 patients with hip fractures are treated each year in the UK. The majority of patients are aged over 65, many have multiple comorbidities and 30-day mortality remains at 8–10%. Cardiovascular, respiratory disease and cognitive impairment are particularly frequent problems and multidisciplinary orthogeriatric input is useful, both pre- and postoperatively.

Surgical repair remains the most effective form of analgesia. It is recognised that outcome can be improved by early surgery and mobilisation. Both morbidity and mortality increase when surgery is delayed beyond 48 hours from admission. To this end, the Department of Health has set a target of 24 hours from decision to operation. The British Orthopaedic Association has suggested surgery should be performed within 48 hours of admission, unless there are medical conditions which can be easily optimised.

The issue of delay for 'optimisation' was highlighted in the 2010 CEPOD report 'An age old problem' which recommended that senior anaesthetic, medical and surgical input is required at this point.

Preoperative assessment should focus on comorbidities and easily reversible pathologies. Around 70% of patients will be ASA 3–4. Preoperative nerve blocks (such as fascia iliaca) can be helpful in alleviating pain whilst waiting for surgery. Preoperative anaemia can lead to perioperative myocardial and cerebral ischaemia and should be treated. Surgery should not be delayed if patients are on antithrombotic agents but a greater perioperative blood loss should be anticipated. Many centres now offer routine echocardiography in this patient group to assess ventricular function and aortic valve status (calcific AS being associated with morbidity in this patient group). However, most anaesthetists would modify their anaesthetic according to clinical suspicion in the absence of an echo.

Patients lacking mental capacity require special consideration and every effort should be made to involve their family and carers in their care. As with elective hip surgery, there appears to be no compelling evidence regarding general versus regional anaesthesia with complication rates and length of stay broadly similar. Clear advantages of regional anaesthesia in the elderly include less postoperative confusion, reduced respiratory complications and reduced perioperative blood loss.

Nerve blocks, such as '3-in-1' (achieves blockade of all three nerves in only 20% of cases), fascia iliaca and lumbar plexus blocks can be used to supplement general anaesthesia. Deep vein thrombosis has a reported incidence of 30–60% following hip fracture without thromboprophylaxis. Low molecular weight heparin should be used both pre- and postoperatively.

Open fractures

Early antibiotic therapy and early debridement have always been the mainstay of treatment for open fractures. Although antibiotics are still given at initial patient assessment, there is now some debate regarding necessity for surgical debridement within 6 hours of injury. Many recent studies have found that there is little increase in infection rates if debridement is delayed until up to 13 hours after injury. Infection is more likely in lower limb open fractures than upper limb. The British Orthopaedic Association currently recommends intravenous co-amoxiclav or cephalosporin within 3 hours of injury.

Compartment syndrome

Compartment syndrome occurs when the pressure within a tissue compartment is persistently raised above 30–45 mmHg. Reperfusion of damaged ischaemic tissue within the compartment results in further increases in pressure (the ischaemia-reperfusion-ischaemia cycle). Incidence is around 4% in tibial shaft fracture and it may be seen following long-bone fracture due to bleeding, oedema or infection within the tissue compartment. Symptoms comprise pain and paraesthesia; however, signs are unreliable. It is a surgical emergency and should be treated promptly with fasciotomy.

There is ongoing debate regarding the suitability of regional anaesthesia in patients at risk of compartment syndrome due to a perception that regional anaesthesia may delay the diagnosis and hence treatment of compartment syndrome. A review in 2009 concluded that there was no convincing evidence of delayed diagnosis in the presence of regional anaesthesia and that clinical diagnosis could be made regardless of the presence of regional blockade. If regional anaesthesia is used in high-risk patients, there should be regular monitoring of the affected limb for signs of tissue ischaemia.

Fat embolism

Fat embolism occurs in 2% of femoral fractures and after 0.1% of hip and knee replacements. It is much more common after multiple trauma (up to 90%). Fatty marrow is released, embolised and causes lung damage. A triad of respiratory compromise, cerebral dysfunction and petaechial haemorrhages is described. Cardiovascular, respiratory and nervous system signs are similar to those with air embolism. Fat emboli may also be seen in the urine, sputum and retinal blood vessels. It may be complicated by secondary infection, acute lung injury, disseminated intravascular coagulation and multiorgan failure. Supportive treatment is needed and fixation of any fractures is performed. Steroids, heparin and aspirin have all been advocated.

Paediatric fractures

Trauma is the leading cause of death in children aged over 1. However, most paediatric fractures are isolated limb injuries, such as supracondylar, radius/ulnar or lower limb long-bone fractures. Concealed haemorrhage following long-bone fracture in a child is often underestimated.

Preoperative assessment should focus on the timing of injury relative to last oral intake and analgesics given since. Rapid sequence induction is often required if the injury occurred within 6 hours of food or if significant amounts of opiates have been given since. Sedative premedication may be required for the anxious child and a multimodal approach should be used to manage pain. Preoperative analgesia can be successfully provided by use of intranasal diamorphine or ketamine in addition to paracetamol and NSAID.

Postoperative analgesia may be provided by regional anaesthetic blocks, judicious use of opiates and the WHO pain ladder. There is a general acceptance that regional anaesthesia may be performed in asleep paediatric patients.

Further reading

Gupta A. Reilly CS. Fat embolism. Br J Anaesth: Contin Educ Anaesth Crit Care Pain Med 2007; 7:148–151.

Association of Anaesthetists of Great Britain and Ireland (AAGBI). AAGBI safety guideline: management of proximal femoral fractures. London; AAGBI, 2012.

Mar GJ, Barrington MJ, McGuirk BR. Acute compartment syndrome of the lower limb and the effect of postoperative analgesia on diagnosis. Br J Anaesth 2009; 102:3–11.

Related topics of interest

- Blood transfusion and salvage (p. 22)
- Elderly patients (p. 64)
- Emergency anaesthesia (p. 70)
- Orthopaedics – elective (p. 174)
- Paediatric anaesthesia – basic concepts (p. 179)
- Paediatric anaesthesia – basic practical conduct (p. 183)
- Pain – acute management (p. 198)
- Polytrauma (p. 217)
- Regional anaesthesia – central and neuraxial blockade (p. 242)
- Regional anaesthesia – plexus and peripheral nerve blocks (p. 247)
- Venous thromboembolism – risk (p. 324)
- Venous thromboembolism – prevention and treatment (p. 320)

Paediatric anaesthesia – basic concepts

Key points

- Appreciation of the significant differences between adult and paediatric physiology is essential to provide safe anaesthesia to paediatric patients
- Hypoxia occurs quickly and will result in bradycardia in neonates and infants
- Apnoea is common in neonates and infants undergoing surgery
- Immature metabolic systems and altered physiology necessitate adjustment of drug dosing in small children

There are many important differences in the anatomy, physiology and pharmacology of adults and children; a detailed description is beyond the scope of this text. This topic focuses on how the clinical practice of paediatric anaesthesia is influenced by these differences.

Airway and respiratory management

- The tongue is relatively large and the upper airway and trachea are easily obstructed by soft tissue compression. An oropharyngeal airway or jaw thrust may be needed and extra care is required when holding a mask. Gastric insufflation occurs at low airway pressures
- The larynx lies at C3-C4 rather than C4-C6, the occiput is large and the airway can become obstructed with overextension therefore head position should be neutral for mask ventilation and laryngoscopy (may require a shoulder roll). The epiglottis is large and floppy and straight blade laryngoscopes are often preferred for infants under one
- The cricoid is the narrowest portion, and the only solid circumferential component of the airway. Minor trauma can cause oedema and postextubation stridor/long-term subglottic stenosis. Uncuffed endotracheal tubes (ETT) are placed

so that there is a small leak in pre-pubertal children. Placement of a cuffed ETT requires a reduction in tube size and therefore internal diameter with a subsequent increase in airway resistance
- The trachea is short (5 cm in the neonate) and precise placement and fixation of the ETT is essential with reassessment of bilateral air entry after repositioning for surgery

Mode of ventilation

- Functional residual capacity (FRC) is low due to the combination of a compliant chest wall and elastic recoil of the lung. Closing volume is large and encroaches on FRC even during normal tidal breathing. FRC decreases significantly during apnoea and anaesthesia, accompanied by airway closure and impaired oxygenation. Infants generally require controlled ventilation during anaesthesia and benefit from high respiratory rates and positive end-expiratory pressure
- Continuous positive airway pressure during mask ventilation prevents airway closure and the collapse of soft tracheal cartilages and tissues in the pharynx and nasopharynx

Prevention of hypoxia

- Neonates have a high oxygen requirement reflected in an alveolar ventilation of twice that of adults (150 mL/kg/min vs. 60 mL/kg/min). The ratio of alveolar ventilation to FRC is high (5:1 vs. 1.5:1 in adults), meaning a reduced ventilatory reserve and more rapid onset of hypoxia during anaesthesia if there is any airway obstruction
- In the early neonatal period, pulmonary arteries remain very sensitive to the vasoconstrictor effects of hypoxaemia, acidosis and serotonin and to the vasodilator effects of acetyl choline

and nitric oxide. If hypoxia occurs, circulation can revert to a transitional state: pulmonary vascular resistance (PVR) increases, the foramen ovale opens and the ductus arteriosus may also re-open so blood bypasses the pulmonary circulation causing a further reduction in arterial oxygenation. Impaired tissue oxygenation also results in acidosis which leads to further increase in PVR. This cycle can complicate any condition causing hypoxia/acidosis, e.g. congenital diaphragmatic hernia, respiratory distress syndrome, cardiac failure, surgical stress or sepsis

- The neonatal response to hypoxia is bradycardia. The neonatal myocardium has less contractile tissue (30% vs. 60%) than the adult and the myofibrils and sarcoplasmic reticulum within the contractile tissue are immature; this means that the myocardium is less compliant when relaxed and generates less tension during contraction. Stroke volume is relatively fixed, thus cardiac output (CO) is rate dependant. Consequently, bradycardia leads to a dramatic fall in CO and is poorly tolerated (**Tables 43** and **44**)
- Awake and normothermic preterm and term infants <1 week in age demonstrate a biphasic response to hypoxia; a brief initial hyperpnoea followed by ventilatory depression. This is not seen in older children and adults who respond with an increase in ventilation. Hypothermic infants and very pre-term infants respond directly with ventilatory depression. Hypoxia may induce 'periodic breathing' in many preterm and some full-term infants. Some preterm infants demonstrate life-threatening episodes of apnoea, which commonly exceed 20 seconds and may be accompanied by bradycardia and desaturation. Apnoeas may be central or obstructive in origin. Pre-term and former pre-term infants up to 60 weeks post-conceptual age, especially those with anaemia, respiratory disease and neurological disease, are at risk from post-operative apnoeas even if they are apnoea-free at the time of anaesthesia. They must be monitored post-operatively. Oxygen is protective against apnoeas
- Pre-term infants are at risk of retinopathy of prematurity (retrolental hyperplasia of blood vessels) associated with a high Pao_2. The risk persists until approximately 8 months of age and oxygen saturations should be maintained between 90% and 96% in at-risk babies

Fluid and electrolyte replacement therapy

- Renal function in the neonate is limited by immaturity of tubular function and an increased renal vascular resistance. There is reduced renal blood flow and glomerular filtration rate (GFR). Adult values are usually achieved by 1 year of age

Table 43 Normal heart rates for children	
Age	**Heart rate (bpm)**
Neonatal	100–170
<1 year	80–160
2 years	80–130
4 years	80–120
6–10 years	75–115
10–14 years	60–105
14–16 years	55–100

Table 44 Normal blood pressure in children	
Age	**Blood pressure (mmHg)**
Preterm	49/24
Term	60/35
<1 month	70/35
<6 months	95/40
4 years	95/55
6–8 years	110/60
8–12 years	115/65
12–16 years	120/65

- The ability to modify the glomerular filtrate for conservation or excretion is impaired, thus sodium losses may be large, particularly in pre-term infants
- Maintenance requirements are covered in the next chapter. A fluid management plan for any child should address three key issues:
  - Fluid deficit present
  - Maintenance requirements
  - Losses due to surgery, e.g. blood loss, '3rd space' losses
- During surgery, these losses should be managed by isotonic fluids in all children over 1 month of age. Hypoglycaemia is more likely in those on parenteral nutrition, receiving dextrose-containing solutions pre-operatively, low body weight (<3rd centile), surgical duration >3 hours and extensive regional anaesthesia. These children should receive dextrose-containing fluids or have blood sugar monitoring during surgery
- Neonates are born 'waterlogged' and then lose 10% of their body weight in the 1st week of life. They therefore require smaller maintenance volumes, increasing over the next few days. Premature/low birth weight babies have a greater surface area:weight ratio, lose more water by evaporation and therefore require more replacement fluid (**Table 45**)

Blood glucose

- Stores of glycogen in the liver and myocardium in the term infant are used during the first few hours of life until gluconeogenesis becomes established. Small-for-gestational age and pre-term infants may have inadequate stores and are very dependent on intravenous infusions to prevent hypoglycaemia (see above)

Temperature maintenance

- Infants lose heat rapidly due to their large surface area:body weight ratio and their lack of heat-insulating subcutaneous fat. Infants rely primarily on non-shivering thermogenesis, which occurs mainly in brown adipose tissue (contains high numbers of iron-containing mitochondria, has a rich blood supply and sympathetic innervation) located between the scapulae, and alongside the great vessels in the thorax and abdomen. This results in large increases in glucose and oxygen consumption, which can cause acidosis. Furthermore hypothermia abolishes the biphasic ventilatory response to hypoxia, resulting in initial ventilatory depression

Drug dosing

- Inhalational agents

Induction of anaesthesia with inhalational agents is more rapid in infants and small children due to the increased alveolar ventilation:FRC ratio, lower blood:gas solubility and tissue:blood solubility and more rapid distribution to vessel-rich groups. Elimination is also more rapid. Minimum alveolar concentration (MAC) is greater in infants than in older children and adults, the reason for this is unknown. There are slight increases at the time of puberty. Note that, unlike other agents, the MAC of sevoflurane is greatest in the term neonate and falls progressively rather than peaking in the infant. Bradycardia can occur in infants during induction with sevoflurane especially with trisomy 21. Significant hypotension can occur if very high concentrations of inhalational agents are given to infants, particularly with controlled ventilation (**Table 46**).

Table 45 Maintenance fluid requirements in children		
	Fluid requirement	Rate
1st 48 hours	10% Dextrose	2–3 mL/kg/h or 40–80 mL/kg/day
Day 3 onwards	10% Dextrose + 0.18 % Saline	4 mL/kg/h or 100–120 mL/kg/day

Table 46 MAC of inhalational agents in different age groups			
	<6 Months	<1 Year	Adult
Halothane	0.8	1.2	0.75
Sevoflurane	3.1	2.5	1.7
Isoflurane	1.6	1.8	1.15
Desflurane	8	11	6.0

- Induction agents

Induction agents act faster in neonates, in part due to the higher proportion of CO going to the brain (25%). Propofol is widely used in children; higher doses are required than for adults (3–5 mg/kg). Pain on injection is common, decreased with addition of lignocaine (1 mg/10 mg propofol). Ketamine maintains blood pressure and is the agent of choice in shocked infants and children

- Neuromuscular blockers

Infants require a relatively higher dose of succinylcholine than adults (2 mg/kg) due to distribution of drug throughout the relatively large extracellular fluid compartment. Bradycardia is common after a single intravenous dose which can be prevented by prior administration of intravenous atropine or glycopyrrolate. Intramuscular administration (4 mg/kg) is effective and has minimal effect on the heart rate

Nondepolarising neuromuscular blockers are given in a similar dose per kilogram as adults (due to a combination of the larger volume of distribution and a greater degree of block for a specific plasma concentration in the infant). Their duration of action however is more variable, probably due to immaturity of muscle fibres and receptor sites.

Elimination of those agents metabolised by the kidneys or liver is prolonged in neonates/infants

- Local anaesthetics

High plasma levels may be reached due to increased tissue blood flow and cardiac output. Metabolism is reduced because of immature enzyme systems and protein binding is less in neonates due to reduced total serum protein concentrations (e.g. a-1 acid glycoprotein). More of the administered drug is thus free in the plasma to exert a clinical effect and reduced doses of drugs are indicated

- Opioids

Neonates have little fat or muscle tissue so drugs normally distributed throughout these tissues will have greater plasma concentrations and prolonged duration of action. The elimination half-life of drugs such as morphine and fentanyl is increased up to a few months of age due to immature conjugation pathways

- Antibiotics

Reduced GFR and tubular secretion capacity require that greater intervals between doses of drugs excreted by the kidneys (most antibiotics) are necessary

Further reading

http://www.apagbi.org.uk/publications/apa-guidelines

Related topics of interest

Paediatric anaesthesia – basic practical conduct

Key points

- Preoperative assessment is an important time to establish a rapport with the child
- Perinatal and developmental history should be included in the preoperative assessment
- Sedative premedication may be useful for children with learning difficulties
- There is an obligation on the anaesthetist to consider child protection issues and concerns must be acted upon

This section covers the practical management of many of the issues explored in the previous topic on paediatric basic concepts.

Safe provision of paediatric services

There have been significant changes to the delivery of paediatric anaesthesia and surgery in the UK in recent years and the correct balance between district general hospitals and centralisation is still being sought. The Royal College of Anaesthetists offers guidance and recommendations for the safe provision of paediatric anaesthetic services.

Preoperative assessment

This is an important time to review the notes and develop a rapport with both child and parents/carer which should not be underestimated. The anaesthetic and analgesic techniques should be discussed in full, any questions answered and further explanations given. Consent (e.g. for suppositories, regional anaesthesia) should be sought (**Table 47**).

Premedication

Topical local anaesthetic cream should be applied if an intravenous induction is being considered (**Table 48**).

Sedation may be indicated plus preoperative analgesia. Common choices for sedation include oral midazolam or

Table 47 Key principles of pre-assessment		
History	**Examination**	**Further action**
Perinatal	Weight	Resuscitation as indicated
Medical – comorbidity and	Baseline observations	Review Investigations
intercurrent illness, e.g. RTI	Airway – note loose teeth/conditions	Request and review other relevant
Anaesthetic (child and family)	predisposing to difficult intubation	investigations
Drugs	Cardiovascular	Optimise medical condition
Allergies	Respiratory	Continue relevant usual drugs
Immunisation status	Abdominal	Formulate anaesthetic plan and convey to
Starvation times	Neurological – baseline level of cognitive	child and parents in age-appropriate way
	function in children with special needs,	Premedication as required
	anxiety level	
RTI; respiratory tract infection.		

Table 48 Comparison of topical local anaesthesia for venous access			
	Ametop	**LMX-4**	**EMLA**
Anaesthetic component	4% Tetracaine	4% Lignocaine	Eutectic mixture of 2.5% lignocaine and 2.5% prilocaine
Onset of action	30–40 minutes	30 minutes	45–60 minutes
Duration of action	4–6 hours	40–60 minutes	2 hours

clonidine; there are pros and cons to both. Oral midazolam is effective more rapidly (approximately 20 mins), produces anterograde amnesia, may reduce postoperative psychological sequelae and does not result in excessive prolonged sedation. However, it has a bitter taste and may cause severe disinhibition and restlessness in some children. Clonidine is effective as a sedative but has a longer onset time (approximately 45 minutes). It may improve intraoperative haemodynamic stability and enhance postoperative analgesia.

Oral ketamine can be used, but is usually reserved for the most challenging behaviour, such as children with severe autism.

Starvation times

Recommended minimum fasting times for children are indicated in **Table 49**.

Useful formulae

Estimated weight of a full-term baby 3–4 kg.
Estimated weight:
  1–12 months: (0.5 × age months) + 4
  1–5 years: (2 × age years) + 8
  6–12 years: (3 × age years) + 7
Tracheal tube size: (Age/4) + 4
Length of tracheal tube:
  (Age/2) + 12 (Term 3–3.5 mm, 9 cm at lips)

Perioperative management

Induction

Parental presence is usual practice in the UK; however, this may not be suitable for all, e.g. if induction occurs in theatre, very sick children, patients declining parental presence or if parental distress is likely to increase the child's anxiety. A ward nurse should be designated to accompany the forewarned parents out of the anaesthetic room once the child is anaesthetised or at the request of the anaesthetist – this is especially important if the parent is present during a rapid sequence induction (RSI).

Induction technique will depend upon the medical needs of the patient and urgency of securing the airway. The need for RSI is suggested by a full stomach, trauma, airway bleeding or gastro-oesophageal reflux disease. An inhalational induction is likely in the patient presenting with stridor, airway obstruction or difficult intravenous access. In other situations the wishes of the child, parent and anaesthetist can be considered.

Maintenance

Volatile agents are commonly used. Total intravenous anaesthesia (using paediatric algorithms) is particularly useful in procedures or patients associated with nausea and vomiting.

Airway

For brief procedures not requiring intubation a facemask and Ayre's T-piece is effective. The laryngeal mask airway (LMA) is commonly used in elective paediatric surgery; however, intubation is generally recommended for neonates for a secure airway and to prevent gastric distension. For surgery requiring muscle relaxation patients are generally intubated. Specifically designed paediatric cuffed endotracheal tubes offer many advantages over the traditional uncuffed tubes and have a good safety profile.

Fluids

Fluid requirements are determined by the pre-existing deficit, maintenance requirements and ongoing losses. In elective cases deficit can be calculated by multiplying the hourly requirement by the starvation period. In emergency cases, hypovolaemia should be corrected with a bolus of 10–20 mL/kg of an isotonic fluid or colloid and reassessed and repeated as necessary

Table 49 Minimal fasting times in children	
Substance	Minimum fasting time (hours)
Clear fluids	2
Breast/formula milk	4
Food/solids/cow's milk	6

according to Advanced Paediatric Life Support guidelines.

Maintenance fluid should be isotonic and, in the majority of cases, without dextrose. Volumes can be guided by the Holliday–Segar formula for children over 4 weeks old; below that, requirements are generally reduced (**Table 50**).

Ongoing losses include estimated occult losses (e.g. evaporative losses from surgical sites) and actual blood loss. In children over 3 months of age the haematocrit may be allowed to fall to 25%, the commonly used transfusion trigger is 70 g/L. However, transfusion should be considered in the context of the clinical situation (cyanotic congenital heart disease patients may need a higher haematocrit), preoperative haemoglobin and likelihood of ongoing blood loss.

Temperature regulation

Attention to detail is important. Strategies to avoid hypothermia include core temperature monitoring, warm theatre, overhead heaters, HME, forced air warmers, warming mattress and warmed fluids.

Emergence

Laryngospasm is the most common problem encountered (particularly in the very young or recent upper respiratory tract infection) and consideration should be given to the risks and benefits of awake versus deep extubation or LMA removal depending upon the clinical situation.

Postoperative care

Cannulae should always be flushed prior to transfer to recovery. Recovery should occur in a specially designed area separated from adult cases, with appropriately trained staff, a clear handover, postoperative instructions and contact details for the responsible anaesthetist be provided (**Table 51**).

Child protection

Duties of the anaesthetist include acting in the best interests of the child, being aware of the child's rights to protection and confidentiality, local child protection mechanisms and the rights of those with parental responsibility. A paediatrician with experience of child protection should be contacted for advice if there are concerns.

Table 50 Holliday-Segar formula for estimating basic IV fluid requirements in children	
Weight (kg)	mL/h
<10	4/kg
11–20	40 + 2/kg for each kg >10
>20	60 + 1/kg for each kg >20

Table 51 Postoperative analgesia and antiemesis			
Complication	Preoperative strategy	Perioperative strategy	Postoperative strategy
Postoperative nausea and vomiting (PONV)	Identification of risk factors: • Age (increased risk >3 years) • Postpubertal female • Previous PONV • Motion sickness • Use of volatile agents • Surgical procedure, e.g. adenotonsillectomy, strabismus correction, otoplasty, plus surgery >30 minutes	• Prophylaxis for high risk cases (ondansetron, dexamethasone) • Propofol, TIVA • Avoidance of precipitants, e.g. opioids, use of regional anaesthesia where indicated • IV fluids to maintain hydration	• Multimodal antiemetic agents • IV fluids • Avoidance of early mobilisation • Avoidance of early oral fluids
Pain	• Identification of high-risk procedures • Preoperative analgesia Psychological preparation	• Multimodal analgesia • Regional analgesia • Adjuncts to spinal local anaesthetics, e.g. clonidine	• Regular pain assessment • Pain team involvement • Multimodal approach • Nonpharmacological strategies, e.g. parental reassurance, play therapy and distraction
TIVA, total intravenous anaesthesia.			

Further reading

The Association of Paediatric Anaesthetists of Great Britain and Ireland. http://www.apagbi.org.uk

Berry J, Waterhouse P. Principles of paediatric anaesthesia. Anaesth Intensive Care Med 2007; 8:169–175.

Clark N, Nolan J. The principles of paediatric anaesthesia. Anaesth Intensive Care Med 2010; 11:205–209.

Royal College of Anaesthetists. Guidance on the provision of paediatric anaesthesia services. Chapter 10. In; Guidelines for the provision of anaesthetic services 2013. London; RCOA publications, 2013.

Related topics of interest

- Paediatric anaesthesia – basic concepts (p. 179)
- Paediatric anaesthesia – neonatal surgery (p. 187)
- Paediatric anaesthesia – pyloric stenosis (p. 191)
- Paediatric emergency airways (p. 194)

Paediatric anaesthesia – neonatal surgery

Key points

- Neonatal physiology is a distinct variant from older patients and evolves on a daily basis
- The margin of error is reduced
- Intraoperative communication with the surgical team is vital

Contrary to historical beliefs, neonates (0–28 days) feel pain and as a result effective anaesthesia is essential for surgical interventions. Recent concerns regarding neuronal apoptosis associated with general anaesthesia in animal models has, however, resulted in a more guarded approach to its use.

The transition from placental support to autologous organ function creates a rapidly changing and challenging physiological model. Key anatomical and physiological differences in the neonate necessitate a tailored approach to their anaesthesia.

- Increased total body water: Neonates are 85% water and have a reduced fat and muscle component. This impacts upon doses required for muscle relaxation and the relative distribution of fat-dispersed agents
- Immature liver function: Although capable of metabolising most agents, metabolism is generally delayed
- Immature renal function: Glomerular filtration rate increases rapidly over the first month. As a result, drug half-lives and fluid requirements can change on an almost daily basis
- Minimum alveolar concentration (MAC) requirements: The MAC for the volatiles increases to a peak at 3–6 months before reducing gradually. Neonatal requirements are greater than those of children above the age of 1. The exception is sevoflurane, for which the MAC in neonates does not change significantly through to 6 months of age
- Blood volume: Although relatively higher (80 mL/kg) than older children, a typical 2 kg neonate only requires a 40 mL blood

loss to lose a quarter of their circulating volume
- Temperature control: Neonates have poor temperature control, quickly becoming hypothermic and coagulopathic
- Delicate airways: A carefully positioned uncuffed endotracheal tube is used for the following reasons:
  - The cricoid ring is the narrowest part of the upper airway
  - The Hagen–Poiseuille equation helps account for the disproportionate reduction in gas flow following small reductions in airway diameter. Cuffed endotracheal tubes require a smaller internal diameter
  - Slight movements of the airway device can compromise the airway through obstruction, endobronchial intubation or unintentional extubation
  - Mucosal pressure from an airway device can compromise tissue perfusion pressure creating subsequent oedema
  - A poor seal and tendency for dislodgement/obstruction usually preclude the use of the laryngeal mask airway in neonates

Congenital diaphragmatic hernia

Abdominal contents herniated into the thorax through a congenital defect. Poor prognostic signs include the liver situated in the chest and antenatally measured lung to head ratio <1. Death is common, with a 20% mortality associated in neonates surviving to surgical repair. The primary danger is pulmonary hypertension secondary to reactive vasculature, lung hypoplasia and ventilatory barotrauma. The main principle of care is delayed surgery after physiological stabilisation.

Perioperative considerations

- Immediate intubation, avoidance of facemask intermittent positive pressure ventilation

- Nasogastric (NG) tube placement
- 'Gentilation' ventilation strategy (avoidance of barotrauma at the expense of permissive hypercapnia and lower postductal O_2 saturation), inhaled nitric oxide, HFOV or ECMO as required
- Inotropic support
- Surgery, after physiological stabilisation. Typically normal mean arterial pressure, preductal O_2 saturation levels of 85–95%, FiO_2 50%, Lactate <3 mmol/L and urine output >2 mL/kg/h
- Reduction of the viscera into the abdomen may cause ventilatory compromise. In the event of increased abdominal pressure an abdominal patch may be utilised by the surgeon
- Kinking of the liver vessels during reduction can precipitate a drop in venous return
- Sudden deterioration may be due to pulmonary hypertensive crisis

Inguinal hernia

It is one of the most common (and surgically challenging) neonatal surgical procedures occurring in 1% of term babies. It can present electively for repair or as an acute emergency with incarcerated or strangulated bowel. Unlike adult hernia repairs a mesh is not employed.

Perioperative considerations

- Often associated with prematurity and the associated respiratory complications
- Spinal anaesthesia is a useful technique for opiate sparing in the apnoea-prone neonate

Postoperative care

- All neonates and infants <54 weeks postconceptual age, will require admission and overnight saturation monitoring due to the increased risk of apnoea
- Caudal anaesthesia is highly effective as an opiate sparing technique

Intestinal obstruction

This is a common reason for an exploratory laparotomy in the neonate. The most common causes include:

- Bowel atresia: Can occur anywhere in the GI tract but typically affects the duodenum (especially in trisomy 21) or the small bowel
- Malrotation and volvulus: A surgical emergency where the position of the bowel predisposes it to twisting and occluding its blood supply. This can result in catastrophic bowel loss within hours
- Hirschsprung's disease: Congenital aganglionosis of the distal intestine causes a functional obstruction, which may require decompressive stoma formation prior to definitive surgery
- Anorectal malformations: The absence of a normal anus leads to obstruction, typically requiring a sigmoid colostomy prior to definitive surgery
- Meconium Ileus: Associated with cystic fibrosis in 90% of cases. The abnormal composition of the meconium due to the chloride channel abnormalities causes a luminal obstruction. On-table enterostomy with bowel washout and often stoma formation are required

Perioperative considerations

- Sepsis, hypovolaemia and electrolyte imbalance
- Abdominal splinting due to distention
- Duodenal atresia and anorectal malformations are associated with cardiac anomalies and often require a pre operative echocardiogram
- High risk of aspiration

Abdominal wall defects

The most common abdominal wall defect is gastroschisis, where the bowel is herniated through the abdominal wall and does not possess a covering. Exomphalos is bowel herniation with a covering and, unlike gastroschisis, is associated with other congenital anomalies. The aim is to reduce the contents into the abdomen either primarily or in a staged procedure using a prosthetic bag (silo) applied over the herniated abdominal contents.

Preoperative considerations

- Hypovolaemia and hypothermia due to the exposed bowel

- Associated cardiac anomalies and hypoglycaemia in exomphalos
- NG decompression is required

Conduct of anaesthesia

- The most critical phase is the reduction of the abdominal contents. Raised intra-abdominal pressure can cause respiratory and organ compromise. Communication between the anaesthetic and surgical team is vital to decide on whether to continue reduction or to convert to silo application
- Secure medium-term intravenous access is mandatory as all gastroschisis patients will require parenteral nutrition

Postoperative care

- Monitor for abdominal compartment syndrome
- Post op ventilation is common

Necrotising enterocolitis (NEC)

NEC is a poorly understood disease resulting in focal- to pan-intestinal wall necrosis in premature infants. Although it can be managed with bowel rest, intravenous antibiotics and supportive care, surgical intervention is required in up to a third of cases. Surgical intervention ranges from percutaneous drainage to laparotomy with extensive bowel resection and stoma formation. Morbidity and mortality is high.

Preoperative considerations

- Prematurity and its associated complications
- Sepsis
- Multisystem failure
- Thrombocytopaenia and coagulopathy
- Hypovolaemia

Conduct of anaesthesia

- Avoid intraoperative hypothermia as this may cause worsening coagulopathy and lead to irreversible liver haemorrhage
- Surgery is often a 'damage control' scenario requiring a rapid operation, followed by stabilisation and second look surgery

Tracheoesophageal fistula and oesophageal atresia

In this condition, abnormal separation of the trachea and oesophagus can result in five possible configurations (**Figure 14**). The most common configuration is oesophageal atresia with a distal fistula accounting for 85% of cases. The neonate typically has respiratory compromise, bubbling at the mouth and it is not possible to pass an NG tube. Diagnosis is confirmed on a plain chest X-ray with the

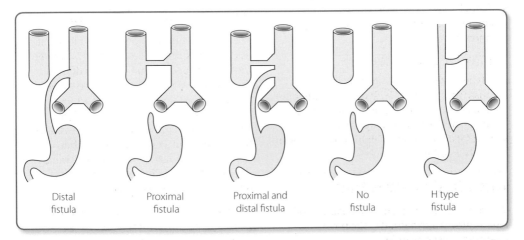

| Distal fistula | Proximal fistula | Proximal and distal fistula | No fistula | H type fistula |

Figure 14 Anatomical classification of tracheo-oesophageal fistula and oesophageal atresia.

NG tube curled in the upper oesophagus. The operative repair can typically wait for semielective repair. Rarely, it is associated with gas trapping in the stomach, leading to abdominal distension, splinting and gastric perforation requiring emergency tracheoesophageal fistula (TOF) ligation.

Preoperative considerations

- Associated cardiac anomalies and right sided aortic arches can be detected on echocardiogram
- Specialised tube suction (known as a Replogle tube) prevents overspill of saliva from the proximal pouch to the lungs
- Avoid noninvasive ventilation as this can exacerbate gas trapping in the stomach

Conduct of anaesthesia

- Tracheal tube positioning, ideally placing the tip distal to the fistula (but avoiding endo-oesophageal intubation) reduces the chance of gas trapping in the stomach
- Preoperative flexible bronchoscopy is often performed to identify the site, size and number of fistulae
- Surgical lung retraction often results in impaired ventilation; frequent surgical breaks may be required to allow rerecruitment

Postoperative

- Postoperative paralysis and ventilation is often employed to protect the oesophageal repair

Further reading

Zisovska E. Anaesthetics safe in neonates. London; World Health Organisation Secretariat, 2012.

Reiss I, Schaible T, van den Hout, L et al. Standardized postnatal management of infants with congenital diaphragmatic hernia in Europe: the CDH EURO Consortium consensus. Neonatology 2010; 98:354–364.

Related topics of interest

Paediatric anaesthesia – pyloric stenosis

Key points

- Pyloric stenosis may be a medical but not a surgical emergency. The classic metabolic derangement is a hypokalaemic, hypochloraemic metabolic alkalosis
- Postoperative monitoring is required due to the risk of postoperative respiratory depression

Disease summary

Infantile hypertrophic pyloric stenosis (IHPS) is a condition, affecting approximately 1 in 400 live births, in which the pyloric portion of the stomach becomes abnormally thickened leading to gastric outlet obstruction. Affected infants usually present between 2 and 3 weeks old and only rarely after 12 weeks old.

Typical presenting symptoms include immediate, postprandial, nonbilious, projectile vomiting with a demand to be refed soon afterwards. There may be weight loss and failure to thrive. Infants are typically diagnosed early but may present with significant dehydration and electrolyte abnormalities, which must be corrected before surgery.

The exact aetiology of pyloric stenosis is unknown but is probably multifactorial including genetic and environmental factors. It is four times more common in males than females and around 30% of cases occur in first-born children. Having a sibling with IHPS confers a 20-fold increase in risk compared to an infant with no affected relatives. There may be an association with administration of macrolide antibiotics either directly to infants under 2 weeks old or to women in late pregnancy or during breastfeeding.

Problems

- Preoperative resuscitation required for metabolic abnormalities and dehydration
- Risk of aspiration on induction
- Risk of postoperative apnoea

Diagnosis

Diagnosis is usually made on the clinical presentation and palpation of an 'olive-like' mass of hypertrophied pyloric muscle at the lateral edge of the rectus abdominis muscle in the right upper quadrant of the abdomen. The mass may be difficult to feel in infants who present early before they are significantly dehydrated and the diagnosis can be confirmed by an ultrasound or an upper GI contrast study.

Treatment

Pyloric stenosis is not a surgical emergency; however, it may be a medical one.

Preoperative resuscitation

Dehydration and metabolic abnormalities are often present and must be corrected before surgical management is undertaken. Vomiting of gastric contents containing sodium, potassium and hydrochloric acid leads to a hypokalamic, hypochloraemic metabolic alkalosis and dehydration, which can be severe.

An intravenous cannula should be placed and blood samples analysed for electrolyte concentrations and acid–base status. Oral feeds should be stopped and a nasogastric tube placed, allowing stomach contents to be aspirated if vomiting continues despite stopping feeds. An assessment of dehydration should be made based on estimated percentage weight loss, urine output and clinical signs such as delayed capillary refill time, loss of skin turgor, sunken fontanelle and apathy.

Infants with moderate to severe dehydration may require 10–20 mL/kg boluses of 0.9% saline to restore circulating volume before continuing fluid replacement therapy with 0.45% saline/5% dextrose at a rate of 4–6 mL/kg/h. When urine output is evident, potassium chloride can be added to the fluids. Electrolytes and pH measurement

Paediatric emergency airways

Key points

- The anaesthetist should be comfortable with the management of laryngospasm, which has an incidence of 2–3% in children
- Removal of the inhaled foreign body (FB) requires clear communication between the anaesthetist and a skilled surgeon. Ninety per cent lodge in a main bronchus
- Post-tonsillectomy bleed can create multiple issues including hypovolaemia, a soiled airway and full stomach
- Paediatric difficult airway guidelines have been published by the Association of Paediatric Anaesthetists and the Difficult Airway Society

Airway management in children is generally straightforward but can occasionally be an extraordinary challenge. Anaesthesia and airway management are required for the vast majority of operations and many nonoperative procedures as children and babies are less likely to be managed with sedation or regional techniques than adults. Sick children requiring airway management also present to emergency departments and to the paediatric intensive care.

In the Royal College of Anaesthetists NAP4 audit, most airway events occurred in children with congenital developmental abnormalities, where airway management was predictably difficult. Unexpected difficulties in airway management also occurred in a small number of healthy children.

A critical incident may arise due to predicted/unanticipated difficult bag-mask ventilation or intubation, upper or lower airway obstruction (including laryngospasm, depressed level of consciousness, infectious causes such as croup, tracheitis, epiglottitis, inhaled FB, retropharyngeal abscess, anaphylaxis, asthma or trauma).

Laryngospasm

Laryngospasm is an exaggeration of the normal glottic closure reflex and is produced by stimulation of the superior laryngeal nerve. Although there is some evidence from animal studies that hypoxia and hypercapnia may have an inhibitory effect on laryngospasm, it is untrue that the vocal cords will open before death occurs.

Classically, laryngospasm presents with a characteristic inspiratory 'crowing' sound. If the obstruction worsens, marked suprasternal recession ('tracheal tug'), use of accessory respiratory muscles and paradoxical movements of the thorax and abdomen may develop. Complete obstruction presents with silent inspiration. If unrelieved, laryngospasm may lead to postobstructive pulmonary oedema and can progress to hypoxic cardiac arrest and death.

Incidence: 8.7/1000 in adults, but 2–3% in children.

Risk factors: patients with pre-existing airways infections, procedures involving airway manipulation, increased secretions, and blood and surgical debris around the glottic area, particularly during light planes of anaesthesia. The management of laryngospasm can be divided into strategies for prevention and for treatment.

Prevention

Clinical experience suggests that intravenous anaesthesia using a propofol-based technique is associated with a lower incidence of complications related to exaggerated airway reflexes, and there is some evidence to support this.

Strategies to prevent laryngospasm at extubation: there is no difference between awake or deep extubation; suction should be performed under direct vision with the patient deeply anaesthetised, to ensure that the upper airway is clear of any debris; further stimulation should be avoided until the patient is awake. Topical lidocaine sprayed onto the vocal cords at induction has been shown to reduce the risk of laryngospasm following short procedures.

Treatment

The sequence of events for treatment of laryngospasm is detailed in **Table 53**.

Table 53 Management of laryngospasm in children		
1.	Call for help 100% oxygen Continuous positive airway pressure Larson's manoeuvre	Larson's manoeuvre – place the middle finger of each hand in the 'laryngospasm notch' between the posterior border of the mandible and the mastoid process whilst also displacing the mandible forward in a jaw thrust
2.	Intravenous propofol 0.25 mg/kg, suxamethonium 0.1 mg/kg	Low-dose propofol may be helpful in early laryngospasm but will not work in severe spasm or total cord closure
3.	Intramuscular suxamethonium 4 mg/kg	Laryngeal tone lost within 30–40 seconds
4.	Intraosseous suxamethonium 2 mg/kg	

Inhaled foreign body

A leading cause of accidental death; occurs most commonly in children aged 1–3 years; majority of cases due to inhaled food items. Ninety per cent lodge in main bronchus, right > left.

Signs and symptoms include: history of choking/aspiration, wheezing, stridor, cough, reduced breath sounds on auscultation, hoarseness, respiratory distress, cyanosis, fever, respiratory arrest. A history of choking is the most reliable predictor of foreign body (FB) aspiration and should prompt evaluation and consideration of bronchoscopy.

Management will depend upon the clinical presentation, the aim is to support oxygenation and ventilation and to prevent and treat complete airway obstruction. Initial management should follow the 'choking child' BLS algorithm. In the case of complete airway obstruction and respiratory failure, resuscitation guidelines should be followed.

Close communication between a skilled surgical and anaesthetic team is vital with respect to planning and equipment required (tracheotomy equipment should be immediately available). The danger of delayed removal (fatal progression of obstruction) outweighs the risk of a full stomach (a large bore OG tube may be passed after induction). Rigid bronchoscopy is the treatment of choice for lower airway FBs:

Induction: (in theatre with ENT surgeon present) maintaining spontaneous ventilation (SV) is common practice. There is a risk of converting proximal partial obstruction to complete obstruction with use of intermittent positive pressure ventilation (IPPV). Induction can be achieved with sevoflurane or a total intravenous technique (propofol + remifentanil). Nitrous oxide is avoided to allow better preoxygenation and to minimise gas trapping. The vocal cords should be sprayed with lidocaine (maximum 3 mg/kg).

Maintenance: Once the rigid bronchoscope is in place, an Ayres T-piece is connected to the side-arm for delivery of oxygen and/or anaesthetic agents. There is no evidence that either SV or IPPV techniques are superior. SV may carry less risk of distal movement of FB and worsening of distal air trapping and may be more suitable for proximal FB. Leakage around bronchoscope may make effective IPPV difficult. IPPV may be more suitable for distal removal. Either technique must avoid coughing/bucking due to intense stimulation of bronchoscope (neuromuscular blockade/deep anaesthesia required). Either technique can use inhalational agent or total intravenous anaesthesia (TIVA). TIVA allows constant level of anaesthesia irrespective of ventilation. Children maintain SV at higher doses of remifentanil than adults.

Removal of FB is a high-risk part of procedure, FB can be snagged/dislodged at cords or larynx and can cause severe or complete airway obstruction. There is little evidence for effectiveness of steroids; many anaesthetists give a single dose to reduce postoperative airway oedema. A postoperative chest X-ray is required to exclude pneumothorax/other abnormality. The majority of children can be discharged home the same day.

Infectious causes

Table 54 provides a comparison of the principle infective upper airway emergencies.

Pain – chronic management

Key points

- Chronic pain affects 1 in 5 adults and 50% suffer significant associated anxiety or depression
- Surgery may both cause and exacerbate chronic pain
- Strong opioids are not the mainstay of chronic pain management – this should revolve around a multidisciplinary team approach and, pharmacologically speaking, simple and atypical nonopioid analgesia

Pain is defined as 'an unpleasant sensory and emotional experience associated with actual or potential tissue damage' (International Association for the Study of Pain [IASP]). Chronic pain is defined as pain lasting >3 months. This is a common condition with a prevalence of 19% in Europe. Chronic pain is associated with characteristic neuroplastic changes resulting in increased sensitivity to painful and nonpainful stimuli. These processes are termed peripheral and central sensitisation and result in abnormal pain sensations including hyperalgesia, allodynia and spontaneous pain. These sensory changes are particularly common in neuropathic pain. This is defined as pain due to a lesion or disease process affecting the somatosensory nervous system.

Significant pain, which interferes with the individual's quality of life, is associated with psychological distress, poor self-rated health, the need for disability or unemployment financial benefit and greater use of health care services. The prevalence of significant anxiety or depression is approximately 50% in patients with chronic pain. Patients with chronic pain present a significant challenge to the anaesthetist, with an increased risk of severe acute postoperative pain, complex polypharmacy, opioid tolerance and psychosocial problems.

As well as the impact of pre-existing chronic pain, surgery itself may result in long-term pain. Chronic postsurgical pain (CPSP) has been defined as 'pain persisting for more than two months following a surgical procedure that is not a continuation of a preoperative pain problem'. It is now accepted that long-term pain following surgery is common (15% following hernia repair or 30–50% following thoracotomy).

Problems

- High-dose opioid use (>180 mg morphine equivalent/24 hours)
- Opioid tolerance, dependence and opioid-induced hyperalgesia may occur
- Postoperative pain perception will be heightened by central sensitisation
- Pharmacological implications and interactions of atypical analgesics
- Modifying the risk of CPSP
- Managing the impact of psychological comorbidity

Clinical features

Take a careful drug history. Note opioid tolerance and the use of atypical analgesics. Assess the presence and number of other chronic pain conditions. Patients with chronic pain often suffer from more than one pain problem. The number of pain problems has been shown to impact negatively on the outcome of surgery. For example, the odds ratio of poor outcome following total knee replacement is >10 for patients with multiple pain problems. Psychopathology may impact on rehabilitation and long-term pain postoperatively. High levels of anxiety may affect induction of anaesthesia. Chronic musculoskeletal pain often worsens following surgery

High levels of anxiety and depression as well as more specific problems such as catastrophising (tendency to overemphasise the chance of the worst outcome) and kinesiophobia (fear of movement) may impact significantly on pain and rehabilitation following surgery. Careful explanation of anaesthetic and analgesic techniques as well as managing patient expectations will ameliorate some of these concerns.

Treatment

Chronic pain is best treated within a multidisciplinary pain clinic adopting a bio-psycho-social model. This includes pharmacological, psychological and physical treatments as well as interventional pain management. Pharmacological treatment of chronic pain includes simple analgesia and atypical analgesics. The use of strong opioids in chronic noncancer pain is controversial and their efficacy may be limited due in part to down regulation of opioid receptors

Anaesthetic management

Induction and maintenance of anaesthesia are not generally affected by chronic pain conditions. However, careful planning is required to avoid analgesic failure in the postoperative period. Multimodal analgesia should be delivered in theatre, including consideration of adjuvant therapy such as ketamine, clonidine or gabapentinoid premedication.

Opioid tolerance and withdrawal

Patients taking high dose opioids must have these continued postoperatively. Postoperative opioid requirement will be significantly higher than expected. For example, increased opioid bolus doses may be required via PCA. If the patient's background opioid analgesia cannot be given by mouth, the equivalent dose may need to be delivered as an opioid infusion. Sudden cessation of opioids will risk withdrawal and should be avoided. Opioid withdrawal presents with sympathetic nervous system activation, flu-like symptoms or worsening of pain.

Although not recommended for use in noncancer pain, some patients with chronic noncancer pain may use opioid patches (fentanyl and buprenorphine). Patches should be continued throughout the perioperative period to avoid significant withdrawal.

Regional anaesthetic techniques may ameliorate the requirement for very high opioid doses postoperatively, with the proviso that background analgesia is continued. Weaning from regional anaesthesia may need to be gradual – favouring catheter-based techniques over single shot blocks. Low dose ketamine infusions (0.1 mg/kg/h) have been shown to reduce opioid tolerance and opioid use post operatively.

Adjuvant analgesics

Adjuvant analgesics (**Table 57**) such as gabapentin or pregabalin have been shown to reduce opioid requirements in the immediate postoperative period. Gabapentin and pregabalin are competitive inhibitors at the $\alpha_2\delta$ subunit of N-type calcium channels. These drugs are renally excreted and reduced doses are required in renal impairment. They are used to manage neuropathic pain and chronic pain conditions resulting from central sensitisation.

Pregabalin has more consistent absorption and acts more quickly in neuropathic pain.

Table 57 Atypical analgesics used in chronic pain management		
Drug class	Drug names	Mechanism
$\alpha_2\delta$ calcium channel ligands	Gabapentin/pregabalin	Competitive central Ca^{2+} channel blockade
Tricyclic antidepressants	Nortriptyline/amitriptyline/imipramine	Central modulation of monoamines
Serotonin norepinephrine reuptake inhibitor (SNRI) antidepressants	Duloxetine	Increased NA/5HT mediated inhibition
Other antiepileptic drugs	Carbamazepine/lamotrigine	Central Na^+ channel blockade
N-Methyl-D-aspartate (NMDA) antagonists	Ketamine	Noncompetitive NMDA receptor blockade
Sodium channel blockers	Lidocaine (topical)	Peripheral local anaesthetic effects
Vanilloid receptor agonists	Capsaicin (cream or 8% patch)	Defunctionalisation of C-fibre afferents

However, gabapentin has the most evidence for efficacy in acute pain. There is increasing evidence that pregabalin may be effective in preventing CPSP. These drugs interact with other sedative medications.

Tricyclic antidepressants such as amitriptyline are usually employed at low doses in the management of chronic pain. Their sedative effects are additive with opioid medication. They interact with drugs such as tramadol or selective serotonin reuptake inhibitor/serotonin and noradrenaline reuptake inhibitor class antidepressants resulting in elevated central levels of serotonin. This may result in serotonergic syndrome, a potentially life-threatening condition presenting with hypertension, hyperthermia, clonus and cerebral irritability.

Prevention of chronic postsurgical pain

Modifiable risk factors for CPSP include severe acute postsurgical pain. Meticulous planning of postoperative analgesia including regional techniques will reduce this risk. Some specific interventions have been shown to reduce CPSP. Pregabalin given perioperatively reduces CPSP following knee joint replacement. Ketamine has also shown long-term analgesic effects from a single dose

Further reading

McGreevy K, Bottros MM, Raja SN. Preventing chronic pain following acute pain: Risk factors, preventive strategies, and their efficacy. Eur J Pain Suppl 2012; 5:365–376.

Pogatzki-Zahn EM, Englbrecht JS, Schug SA. Acute pain management in patients with fibromyalgia and other diffuse chronic pain syndromes. Curr Opin Anaesthesiol 2009; 22:627–633.

Related topics of interest

Patient transfer and transport

Key points

- Any transfer is potentially hazardous for all concerned
- Preparation is the key to mitigating risks
- For the patient; think of what is happening to them now, what will happen and what could happen, then plan each by ABCDE
- For yourself; take care of personal safety, comfort, clinical support and consider insurance

Transfers consist of generic clinical considerations but also many logistical and systems elements which by their nature are very locally-specific. For these aspects, systems within the UK are used for illustration here. A transfer, either within or between hospitals, is one of the most hazardous interventions to which we electively expose our patients. All the hazards of the journey have, until comparatively recently, been compounded by a failure to acknowledge the dangers. Consequently inexperienced junior staff have traditionally accompanied these patients. Recent unpublished data revealed 10% of intrahospital transfers for CT scans were complicated by life-threatening incidents including profound hypotension, arterial line disconnection and pathological pupil dilatation. The preparation and mindset should be the same for intrahospital transfers (e.g. from ICU to the CT scanner) and interhospital transfers (e.g. between ICUs in two different hospitals). The increased distance and clinical isolation of an interhospital transfer increase the risk but the potential problems are almost the same. Such an approach fosters good practice for the shorter trip and avoids haphazard planning for different trips, e.g. ICU-CT, ICU-MRI, and ICU-ICU.

Problems

These can be divided into generic concerns and journey-specific concerns. The themes are raised as an overview with examples and should not be treated as exhaustive checklists.

Generic concerns

These are usefully divided into three categories and then, within each, an ABCDE approach will usually suffice to cover all issues.

- What is happening now? For example, intubated, ventilated and sedated patient for transfer
  - a. Airway/breathing:
    - i. Transfer ventilator familiar and functioning
    - ii. Patient established on transfer ventilator with satisfactory ABG
    - iii. Adequate relaxant drugs packed
  - b. Circulation/disability:
    - i. Adequate vasoactive and sedative drugs, fluids etc.
    - ii. All vascular access patent, reliable and secured
    - iii. Patient adequately sedated for increased stimulus of trolley movement
  - c. Exposure:
    - i. Patient secure in the bed and not excessively exposed (temperature, dignity)
    - ii. No equipment resting on the patient
    - iii. No pressure areas at risk
- What will happen? For example, what will you have to deal with at some point on the trip?
  - d. Airway/breathing:
    - i. Calculated adequate oxygen for the trip
    - ii. Power supply for ventilator on longer trips
  - e. Circulation/disability:
    - i. Large-bore access available for contrast infusion if going to CT
    - ii. Strategy in place for intracranial pressure (ICP) management when brain injured patient positioned supine
  - f. Exposure:
    - i. Temperature probe in situ and extra blankets for long journey
    - ii. Extra adhesive tape to resecure C-spine and enough personnel for

log-rolling if taking a trauma patient to CT

- What could happen? The most difficult – all the possible problems
  g. Airway/breathing
     i. All equipment and drugs to reintubate
     ii. Means to hand-ventilate in case of O_2 +/– ventilator failure
     iii. Spare inner tube for tracheostomy
  h. Circulation/disability
     i. Drugs to manage cardiovascular collapse/arrest
     ii. Blood products where applicable
     iii. Osmotherapy for ICP crises
     iv. Equipment to replace vascular access
  i. Exposure
     i. Are you exposed? – know how to get help

Journey-specific concerns

These relate to either destination or transport.
- Destination
  a. MRI – compatible equipment, safety checklist complete for patient and staff, familiar with location and equipment, scanner booked and empty/ready
  b. CT – female patient's pregnancy status checked, concerns regarding contrast agents (allergy status, renal function known)
  c. Other hospitals – bed confirmed, patient clinically accepted, phone number for receiving unit, know where to go when you get there, do relatives know?
- Transport (**Table 58**)
  d. Is it booked, when is it due?
  e. What staffing and equipment will be onboard?
  f. Will there be power for electrical equipment?
  g. Are you familiar with the layout?
  h. You – are you insured, do you get motion sickness, have you had a personal break, are you suitably dressed?

Other issues
Preparedness

Invariably there is some degree of urgency with most transfers with the exception of repatriation to a patient's home hospital for example. In order to achieve rapid and effective transfer of patients to definitive care whilst maintaining high safety margins, staff must be well prepared.
- Take the time to familiarise yourself with the transfer equipment used in your hospital
- Regularly check kit to ensure it will be complete and in working order when needed
- Get help with transfer preparation – there are many tasks to be achieved quickly
- Use checklists to reduce the chance of overlooking details during pretransfer preparation

Table 58 Options for interhospital transfer in the UK		
	Advantages	**Disadvantages**
Land ambulance	24-hour availability Door-to-door Easy to divert/pull over	Motion sickness May be slower May be less smooth Can be diverted on return journey
Air ambulance	Relatively fast Virtually door-to-door Comparatively smooth	Tight space Noisy Vibration, flicker vertigo Weight limits Limited by light and weather
Military helicopter	24-hour operations Relatively fast and smooth Flies in almost all conditions Can carry large amounts of personnel/equipment with a patient	Limited landing sites (size and weight of aircraft) Comparatively dark in cabin even during daylight hours More vibration/noise but less flicker effect Risk of hypothermia, due to low ambient temperature

Personal safety and comfort

To perform at their best in a strange environment, staff must be mindful of their limits and comfortable in their surroundings.

- Are you clinically capable to care, single-handedly, for the patient you are being asked to transfer?
- Have you had specific training in transfers? Intensive Care Society guidelines recommend all transfers are undertaken by ST3+ Doctors with specific transfer training
- Avoid transfers if you suffer truly incapacitating motion sickness
- Ensure you have been to the toilet before you leave and have eaten something recently
- Be properly dressed in warm clothes and shoes (not scrubs and theatre shoes)
- Take money (food, alternative transport home) and a mobile phone (clinical advice etc.)
- Always do as instructed by the ambulance crew or aircrew from an operational standpoint – they will keep you safe. You are strongly advised to make sure you have personal injury insurance for such trips; membership of certain professional organisations, e.g. Intensive Care Society and AAGBI typically include this cover

Further reading

Association of Anaesthetists of Great Britain & Ireland. Transfer of patients with brain injury. London: AAGBI, 2006.

Intensive Care Society. Guidelines for the transport of the critically ill adult, 3rd edn. London: ICS, 2011.

Martin T (ed.). Aeromedical transportation: a clinical guide, 2nd edn. Aldershot: Ashgate Publishing, 2006.

Related topics of interest

Perioperative fluid management

Key points

- Fluid administration is not a benign therapy – significant morbidity and mortality can result from inappropriate treatment
- Careful assessment of patients' fluid status and requirements are required for safe anaesthesia
- Regular reassessment of haemodynamic trends and the response to fluid is key to optimising intravascular filling

Appropriate fluid management in the perioperative period is key to ensuring optimal postoperative patient outcomes. Both hypovolaemia and fluid overload are associated with significant morbidity, and excessive administration of certain fluids may lead to electrolyte and acid–base abnormalities as well as impaired coagulation and renal function. The volumes and nature of intravenous fluid administered to patients undergoing surgery should be guided by:

- An estimate of any deficit in intravascular volume and composition
- The anticipated volume and type of fluid loss both ongoing during surgery and predicted postoperatively
- Interpretation of physiological responses to fluid administration

The aim is to optimise each individual patient's cardiovascular status with judicious fluid administration so they lie on the shoulder of their Frank–Starling curve.

Preoperative considerations

Elective surgery patients normally only have a minimal fluid deficit on arrival to theatre. They are permitted clear oral fluids until 2 hours before induction of anaesthesia and 'Enhanced Recovery After Surgery' (ERAS) programmes encourage carbohydrate drinks on the morning of surgery and discourage the use of strong osmotic bowel preparation.

In contrast, many emergency cases have a significant fluid deficit and therefore a careful evaluation of their fluid status should be made. Reasons for fluid depletion include:

- Increased losses: nausea and vomiting, diarrhoea, bleeding, drug therapy (e.g. diuretics), pyrexia, burns and drains
- Inadequate intake: prolonged fasting (including the period prior to presentation to hospital), inability to tolerate oral intake or uncertainty surrounding the timing of a patient's theatre slot
- Redistribution losses of circulating volume: sepsis, pancreatitis and other causes of systemic inflammatory response syndrome

Assessment of hydration should consist of:

- A detailed medical and surgical history
- An examination including peripheral and central capillary refill, heart rate, blood pressure, mucus membranes, respiratory rate, urine output and the presence of thirst (indicating ~10 mL/kg dehydration)
- A review of trends in physiological observations, fluid and drug charts. The patient's age, gender, body mass index and associated comorbidities need to be taken into account
- Full blood count and urea and electrolytes, with an estimate of glomerular filtration rate for the chronic kidney disease patient
- An arterial blood gas should be considered to measure lactate and base excess

Patients who have marked intravascular depletion preoperatively should have a period of resuscitation prior to the induction of anaesthesia to reduce cardiovascular instability. The duration of this resuscitation is dependent on the urgency of the surgery, the underlying pathology and the response to therapy. It should be 'goal directed', i.e. targeted towards individualised haemodynamic parameters and blood results (e.g. arterial lactate concentration).

Intraoperative considerations

The stress response to surgery promotes a shift of fluid from the circulating volume into the extracellular space. This is more pronounced in prolonged surgery, particularly in the emergency setting and surgery involving significant tissue trauma (e.g. gastrointestinal). Intraoperative haemorrhage may exacerbate this. Occult hypovolaemia is common. Splanchnic vasoconstriction allows blood pressure and pulse to be maintained as compensation but at the expense of gut perfusion.

For elective cases of short duration where minimal stress response is anticipated, up to a litre of either Hartmann's solution or 0.9% saline is recommended. There is evidence that this reduces postoperative nausea and vomiting rates. It aids the delivery of intravenous medications into the blood stream and maintains cannula patency.

During longer, more complex surgery intravenous fluid administration should be specifically tailored to the individual patient requirements, and be dynamically reviewed at regular intervals. Considerations will be:

- The present volume status, cardiovascular reserve and fluid responsiveness of the patient
- The type of surgery
- An estimate of ongoing operative losses (evaporation, redistribution, urine output, bleeding and drains)
- The effect of any neuraxial blockade that promotes venodilatation and vasoparesis leading to relative hypovolaemia owing to an increased intravascular compartment

Invasive blood pressure monitoring is strongly recommended for procedures involving large fluid shifts, those at risk of major haemorrhage and patients with significant comorbidities. It provides beat-to-beat blood pressure monitoring, allows frequent blood sampling and can be used for pulse contour analysis (to estimate cardiac output).

Intraoperative fluid management technologies (e.g. oesophageal Doppler and lithium dilution cardiac output monitoring) may help to individualise fluid therapy and are recommended in the UK for example, by NICE and the NHS Technology Adoption Centre for 'high risk' patients. Examples are emergency body cavity surgery, prolonged elective surgery likely to be associated with a pronounced surgical stress response and patients with significant comorbidities that may affect their ability to maintain adequate organ perfusion.

Type of fluid administered

- Excessive amounts of 0.9% saline are not recommended; risk of hyperchloraemic acidosis
- Starches are not recommended due to recent studies demonstrating an increase in mortality and renal failure associated with their use particularly in sepsis
- Particular attention should be given to the risks of iatrogenic hyponatraemia in children receiving intravenous fluid therapy and solutions containing a low concentration of sodium should be avoided
- Packed red cells: the benefits of transfusion through oxygen carrying capacity may be offset by transfusion related complications. The TRICC study suggests that critically ill patients without ischaemic heart disease can tolerate a haemoglobin down to 70 g/L. However, there is evidence that a haemoglobin level >100 g/L may be desirable in sepsis

Postoperative considerations

Oral intake of fluid is the route of choice and therefore patients who are able to eat and drink soon after surgery should be encouraged to do so and intravenous fluids discontinued. Where enteral intake is restricted or impaired or where ongoing fluid losses are likely, intravenous fluid may be prescribed for the immediate postoperative period. This amount should be limited to the minimum required and should be reviewed regularly. If there is likely to be a significant or unpredictable ongoing fluid requirement or the patient has multiple comorbidities implying a reduced cardiovascular reserve, it is prudent to consider admission to a high dependency area.

Special cases

Paediatrics: for routine elective surgery without risk of major fluid shifts and blood loss, between 10 and 20 mL/kg is normally given.

Liver resection surgery: a high central venous pressure in patients undergoing liver resection is associated with increased intraoperative blood loss. Fluid administration is restricted (as tolerated by the patient) to achieve a low inferior vena caval pressure until completion of the resection. This is balanced against the need to maintain an adequate cardiac output and minimise the risk of air embolus.

Thoracic surgery: liberal fluid management has been shown to be an independent risk factor for acute lung injury following thoracic surgery.

A restrictive perioperative fluid regimen is adopted.

Neurosurgery: cerebral oedema should be avoided. A restrictive perioperative fluid regimen is preferred.

Renal transplant surgery: the main aim is to ensure adequate renal perfusion for the transplanted kidney and a more liberal fluid strategy is normally adopted to achieve this.

Further reading

Della Rocca G, Pompei L. Goal-directed therapy in anesthesia: any clinical impact or just a fashion? Minerva Anestesiol 2011; 77:545–553.

Grocott MP, Mythen MG, Gan TJ. Perioperative fluid management and clinical outcomes in adults. Anesth Analg 2005; 100:1093–1096.

National Institute for Health & Care Excellence. CardioQ-ODM oesophageal Doppler monitor (MTG 3). London: NICE, 2011.

Pearse RM, Ackland GL. Perioperative fluid therapy. Br Med J 2012; 344:e2865.

Related topics of interest

Phaeochromocytoma

Key points

- Hypertensive end-organ damage, including cardiomyopathy, must be assessed prior to surgery
- Adequate medical treatment before surgery to temper the effects of the tumour is essential and improves outcome
- The most commonly secreted neurotransmitters are adrenaline, noradrenaline and dopamine
- Perioperative cardiovascular instability should be anticipated and managed with appropriate short-term agents
- Hypertension may persist well into the postoperative period

Phaeochromocytomas are catecholamine-secreting tumours that arise from chromaffin cells in the adrenal medulla or from extra-adrenal sympathetic ganglia in the chest, abdomen or pelvis. Extra-adrenal tumours are known as paragangliomas. Phaeochromocytoma is referred to as the 10% tumour, with approximately 10% occurring extra-adrenally, 10% familial, 10% bilateral and 10% malignant.

They usually present with severe sustained or paroxysmal hypertension and other symptoms and signs of sympathetic activation such as sweating, anxiety, headaches and palpitations. Sustained catecholamine secretion can cause hypertensive encephalopathy or cardiomyopathy; affected individuals may present with pulmonary oedema. Some phaeochromocytomas are asymptomatic presenting as an incidental finding of an adrenal mass on imaging or at laparotomy. Mortality is much higher for tumours presenting as a hypertensive crisis during other surgery. Phaeochromocytoma presents most frequently in the fourth decade and are equally common in men and women.

Adrenaline, noradrenaline or dopamine may be secreted and diagnosis is confirmed by measurement of urinary catecholamines and their metabolites, in particular, vanillylmandelic acid. Abdominal and pelvic CT or MRI scanning is used to locate the tumour and will identify 97%. The remaining 3%, located outside of the abdomen or pelvis, may be identified using radioisotope studies. Treatment is by open or laparoscopic resection of the tumour following appropriate medical management.

Problems

- Tumours are uncommon and often unfamiliar to the anaesthetist
- Haemodynamic effects of undiagnosed untreated tumours can present during unrelated surgery
- Adequate pre-operative treatment is necessary to reduce perioperative mortality
- Perioperative release of catecholamines may require specific treatment strategies

Anaesthetic management

Preoperative assessment

Clinical assessment should focus on cardiovascular status and identification of hypertensive end-organ damage. ECG may show evidence of ventricular hypertrophy, arrhythmias or ischaemia. Echocardiography is required to assess myocardial function and evidence of catecholamine induced cardiomyopathy, which may occur in up to 50% of patients. Blood tests may reveal a raised haematocrit due to depleted intravascular volume, hyperglycaemia and renal impairment.

Preoperative preparation

Medical therapy prior to tumour resection intends to control persistent hypertension, prevents hypertensive crises and expands the depleted intravascular volume. The most common regimen comprises combined α- and β-adrenergic blockade but other regimes include calcium channel blockers and metyrosine, an inhibitor of catecholamine synthesis.

Phenyoxybenzamine is a long-acting nonselective irreversible alpha-blocker and is usually started 10–14 days prior to surgery to prevent the response to excess catecholamine release and restore normovolaemia and myocardial function. It has a long half-life (24 hours) and irreversible action, which can contribute to postoperative hypotension.

As a nonselective alpha-blocker, phenoxybenzamine also blocks α_2 receptors, which can lead to tachyarrhythmia. This is controlled by the addition of a beta-blocker. Beta-blockade should *never* be started prior to establishing alpha-blockade since the attenuation of β_2-mediated vasodilation will cause further hypertension.

Other short-acting, selective α_1-adrenergic blocking drugs, e.g. prazosin or doxazosin, are sometimes preferred to phenoxybenzamine due to reduced side effects. However, since they have a competitive action, clinical effects may be overcome by large catecholamine surges during surgery.

Perioperative management

Benzodiazepine premedication may be appropriate to reduce anxiety-related release of catecholamines. Large-bore intravenous access, arterial blood pressure monitoring and central venous access are required to monitor and treat intraoperative cardiovascular instability. Cardiac output monitoring should be considered, particularly if significant myocardial dysfunction has been identified preoperatively. Perioperative transoesophageal echocardiography has been used in severe cases.

Induction and maintenance of anaesthesia can be undertaken with intravenous or inhalational agents. Drugs that sensitise the myocardium to catecholamines, e.g. older volatile agents, or those that cause histamine release, e.g. atracurium or morphine, should be avoided.

Regional analgesia may be appropriate for an open surgical approach and will reduce catecholamine surges due to surgical stimulation. Neuraxial block will not prevent the effects of tumour handling and may complicate management of intra- and postoperative haemodynamics. For a laparoscopic approach, fentanyl, alfentanil or remifentanil are suitable analgesics, with the latter enabling rapid titration to cardiovascular changes.

Intraoperative catecholamine surges should have minimal effect following adequate preoperative preparation; however, the anaesthetist should have a strategy for managing sudden changes in cardiovascular parameters. These most commonly occur during laryngoscopy, positioning, peritoneal insufflation and tumour handling.

Hypertension can be managed with a short-acting alpha-blocker such as phentolamine or an arteriovenodilator such as sodium nitroprusside. Tachycardia can be controlled with a short acting beta-blocker, e.g. esmolol. Hypotension is managed by discontinuing antihypertensive infusions and titrating fluid boluses. A noradrenaline infusion may be required. Magnesium sulphate has been used successfully in a number of case reports and may have a place in stabilising fluctuations in blood pressure.

Postoperative care

Initial postoperative care should be undertaken in a critical care setting to allow close monitoring and control of cardiovascular parameters. Hypertension may persist for several days after surgery until catecholamine levels return to normal and it may be necessary to continue antihypertensives for this period. Hypotension is less common, although there may be residual alpha-blockade or a requirement for further volume expansion.

Blood glucose levels should be closely monitored after tumour removal as patients are at risk of hypoglycaemia due to a reduction in catecholamine-mediated glycogenolysis. Steroid replacement therapy will be necessary if the patient has undergone bilateral adrenalectomy.

Further reading

Pace N, Buttigieg M. Phaeochromocytoma. Br J Anaesth Contin Educ Profess Develop Rev 2003; 3:20–23.

Prys-Roberts C. Phaeochromocytoma – recent progress in its management. Br J Anaesth 2000; 85:44–57.

Shawcross R, Moore J. Recognition and management of phaeochromocytoma. Anaesth Intensive Care Med 2011; 12:442–445.

Young W, Kaplan N. Treatment of phaeochromocytoma in adults. In: Martin K, Duda R (Eds), UpToDate 2013. http://www.uptodateonline.com. (Accessed May 2013.)

Related topics of interest

- Cardiac dysrhythmia (p. 37)
- Endocrine disease (p. 72)
- Hypertensive disease (p. 89)

Plastic surgery

Key points

- Flap survival is typically >95% but flap failure can be catastrophic
- Meticulous cardiovascular manipulation is key to optimal anaesthetic management
- Careful observation of the flap is required postoperatively – a high-dependency environment may be required for this

Plastic surgery is one of the true remaining 'general surgical' specialties, potentially involving any body region and a variety of tissue types. This topic focuses on free flap and reconstructive plastic surgery. Burns are discussed in *Burns*. Craniofacial and cosmetic procedures are beyond the scope of this book.

The commonest indications for these procedures are tumour resections or trauma. Meticulous attention to detail is required in the anaesthesia for these cases, with a sound application of cardiovascular physiology in particular. In established centres, flap survival is >95%. Flap failure can be catastrophic; reconstructive options are more complex and carry greater risks of subsequent failure. Most of the factors determining success are in the purview of the surgeons but many are modifiable by the anaesthetist (**Table 59**).

Problems

Preoperative/patient related:
- Trauma patients
  - Other injuries, especially head injury
  - Sepsis
  - Bleeding and coagulopathy

- Oncology patients
  - Effects of recent chemotherapy
  - Head and neck patients:
    - Difficult airway (scarring, radiotherapy, tumour obstruction/infiltration)
    - Smokers (respiratory disease, ischaemic heart disease)
    - Often elderly (comorbid, poly-pharmacy)
  - Breast cancer patients
    - Anxiety

Intraoperative:
- Profuse bleeding possible with most procedures
- Two operative sites (donor, graft); analgesia, positioning, access, heat/fluid loss
- Prolonged surgery (pressure area care, venous thrombosis, hypothermia)
- Requirement for cardiovascular monitoring and manipulation

Postoperative:
- Flap failure (secondary ischaemia) – **Table 59**
- Pain control
- Blood loss

Investigations

Patients should be preassessed in the usual manner and minimum blood tests include full blood count, biochemistry, coagulation screen and group and save. There is a potential requirement for blood transfusion

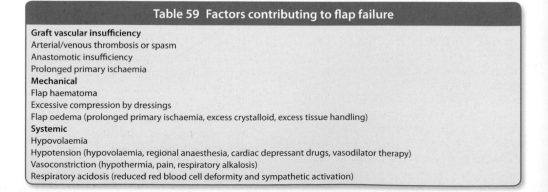

Table 59 Factors contributing to flap failure
Graft vascular insufficiency
Arterial/venous thrombosis or spasm
Anastomotic insufficiency
Prolonged primary ischaemia
Mechanical
Flap haematoma
Excessive compression by dressings
Flap oedema (prolonged primary ischaemia, excess crystalloid, excess tissue handling)
Systemic
Hypovolaemia
Hypotension (hypovolaemia, regional anaesthesia, cardiac depressant drugs, vasodilator therapy)
Vasoconstriction (hypothermia, pain, respiratory alkalosis)
Respiratory acidosis (reduced red blood cell deformity and sympathetic activation)

and an electronic cross-match should be available. Investigations relevant to an individual's comorbid state should also be organised.

Anaesthetic management

Preoperative

Complete a thorough preassessment, particularly of the airway in head and neck cases. Vascular access sites should be planned in conjunction with the surgeon to avoid operative sites. Large-bore intravenous access and an arterial line will form the minimum, particularly for free-flap procedures; central venous access for drug administration and central venous pressure trend monitoring will be useful in larger procedures. Core and peripheral temperature monitoring along with forced-air warming and warmed intravenous fluids should commence prior to induction of anaesthesia. Anaesthetic room and theatre ambient temperature should be raised to 22–24°C. Pneumatic calf compression is recommended for deep vein thrombosis prophylaxis and a urinary catheter will be required. Positioning is important due to length of the procedure.

General anaesthesia will typically be required given the length of surgery and particularly in upper body procedures. Total intravenous anaesthesia offers some advantages – propofol and remifentanil both offer rapid offset (particularly relevant in the lengthy procedure) and smooth emergence as well as vasodilation. Propofol probably causes some reduction in platelet aggregation, reducing the risk of microthrombosis. Remifentanil reduces the stress response to surgery. Volatile anaesthesia, usually in conjunction with remifentanil, also represents a reasonable option.

The sympathetic blockade and intense analgesia of regional anaesthesia techniques are useful for enhancing graft perfusion, provided that blood pressure is not permitted to fall. This effect is particularly useful in the first 12–24 hours when graft perfusion may only be 50% of its final, established levels; this favours catheter techniques where possible. Airway technique will be dictated not only on a case-by-case basis according to the usual factors but also, in certain cases, the proximity of the surgical site to the airway.

Intraoperative

During raising of the flap, relative hypotension is useful to limit bleeding. During the reimplantation phase, attention should be paid to the elements of the Hagen–Poiseuille equation, which loosely models (blood is a non-Newtonian fluid) those factors affecting microcirculation:
Where Q is flow, P is arteriovenous pressure gradient, r is vessel radius, μ is viscosity, L is length of vessel.

$$Q = \frac{\pi \Delta P r^4}{8\,\mu L}$$

The aim is a low systemic vascular resistance and high cardiac output to generate a wide pulse pressure. Localised vasospasm can be reduced by:
- Reduction in core-peripheral temperature gradient to <1°C
- Normocarbia
- Optimal analgesia
- Optimum fluid loading

Potent vasodilators (e.g. sodium nitroprusside and hydralazine) should be avoided as profound hypotension and a steal phenomenon can threaten graft perfusion. Target a haematocrit of 30% (certainly no higher than 40%) to maximise oxygen carrying capacity for an adequately reduced viscosity. Excess fluid contributes to flap oedema, particularly as the flap lacks intact lymphatic drainage. Alpha-agonist vasopressors should generally be avoided in these patients as vasoconstriction jeopardises the graft. Inodilators such as dobutamine may be of use in conjunction with judicious fluid titration.

Postoperative care

These patients require smooth emergence, possibly facilitated by such techniques as deep extubation, conversion to a laryngeal mask airway or continuation of low-dose remifentanil during the extubation phase. Coughing, retching and vomiting risk suture line rupture and increased venous pressures, which threaten the graft.

Multimodal analgesia and antiemetics are always required. NSAIDs should be avoided due to the risk of flap haematoma. Postoperative shivering doubles tissue oxygen requirements, increases catecholamine release and triggers vasoconstriction, all of which threaten the graft significantly: intravenous pethidine or clonidine is useful.

These patients require high-dependency care as a minimum. Targeted management (**Table 60**) should continue to replicate most of the goals of intraoperative management. Regular observation of the flap is vital to detect secondary ischaemia as early as possible (primary ischaemia – from flap elevation to reimplantation, secondary ischaemia – any point following revascularisation of the implanted flap). Guidelines on oncoplastic breast reconstruction from the British Association of Plastic Reconstructive & Aesthetic Surgeons (BAPRAS), for example, give detailed guidance on this.

Table 60 Postoperative goals	
Temperature	Normothermia, core-periphery gradient <1°C
Haematocrit	30%
Cardiovascular	High cardiac output, wide pulse pressure
Urine output	>1 mL/kg/h
Regular flap observations	See BAPRAS guidance

Further reading

Adams J, Charlton P. Anaesthesia for microvascular free tissue transfer. Br J Anaesth: Contin Educ Profess Develop Rev 2003; 3:33–37.

British Association of Plastic Reconstructive and Aesthetic Surgeons (BAPRAS/ABS). Oncoplastic breast reconstruction; Guidelines for best practice. London: BAPRAS/ABS, 2012.

Krassnitzer S. Anaesthesia for reconstructive surgery. Anaesth Intensive Care Med 2012; 13:131–134.

Related topics of interest

Polytrauma

Key points

- Use of permissive hypotension can improve outcomes
- Blood products should be used as primary resuscitation fluids
- Damage control surgery improves outcomes

Injury is the most common cause of morbidity and mortality in adults and young children in the developed world. The most common cause of trauma in the UK is road traffic collisions. Recent evidence suggests that in-hospital mortality is 20% higher in the UK than in the US. Consequently, there has been a drive to create specialist regional trauma centres in the UK, as specialist care improves outcome and implementation of trauma systems significantly reduces mortality.

Trauma is classified as blunt or penetrating. Whilst there is some difference in management, many themes are common to both. The use of a dedicated trauma response, led by senior staff, may improve outcomes. The anaesthetist is a key member of this multidisciplinary team.

Problems

- Anaesthesia in an unstable patient
- Resuscitation goals will be dependent on the injury and may change rapidly as the clinical picture develops
- Coagulopathy in trauma

Anaesthetic management

Airway

Poor airway management in trauma continues to be highlighted as an avoidable cause of morbidity and mortality. Maintaining a patent airway is critical to outcome. Use of nasopharyngeal airways has been discouraged due to the risk of misplacement in base of skull fracture, but with careful placement, many experts would advocate their routine use in trauma on a risk–benefit basis.

Rapid sequence induction is indicated to reduce the risk of aspiration in patients with a Glasgow Coma Scale (GCS) <9. Patients who are cerebrally agitated with a GCS of 13–14 have a 12.5% incidence of abnormal head CT requiring neurosurgical intervention. Intubation may be required to facilitate management of the agitated patient, provide adequate ventilation in chest trauma, allow procedures to be performed or for humane management of the severely injured patient.

Intubation should always be with in-line cervical spine immobilisation. Single episodes of hypoxia (Sp_{O_2} <90%) or hypotension (systolic blood pressure, SBP, <90 mmHg) are major predictors of poor outcome in traumatic brain injury, and should be avoided at all costs. Provision should be made for a difficult airway, including the means to establish a surgical airway if required.

There is no perfect induction agent for trauma. Etomidate has relatively less impact on cardiovascular stability, but suppresses cortisol synthesis with an associated increase in mortality. Ketamine is associated with raised intracranial pressure, but current evidence suggests that there may be some neuroprotective benefit. Thiopentone and propofol are familiar agents to most and decrease cerebral metabolism, but also frequently cause hypotension.

Either suxamethonium or rocuronium can be used for muscle relaxation. Cricoid pressure may worsen the view at laryngoscopy, and should be removed to facilitate intubation if necessary. Raised intracranial pressure in traumatic brain injury is harmful, and use of adjuvant agents on induction may attenuate the effects of laryngoscopy. Fentanyl (3 µg/kg) and lidocaine (1.5 mg/kg) given intravenously over 1 minute and 3 minutes before induction have both been used.

Breathing

Pneumothoraces are frequent and may become tension pneumothoraces, particularly in the ventilated patient. Treatment by insertion of a large bore cannula in the second intercostal space in the midclavicular line may fail due to inadequate length, blockage or kinking of the cannula. Unless signs of impending tension – SpO_2 <92% or SBP <90 mmHg a chest X-ray should be performed before intervention. A chest drain remains the gold standard treatment.

Small pneumothoraces diagnosed on CT may not require treatment in spontaneously ventilating patients. In severe chest trauma, a double lumen tube may be indicated. Patients should be ventilated using standard protective lung strategies.

Circulation

Haemorrhage is a major cause of death following polytrauma. Initial resuscitation is directed at preventing further blood loss. Minimising movement of the patient (e.g. 10° log rolls only when moving the patient from the ambulance stretcher) will reduce the risk of clot disruption. Splinting major long bone or pelvic fractures, applying direct pressure to bleeding wounds or in more extreme circumstances, application of a tourniquet will all help reduce blood loss.

Active bleeding is not always obvious. Pulse, blood pressure and respiratory rate are neither sensitive nor specific for haemorrhagic shock. Young people may lose up to 30% of their circulating volume with little change in their vital signs. Other indicators of tissue hypoperfusion should be sought: altered cerebration, decreased urine output, raised lactate, metabolic acidosis. Early identification of occult shock (cryptic or compensated shock) can improve outcome.

Most causes of shock in polytrauma will be haemorrhagic, but obstructive (tamponade or pneumothorax), myocardial and neurogenic shock should be excluded. The use of focused echocardiography in the periresuscitation period is gaining popularity as an increasing number of emergency physicians and anaesthetists obtain basic echo training. The aim is to diagnose potentially treatable causes of cardiac arrest such as cardiac tamponade. Large volumes of fluid administration should be avoided due to a resultant transient rise in blood pressure, which may disrupt clot formation, dilute clotting factors and result in dilutional anaemia as well as reducing

core temperature. In penetrating disease, there is guidance to aim for a blood pressure compatible with normal cerebration, or a SBP of 70–90 mmHg, until haemostatic control is achieved. In blunt trauma with no associated head injury, a SBP of 90 mmHg is acceptable.

These parameters should be maintained until the patient is stabilised either in theatre or in the angiography suite. The use of angiography in major trauma is gaining recognition; however, it depends on the immediate availability of an interventional radiology suite/team. In addition, from a technical viewpoint, not all pathology is readily identifiable by angiography and many pathologies are not amenable to angiographic therapy. 'Damage control surgery' aims to limit initial surgical intervention to haemorrhage control and reduction of contamination. The aim is to allow restoration of normal patient physiology as quickly as possible in the ICU, before returning to theatre for definitive treatment. This approach is associated with improved outcomes.

Following definitive haemorrhage control, goal directed resuscitation to maintain optimal organ perfusion should be resumed. Blunt trauma with head injury is controversial, as hypotension is associated with worse neurological outcomes. An acceptable compromise is to aim for a SBP of 100–110 mmHg.

Coagulopathy in trauma

It has long been thought that coagulopathy is due to clotting factors being lost (haemorrhage and consumption), diluted (fluid resuscitation) and deactivated (acidosis and hypothermia). It is worthy of note that correction of pH alone (through use of bicarbonate) does not immediately reverse acidosis-induced coagulopathy. Recent studies have shown that hypoperfusion and tissue damage can cause early systemic anticoagulation and hyperfibrinolysis. Patients with acute traumatic coagulopathy have a fourfold mortality compared with those without.

'Damage control resuscitation' originates from military outcome studies from Afghanistan and Iraq. Studies have shown an improvement in mortality rates following the administration of fresh-frozen plasma and packed red blood cells in a 1:1 or 1:2 ratio to correct hypovolaemia.

Thromboelastography may be the most accurate guide to administration of blood products. The CRASH-2 study advocates the use of tranexamic acid within 3 hours of the initial injury.

Further reading

Harris T, Davenport R, Hurst T, et al. Improving outcome in severe trauma: trauma systems and initial management – intubation, ventilation and resuscitation. Postgrad Med J 2012; 88:588–594.

Harris T, Davenport R, Hurst T, et al. Improving outcome in severe trauma: what's new in ABC?

Imaging, bleeding and brain injury. Postgrad Med J 2012 doi:10.1136/postgradmedj-2011-130285.

Report by the comptroller and auditor general. HC213 Session 2009-2010. Major Trauma Care in England. London; National Audit Office, 2010.

Related topics of interest

- Blood physiology (p. 19)
- Blood transfusion and salvage (p. 22)
- Neuroanaesthesia – traumatic brain injury (p. 131)
- Patient transfer and transport (p. 205)
- Respiratory – acute respiratory distress syndrome (p. 256)
- Spinal cord injury (p. 281)

The above recommendations suggest fasting is not necessary for minimal or moderate sedation. In cases where the patient is not starved, take into account the urgency of the procedure, the intended depth and duration of sedation, and the individual patient risk factors for aspiration. In high-risk cases consider delaying the procedure, reducing depth and/or duration of sedation, giving antacid medications and prokinetics and performing RSI or undertaking regional anaesthesia. There is, however, an acknowledged lack of consensus on the best way to proceed in such cases, even amongst experts.

Children may require sedation for a wide range of procedures and investigations. Current NICE guidance for sedation of children in the UK recognises a distinction between painful and painless procedures. For painless procedures, e.g. MRI, midazolam is recommended (chloral hydrate recommended for children under 15kg). Sevoflurane or intermittent boluses of propofol are considered second line. For painful procedures, local anaesthesia is encouraged alongside sedative techniques. Nitrous oxide in oxygen or oral/intranasal midazolam is first line, ketamine or parenteral midazolam with/without fentanyl is second line and propofol with/without fentanyl is third line along with other possible techniques. Other guidance, e.g. for training and monitoring, is broadly similar to that required for adult sedation.

Anaesthetic management

Preassessment, including that of the airway, starvation status and comorbidities should be as for general anaesthesia. Inadequate preassessment is a well-recognised contributor to complications.

Commonly used agents are in **Table 68** – choose agent(s) and dosing regimen based on:

- Intended depth and duration of sedation
- Whether the procedure is painful or painless
- Patient comorbidities and risk of complications

Ensure appropriate monitoring, assistance and resuscitation facilities including capnography and a tipping trolley. Supplemental oxygen is recommended for all patients undergoing moderate, deep or dissociative sedation. If giving adjunctive analgesia alongside sedative agents the risk of respiratory depression is increased. Give the analgesic and await peak effect before giving the sedative medication. Ensure recovery from sedation is complete before discharge, especially in areas without a dedicated postanaesthesia care unit. In the elderly, start with lower initial doses and give less frequent boluses. These patients have a higher chance of complications.

Special circumstances

Endoscopy: Guidelines exist for sedation in patients undergoing upper and lower GI endoscopy. Oesophagogastroduodenoscopy is painless and often well tolerated under local anaesthesia combined with small doses of midazolam. Colonoscopy is more uncomfortable and may necessitate intravenous opioid, e.g. fentanyl (>100 µg is rarely required). Patients having emergency procedures may have multiple comorbidities, full stomachs and may be haemodynamically unstable. Great care must be taken in providing sedation in these circumstances, and formal RSI in a controlled environment may be preferable.

Dentistry: Due to a number of historical adverse events associated with dental anaesthesia, there are now strict guidelines in this setting. It is no longer considered acceptable to provide general anaesthesia in the setting of a dental surgery in the UK, and dentists wishing to provide operator/sedater services must be able to demonstrate suitable facilities, appropriate training and competence.

Table 68 Common sedative agents compared			
Agent	Indications for use	Advantages	Disadvantages
Fentanyl	Analgesia	Rapid onset Potent analgesia	Increased incidence of respiratory depression especially with other agents
Remifentanil	By infusion as sole analgesia or in conjunction with propofol for moderate/deep sedation	Profound analgesia Noncumulative (ideal for long procedures) Low risk of disinhibition	High risk of respiratory depression in excessive doses Bradycardia
Nitrous oxide	Inhaled analgesia (50:50 with oxygen, Entonox) Moderate sedation and analgesia (70:30 with oxygen via anaesthetic system)	Rapid onset/offset Wide margin of safety Patient-controlled via mouthpiece or mask	Environmental issues (scavenging, pollution) May predispose to nausea and vomiting
Sevoflurane	Inhalation sedation especially in paediatric practice	Rapid onset/offset in short procedures Minimal respiratory depression	Environmental issues Requires anaesthetic system Expensive
Propofol	Intravenous (IV) sedation as bolus or infusion	Rapid onset/offset Antiemetic	Wide interpatient variability in dose requirement Pain on injection High-risk respiratory depression
Midazolam	Short-acting benzodiazepine for IV, PO, intranasal or buccal sedation	Relatively wide margin of safety Inexpensive Familiarity amongst wide variety of sedation practitioners	Time to peak onset often underestimated (up to 5 minutes) Cumulative with repeated dosing (best for short procedures) May be up to 8 times more potent when combined with opioid Most likely to result in disinhibition
Ketamine	Phencyclidine derivative, producing dissociative sedation. Used in many parts of the world as sole anaesthetic agent.	Generally safe when used as sole agent Profound analgesic Maintains cardiac output, respiratory function and oropharyngeal reflexes even during deep sedation/GA	May result in emergence phenomena (much less common in paediatric population) High incidence nausea and vomiting following use Difficult to assess depth of sedation as verbal contact often lost with even small doses

Further reading

Academy of Medical Royal Colleges. Implementing and ensuring safe sedation practice for healthcare procedures in adults. [Online] http://www.rcoa.ac.uk/system/files/PUB-SafeSedPrac.pdf [2013]. London: AoMRC, 2010.

National Institute of Health & Care Excellence. CG112. Sedation for diagnostic and therapeutic procedures in children and young people. London: NICE, 2010.

Safe Sedation of Adults in the Emergency Department. [Online] http://www.rcoa.ac.uk/system/files/CSQ-SEDATION-ED2012.pdf [2013]. London: RcoA, 2012.

Related topics of interest

• Dental anaesthesia (p. 54)

• Paediatric anaesthesia – basic practical conduct (p. 183)

Regional anaesthesia – central neuraxial blockade

Key points

- Spinal and epidural anaesthesia convey a wide variety of benefits to perioperative care
- Particular care should be taken regarding neuraxial procedures and anticoagulation
- Although rare, some complications can have devastating consequences
- Epidural haematoma is a neurosurgical emergency and should be treated immediately
- The NAP3 audit has provided key evidence of the safety of neuraxial blockade

Central neuraxial blocks (CNBs) include spinal, epidural and combined spinal epidural techniques. They can be used alone (avoiding potential complications of general anaesthesia), with sedation, or in addition to general anaesthesia to provide prolonged high-quality analgesia for a variety of indications.

The segmental nerves in the thoracic and lumbar region contain somatic sensory, motor and autonomic (sympathetic) nerve fibres. Sensory and autonomic fibres have a smaller diameter and are more easily blocked than larger motor fibres.

Potential benefits of CNBs

- Improved pain relief in comparison with intravenous opiates
- Reduced respiratory complications and failure due to infective and noninfective causes
- Reduced cardiovascular complications. Arrhythmia may be reduced due to a reduction in circulating catecholamines. There is evidence that postoperative myocardial infarction is reduced
- Early return of normal gastrointestinal function
- 'Enhanced recovery' after major gastrointestinal and orthopaedic surgery
- Reduced stress response to surgery, demonstrated by reductions in serum adrenaline, noradrenaline, cortisol and glucose. A reduction in perioperative stress attenuates immunosuppression
- Reduced surgical blood loss and transfusion requirement
- Improved prevention of thromboembolic complications. Reduction in deep vein thrombosis and pulmonary embolism by about 50%
- Better tissue oxygenation and perfusion. Attenuation of the stress response and vasodilatation may improve tissue perfusion and oxygenation, improving wound healing and reducing wound infection

Indications

- Obstetric procedures including caesarean section, assisted delivery and manual removal of placenta
- Surgery to the lower limbs, particularly hip and knee surgery
- Surgery to the perineum or lower abdomen including total abdominal hysterectomy
- Analgesia for abdominal surgery, combined with general anaesthesia
- Epidural block can also be used for cardiac and thoracic surgery, e.g. thoracotomy

Contraindications

Absolute

- Patient refusal
- Allergy to local anaesthetic
- Sepsis at the site of injection
- Uncorrected hypovolaemia
- Coagulopathy
- Raised intracranial pressure
- Potential for severe blood loss, e.g. placenta accreta

Relative

- Cardiovascular disease such as fixed cardiac output states, e.g. aortic stenosis. Patients with severe heart disease may

not tolerate associated haemodynamic changes
- Infection distant from the site of injection
- Unknown duration of surgery may prohibit the use of spinal anaesthesia alone
- Neurological disease, e.g. multiple sclerosis. Some authors postulate that there is a risk exacerbating pre-existing neurologic defects

Complications

The Royal College of Anaesthetists NAP3 project provides some of the best evidence available regarding serious complications associated with neuraxial anaesthesia.

Very common (1 in 10) or common (1 in 100)

- Urinary retention
- Hypotension is usually due to vasodilation as a result of the sympathetic block. The circulatory system should be actively managed with intravenous fluids and vasopressor drugs to avoid complications of hypotension and cardiovascular collapse. Vagal overactivity may also be implicated

- Effects of intrathecal and epidural opioids: pruritis can result in widespread itching. Opioids also risk respiratory depression, sedation and confusion. These side effects can be treated with intravenous naloxone
- Nausea and vomiting
- Inadequate analgesia or failure
- Post dural-puncture headache has an approximate incidence of 1.5%. The risk from spinal needles decreases with small diameter, atraumatic needles

Rare (1 in 10,000) or very rare (1 in 100,000) complications

- Local anaesthetic toxicity
- Nerve and spinal cord injury. The incidence of permanent harm is approximately 1 in 100,000. In most cases symptoms improve or resolve within a few weeks or monthss
- Vertebral canal haematoma. Diagnosis and treatment is necessary within 8–12 hours to prevent paraplegia. Early diagnosis necessitates epidural analgesic regimens that minimise the degree of lower limb nerve block so that early features of neurological deficit can be identified. Incidence is 1 in 20,000

Table 69 Implications of some common anticoagulant medications on neuraxial anaesthesia		
Anticoagulant	Minimum time between last dose and block	Minimum time after block for next dose
Aspirin	No delay required	No delay required
Heparin- Unfractionated- prophylactic Unfractionated-treatment Low Molecular weight-prophylactic Low molecular weight-treatment	 4 hours 4 hours (check APTT) 12 hours 24 hours	 1 hour 4 hours 4 hours 4 hours
Clopidogrel	7 days	No delay required for block*
Fondaparinaux	At least 36 hours	12 hours
Non-steroidal anti-inflamatory drugs	No delay required	No delay required
Tirofiban	8 hours	No delay required
Rivaroxiban	21 hours**	5 hours**
Warfarin	INR<1.5	1 hour

*No delay required for block, but 6-hours suggested from catheter removal until next dose
**Epidurals not recommended with concurrent Rivaroxaban therapy
Broadly speaking, timing of epidural catheter removal is similar to the timing for blocks noted in the table.
Adapted from Harrop-Griffiths W, Cook T, Gill H et al. Regional Anaesthesia and patients with abnormalities of coagulation (2013). Anaesthesia;68:966-72

there is little supportive evidence. An epidural blood patch 24–48 hours post dural-puncture can cause a tamponade effect in the epidural space, increase intracranial pressure and prevent further CSF leak. The chance of symptom relief from a single epidural blood patch is approximately 50% and a further epidural blood patch may be required in up to 40% of patients. A second patch carries a similar chance of success.

Further reading

Association of Anaesthetists of Great Britain and Ireland (AAGBI). Safety Guideline- Management of local anaesthetic toxicity. London; AAGBI, 2010.

Association of Anaesthetists of Great Britain and Ireland (AAGBI). Best practice in the management of epidural analgesia in the hospital setting. London; AAGBI, 2011.

Cook TM, Counsell D, Wildsmith JAW. Major complications of central neuraxial block: Report on the Third National Audit of The Royal College of Anaesthetists. Br J Anaesth 2009; 102:179–190.

Wiles MD, Nathanson MH. Local anaesthetic adjuvants – future developments. Anaesthesia 2009; 65:22–37.

Harrop-Griffiths W, Cook T, Gill H, et al. Regional anaesthesia and patients with abnormalities of coagulation. Anaesthesia 2013; 68:966-972.

Related topics of interest

Regional anaesthesia – plexus and peripheral nerve blocks

Key points

- Ultrasound location has improved the reliability of regional anaesthesia (RA)
- There is an increasing trend for surgical procedures to be performed under regional block alone
- Local anaesthetic maximum doses should be adhered to. The anaesthetist must be familiar with the management of inadvertent toxicity

RA can be used alone, or in conjunction with sedation or general anaesthesia (GA). Proximal plexus blocks allow anaesthesia of an entire limb, whilst more distal blocks of individual nerves can be used separately, or in combination, for both anaesthesia and postoperative analgesia. Peripheral anaesthesia can broadly be thought of as targeting either particular nerves/plexuses or fascial planes through which nerves run. Common sites for regional nerve blocks are indicated in **Table 72**.

Running entire operating lists of procedures performed under regional block can increase efficiency and safety. The logistics of such a list allow for a patient to receive their 'block', whilst the preceding patient is undergoing surgery.

Indications

RA has several potential advantages
- Avoidance of GA
- Many patients prefer regional to GA often because of previous adverse experiences of GA. In patients with severe comorbidities, RA may allow surgical procedures to proceed which would not be possible under GA, or for operations to be performed as daycases rather than in-patients
- Postoperative analgesia
- RA provides excellent postoperative pain relief after major operations, such as shoulder or knee arthroplasty. It allows

Table 72 Common peripheral nerve blocks	
Nerve block	**Comments, suitable surgeries**
Peribulbar, sub-Tenon's	Cataract and vitreoretinal surgery

Brachial plexus
   Interscalene
   Supraclavicular
   Axillary
	
	Shoulder surgery
	Forearm and hand surgery, often misses the ulnar nerve
	Forearm/hand surgery, does not always relieve tourniquet pain

Forearm peripheral nerves: radial, median, ulnar	Accessible at multiple sites along the upper limb. Suitable for forearm and hand surgery
Paravertebral	Chest wall surgery, breast surgery. Small risk of pneumothorax
Transversus abdominis	Abdominal and pelvic surgery. A posterior approach may be more effective
Rectus sheath	Indwelling catheters useful for midline incision analgesia. Gaining popularity as a viable alternative to epidural use
Lumbar plexus	Good for hip surgery, but risks epidural spread
Ilioinguinal/iliohypogastric	Groin surgery
Penile	Circumcision and penile surgery
Femoral, subsartorial	Knee surgery and medial aspect of the lower limb
Sciatic, popliteal	Hip surgery, foot and ankle surgery
Ankle	Forefoot surgery

for avoidance of the side effects of opioid analgesics, such as respiratory depression, nausea and drowsiness

Contraindications

Absolute contraindications

- Patient refusal (informed consent is essential)
- Known allergy to local anaesthetic agents
- Skin infection over the proposed block site

Relative contraindications

- Risk of nerve injury
  - In patients undergoing exploration of an acute nerve injury, or procedures with a significant risk of iatrogenic nerve injury, e.g. humeral or elbow surgery, RA can delay the postoperative assessment of nerve function and confuse the aetiology of any persisting neuropathy
- Risk of compartment syndrome
  - There remains concern that dense postoperative anaesthesia of a limb at risk of postoperative compartment syndrome may delay its diagnosis and management. This was not borne out in a review of the literature in 2009
- Planned early mobilisation
  - Motor weakness of a limb may delay discharge from a day surgery unit, or prevent early mobilisation following major arthroplasty
- Anticoagulant or antiplatelet agents
  - The risk of peripheral RA in the presence of anticoagulation is less than that of neuraxial blockade. It is hard to quantify due to the many variables involved, such as the anticoagulant used, the proposed nerve block, patient comorbidities and associated GA risk. Whilst firm rules regarding RA in the presence of anticoagulation are impractical, the AAGBI has produced a consensus document as a guide
- Block-specific contraindications
  - The side effects of some blocks render them relatively contraindicated in certain patients. For example, the ipsilateral phrenic nerve paralysis invariably resulting from interscalene

brachial plexus blocks may provoke respiratory distress in some patients with chronic chest disease

Continuous nerve infusion catheters

Placement of catheters for the continuous or bolus infusion of local anaesthetics has gained recognition as an effective method to provide ongoing postoperative analgesia. Catheters are often positioned using ultrasound guidance. An aseptic technique is essential and they must be tested to ascertain correct positioning prior to discharge to the ward. Complications include failure/ dislodgement, local anaesthetic toxicity, inadvertent intravascular/intrathecal placement and infection.

Practical aspects of RA

Surroundings

RA should be performed in a well-equipped anaesthetic room, with full monitoring and intravenous access established. Airway management and resuscitation equipment, including lipid emulsion (see below) must be immediately available. A fully trained assistant should be present.

Awake or asleep?

As with neuraxial anaesthesia controversy exists regarding performing RA on anaesthetised patients. General consensus favours an awake or consciously sedated patient, able to communicate any sensations of pain or paraesthesia that may indicate inadvertent intraneural injection of local anaesthesia.

Nerve localisation

Nerves are commonly localised in three ways:
- Landmark techniques. Best suited to distal peripheral nerve blocks, e.g. the ankle block
- Nerve stimulation. An insulated needle is used with an electric nerve stimulator to elicit a motor response when the needle tip is in close proximity to the target nerve
- Ultrasound localisation. Ultrasound is increasingly popular in RA as it allows

direct visualisation of the nerve, the approaching needle and the spread of local anaesthetic around the target

Local anaesthetic action

The choice, concentration and volume of local anaesthetic determine the speed of onset and duration of RA. Local anaesthetics are weak bases, consisting of a hydrophobic and hydrophilic group coupled by either an ester or amide bond. Ester local anaesthetics, such as cocaine, are less stable in solution, and produce a potentially allergenic metabolite. Consequently, amides, such as lidocaine, are the more commonly used agents. Local anaesthetics reversibly inhibit the transmission of nerve impulses by disrupting the cell's resting membrane potential. This is achieved primarily by blockade of sodium ion channels. The local anaesthetic molecules pass through the nerve cell lipid membrane into the axoplasm, where, after ionisation, they bind to transmembrane sodium channels, rendering them inactive.

Complications

Nerve injury

- Nerve injury following RA can result from direct trauma by the needle, haematoma formation or subsequent infection. A recent meta-analysis and evidence review estimates the risk of transient neuropathy postperipheral nerve block at 3%, with only one case remaining unresolved in

the 16 studies with 12 months follow-up. Elsewhere, serious neurological complications following peripheral block is often quoted as 1:5,000-1:30,000

Local anaesthetic toxicity

Presentation

- Absorption of excess local anaesthetic into the systemic circulation can lead to disruption of brain and cardiac membrane potentials. Subsequent CNS complications range from perioral paraesthesia, through to unconsciousness and seizures. Cardiac dysrhythmias may deteriorate to reactive ventricular tachycardia and cardiac arrest

Management

- The injection of local anaesthetic should be stopped immediately and cardio respiratory support provided along the standard ABC pathway
- Seizures should be controlled with benzodiazepines, thiopentone or propofol
- Cardiac arrest should be managed according to Resuscitation Council ALS guidelines but with the important addition of lipid rescue therapy. Lipid emulsion (e.g. Intralipid) 20% should be administered, initially as a 1.5 mL/kg bolus followed by a 15 mL/kg/h infusion. If no response is seen after 5 minutes a further bolus doses should be given, and the infusion rate doubled. A third and final bolus dose can be given if no response is seen after 10 minutes

Further reading

Brull R, McCartney CJL, Chan VWS, et al. Neurological complications after regional anaesthesia: contemporary estimates of risk. Anesth Analg 2007; 104:965–974.

Cave G, Harrop-Griffiths W (chair), Harvey M, et al. AAGBI Safety Guideline: Management of Severe Local Anaesthetic Toxicity. London; AAGBI, 2010.

Harrop-Griffiths W, Cook T, Gill H, et al. Regional anaesthesia and patients with abnormalities of coagulation. Anaesthesia 2013; 68:966-972.

Related topics of interest

Renal disease – acute kidney injury

Key points

- Acute kidney injury (AKI) has replaced the term acute renal failure
- Eighty per cent of AKI is prerenal in aetiology, often due to renal hypoperfusion
- Consideration of altered drug pharmacokinetics is of great significance in patients with AKI
- Fluid and electrolyte status should be carefully assessed prior to anaesthesia if AKI is suspected

AKI has now replaced the term acute renal failure. Clinically, AKI is characterised by a rapid reduction in kidney function resulting in a failure to maintain fluid, electrolyte and acid–base homoeostasis. Over recent years there has been increasing recognition that relatively small rises in serum creatinine in a variety of clinical settings are associated with deleterious outcomes – increases in mortality, morbidity, postoperative complications and hospital length of stay (**Table 73**).

The 'eGFR' is not valid in AKI, as the serum creatinine lags significantly behind changes in renal function – make an individual assessment of current renal function by assessing fluid status, urine output and biochemistry results trends.

AKI is common amongst unplanned hospital admissions, and complicates the postoperative course of many surgical patients. Up to 20% of critically ill patients will have an episode of AKI, and AKI necessitating renal replacement therapy (RRT) occurs in around 5% of all ICU admissions. RRT is more frequently required when AKI complicates multiorgan failure; mortality rates may rise as high as 80%, depending on the population studied.

- The majority (~80%) of cases of AKI are due to prerenal factors, particularly renal hypoperfusion. This is usually preventable, and should resolve with improvement in fluid status
    - It is, however, common to have a number of simultaneous insults (e.g. sepsis and hypotension in an elderly patient with a degree of chronic kidney disease (CKD) who takes an ACE-inhibitor)
- Obstruction of the urinary tract accounts for about 15% of AKI
- The remaining few percent are due to 'renal' causes

In prerenal AKI, the ability to concentrate urine should be preserved, reflected as high urine osmolality, low urinary sodium concentration, and low fractional excretion of sodium or urea (FE_{Na} and FE_{Urea}). In established acute tubular necrosis (ATN), the ability to concentrate urine is lost, and both FE_{Na} and FE_{Urea} will be high. Urinary electrolytes should be interpreted with caution in the elderly or those with CKD, who may have a reduced capacity to concentrate urine, and are invalid in patients taking diuretics.

Problems

Patients with AKI may present a considerable challenge to the anaesthetist:

Table 73 AKI staging system – AKI is present when either the creatinine or urine output criteria are met		
Stage	Serum creatinine	Urine output
1	Rise of ≥26 µmol/L within 48 hours Or rise to ≥1.5–1.9 x baseline within 1 week	<0.5 mL/kg/h For >6 consecutive hours
2	Rise to ≥2.0–2.9 x baseline	<0.5 mL/kg/h For >12 hours
3	Rise to ≥3.0 x baseline Or rise to ≥354 µmol/L Or commenced on renal replacement therapy, irrespective of stage	< 0.3 mL/kg/h For > 24 hours Or anuria for 12 hours

- Fluid balance may be deranged, either as a cause or consequence of AKI. Mechanisms of homeostasis are dysfunctional
- There may be acidosis with substantial biochemical abnormalities and a catabolic state
- The underlying disorder may have significant comorbid features that impact on the conduct of anaesthesia or surgery
- In some situations, the AKI may be improved by surgery, or surgery is necessary despite the increased risks associated with AKI. Otherwise cases should be deferred until renal function is optimised

Anaesthetic management
Altered drug pharmacokinetics

- Renal failure has significant effects on pharmacokinetics, and many drugs require reduction in dosage, frequency or both, depending on the severity of renal dysfunction. Some drugs are contraindicated (e.g. NSAIDs)
  - Reduced renal clearance of (predominantly) polar, water-soluble compounds
  - Hypoalbuminaemia leads to reduced protein binding
  - Metabolic acids compete for protein binding sites, increasing free fraction of drug
  - Impaired salt and water excretion
  - Increased half-lives of drugs metabolised by the kidney

Preoperative assessment

- Preoperative renal dysfunction increases risk of postoperative complications
- Premorbid factors associated with postoperative AKI
  - Increasing age, female sex, cardiovascular disease and heart failure, diabetes, CKD, chronic liver disease and jaundice, multi-system trauma, shock states
  - Nephrotoxic medications
  - Major surgery, cardiopulmonary bypass, surgery involving pelvis or aortorenal vasculature, significant blood loss anticipated, peritoneal contamination

- Assess personally with regard to intravascular volume status
- In established AKI, consider timing of anaesthesia with regard to RRT
- Consider pre-operative optimisation in ward or critical care area and/or scheduled postoperative admission to critical care
- Counsel your patient with regard to their increased risk of postoperative complications

Conduct of anaesthesia

- Prevent perioperative AKI by preserving renal perfusion and tissue oxygenation, whilst minimising nephrotoxicity
- Consider invasive blood pressure and central venous pressure monitoring, urinary catheter +/– CO monitoring. Care should be taken to optimise fluid balance as it can be difficult to remove excess fluid from overloaded patients
- In patients at risk of permanent renal failure, avoid vascular access in non-dominant arm and both subclavian veins
- Avoid crystalloids with supplemental potassium. Starch-based colloids are contraindicated
- Avoid spontaneous respiration in acidotic patients
- Platelet dysfunction and coagulation abnormalities may increase risks of regional anaesthesia
- There is a slightly increased effect of thiopentone; however, propofol is unaffected
- Isoflurane is first line although there is no evidence of harm from compound A with sevoflurane use; There is a theoretical risk of fluoride toxicity with enflurane so its use is discouraged in this setting
- Beware of pre-operative hyperkalaemia if suxamethonium use anticipated
- Atracurium (or cisatracurium) is first line; rocuronium and vecuronium have increased duration of activity and there is significant accumulation of pancuronium
- Neostigmine effect is prolonged
- There is accumulation of morphine metabolites (morphine-6-glucuronide). Fentanyl, alfentanil and remifentanil can be used safely

Postoperative care

- Consider planned admission to critical care environment
- Monitor intravascular fluid status and urine output
- Do not give dopamine or furosemide to prevent AKI – they are ineffective
- Remeasure electrolytes
- Use fentanyl patient-controlled analgesia in preference to morphine

Further reading

Lewington A, Kanagasundaram S. Clinical practice guidelines: acute kidney injury. Petersfield; The Renal Association, 2011.

Ashley C, Currie A (Eds). Renal Drug Handbook, 3rd edn. London; Radcliffe Publishing Ltd, 2009.

Related topics of interest

- Diabetes (p. 56)
- Elderly patients (p. 64)
- Renal disease – chronic kidney disease (p. 253)

Renal disease – chronic kidney disease

Key points

- The degree of renal impairment is usually estimated from the serum creatinine in chronic disease
- Chronic kidney disease (CKD) affects multiple systems, particularly the cardiovascular system
- Patients receiving renal replacement therapy are usually operated on 4–24 hours postdialysis. Care should be taken with fluid loading
- Actual and future dialysis vascular access sites should be protected

CKD describes the state of abnormal kidney function or structure. Abnormal function is defined as a reduced glomerular filtration rate (GFR), which is usually estimated from serum creatinine, measured on at least two occasions, over at least 3 months.

CKD therefore ranges from systemically well patients with mild abnormalities in renal anatomy to established renal failure on dialysis or a functioning renal transplant (**Table 74**). Patients with substantial CKD may have a significant past medical history, take a number of medications and have systemic complications which all increase the risks of anaesthesia and surgery.

CKD affects in the region of 6000 per million population in the UK. Currently greater than 51,000 adult patients (800 per million population) are in receipt of a functioning renal transplant or are on maintenance dialysis for established renal failure (48% transplant, 44% haemodialysis, 8% peritoneal dialysis). Treatment of this group accounts for over 2% of the NHS budget.

Problems

CKD is a major risk factor for the development of postoperative complications, including AKI.

- Creatinine clearance (estimated by the Cockroft–Gault's method) is one of the components of the EUROSCORE-2, for predicting early mortality following cardiac surgery
- Renal function is a factor in the Glasgow Aneurysm Score and Hardman Index for predicting survival after ruptured aortic aneurysm
- Serum urea features in the Ransom Pancreatitis criteria, SAPS and POSSUM score
- Serum creatinine is a factor in the Lee Revised Cardiac Risk Index, APACHE, ICNARC, SOFA and MODS calculations

CKD is often caused by underlying medical conditions, which might include:

- Hypertension
- Atheromatous vascular disease
- Diabetes mellitus
- Reflux nephropathy and obstructive uropathy

Table 74 CKD staging system		
Stage	GFR (mL/min/1.73 m^2)	Description
1	≥90	Normal or increased GFR, but with other evidence of kidney damage* or abnormal anatomy
2	60–89	Slight decrease in GFR, with other evidence of kidney damage* or abnormal anatomy
3a	45–59	Moderate decrease in GFR, with or without other evidence of kidney damage*
3b	30–44	
4	15–29	Severe decrease in GFR, with or without other evidence of kidney damage*
5	<15	Established renal failure

*Other evidence of kidney damage would include persistent microscopic haematuria (of renal origin), proteinuria, biopsy-proven glomerulonephritis, focal renal scarring on imaging.
CKD, chronic kidney disease; GFR, glomerular filtration rate.

- Genetic disorders, including polycystic kidney disease and Alport's syndrome
- Autoimmune disorders, such as systemic lupus erythematosus, systemic vasculitis and Goodpasture's syndrome

CKD is also associated with the development of pathophysiological changes affecting almost every organ system. These include:

- Increased risk of cardiovascular disease
  - Accelerated atherosclerosis, left ventricular hypertrophy, vascular calcification, cardiac conduction abnormalities, hypertension, salt and water retention, altered lipoprotein metabolism, calcification of heart valves
  - Pericarditis, pulmonary oedema and pleural effusions
- Chronic metabolic acidosis
  - Negative nitrogen balance, muscle wasting, growth retardation in children and bone resorption
- Musculoskeletal system
  - Impaired calcium and phosphate homeostasis, renal osteodystrophy, hyperparathyroidism and osteoporosis
- GI system
  - Delayed gastric emptying, increased gastric acidity, malnutrition, anorexia and vomiting
- Immune system
  - Increased susceptibility to both bacterial and viral infections, decreased immune response to antigenic stimuli
  - Immunosuppression (to treat primary renal disease, or for transplantation)
- Haemostasis and coagulation
  - Anaemia, platelet dysfunction
- Fluid and electrolyte homeostasis
  - Hyperkalaemia, acidosis, hyperphosphataemia, hypocalcaemia, chronic volume overload, fixed maximal urine output and reduced urinary concentrating ability
- Nervous system
  - Autonomic neuropathy – reduced baroreceptor sensitivity, sympathetic hyperactivity, parasympathetic dysfunction
  - Peripheral neuropathy, uraemic encephalopathy, cerebral small vessel ischaemia

Anaesthetic management

Altered drug pharmacokinetics

- Renal failure has significant effects on pharmacokinetics which have already been discussed in the preceding chapter

Preoperative assessment

- Preoperative renal dysfunction increases risk of postoperative complications
- Determine the cause of renal failure, as that disease may have manifestations elsewhere
- Assess personally with regard to intravascular volume status – for dialysis patients check current and 'dry' body weights, daily fluid allowance and interdialytic weight gain
- Avoid preoperative dehydration
- Check biochemical and haematological parameters, ECG, chest X-ray
- Control hypertension
- In established renal failure, consider timing of anaesthesia with regard to dialysis schedule and technique
  - 4–24 hours posthaemodialysis is usual (consider heparin-free dialysis perioperatively)
  - Peritoneal dialysis continues until theatre, but ensure patient fully drains out peritoneal dialysis fluid prior to arriving in anaesthetic room
- Consider scheduled postoperative admission to critical care area
- Counsel the patient with regard to their increased risk of postoperative complications
- For all dialysis patients and transplant recipients, ensure Nephrology team are aware of planned surgery

Vascular access

- Haemodialysis necessitates excellent vascular access; where dialysis is permanent, this access becomes a lifeline

- Complications of vascular access have substantial effects on patient morbidity and mortality
- Protect current or potential future access sites by avoiding venepuncture and cannulation
- BP cuffs should not be used on the fistula arm
- In patients at risk of permanent renal failure, avoid vascular access in nondominant arm and both subclavian veins

Conduct of anaesthesia

- The conduct of anaesthesia is similar to that of acute kidney injury and is covered in the preceding chapter

Postoperative care

Considerations for postoperative care are the same as for acute kidney injury. The following additional points should be considered.

- Continue any long-term immunosuppressants postoperatively (with appropriate dose adjustments if converting from oral to intravenous therapy)
- Remember that postoperative complications (e.g. acute cardiac dysfunction, haemorrhage, systemic inflammatory response syndrome, sepsis and hypotension) may have a much greater impact on renal function than intraoperative conditions

Further reading

Craig EG, Hunter JM. Recent developments in the perioperative management of adult patients with chronic kidney disease. Br J Anaesth 2008; 101:296–310.

Jones DR, Lee HT. Surgery in the patient with renal dysfunction. Med Clin N Am 2009; 95:1083–1093.

Webb ST, Allen SD. Perioperative renal protection. Br J Anaesth: Contin Educ Anaesth Crit Care Pain Med 2008; 8:176–180.

Related topics of interest

- Diabetes (p. 56)
- Elderly patients (p. 64)
- Renal disease – acute kidney injury (p. 250)

Respiratory – acute respiratory distress syndrome

Key points

- Acute respiratory distress syndrome (ARDS) is not a diagnosis and treatment must include that of the underlying cause
- Ventilatory strategies are the current cornerstone of supportive care
- Anaesthetic management should include consideration of delaying surgery and close liaison with the intensive care unit (ICU) team and senior surgeon

ARDS is an inflammatory process in response to an intrapulmonary or extrapulmonary pathology. The previous 1994 definition of a spectrum from acute lung injury (ALI) to ARDS has recently been superseded following an international expert consensus panel meeting during the 2011 24th Annual Congress of the European Society of Intensive Care Medicine (**Table 75**). ALI is no longer a defined condition as this term was frequently misused to describe a mild form of ARDS and underplay the significance of the disorder. ARDS occurs in around 7% of ICU admissions and 16% of ventilated patients. Hospital mortality ranges from 10% to 60% depending on the severity and aetiology of the condition although more than half of those presenting with a mild form will progress to severe ARDS. Mortality has improved during the last 15 years.

Aetiology can be divided into pulmonary and extrapulmonary causes. The commonest precipitants are sepsis and pneumonia but any injury, disease or process with the potential to result in exposure of the lungs to inflammatory mediators can cause ARDS. The disease progresses through three broad phases:

- *Exudative (0–4 days):* alveolar/capillary endothelial injury leading to proteinaceous leak into the alveolar space and migration of macrophages and neutrophils. Cytokine and oxygen free radical production leads to pneumocyte damage
- *Proliferative (1–3 weeks):* alveoli filled with cellular debris, fibrin and oxidants leading to hyaline membrane formation and loss of surfactant
- *Fibrosis (3–4 weeks):* phagocytosis of debris, collagen deposition

The mainstay of treatment is that of the underlying disease, which underlines the importance of recognising ARDS as a secondary syndrome and not a primary diagnosis. A number of therapeutic approaches have been proposed over the last 40 years since the condition was first described. The following include accepted treatments, promising innovations or those of particular significance on the list of disproven therapies:

- Low tidal volume ventilation. Several studies, most notably the ARDSNet study, have reported mortality benefit from this strategy and this is probably the most accepted intervention for ARDS. 6 mL/kg (Ideal Body Weight) tidal volume reduces the incidence of volutrauma (worsening lung inflammation due to overdistension) and barotrauma (lung

Table 75 2012 Berlin definition of ARDS		
All require • Acute onset within 1 week of a known clinical insult or new/worsening respiratory symptoms. • Bilateral opacities on chest X-ray or CT — not wholly explained by effusions, lobar/lung collapse, or nodules. • Respiratory failure not fully explained by cardiac failure or fluid overload. This may need objective assessment (e.g. echocardiography) to exclude hydrostatics oedema if no risk factors are present.		
MILD	**MODERATE**	**SEVERE**
PaO_2/FIO_2 ratio 201-300 mmHg PEEP or CPAP ≥5 cmH$_2$O.	PaO_2/FIO_2 ratio <200 mmHg PEEP ≥5 cmH$_2$O.	PaO_2/FIO_2 ratio <100 mmHg PEEP ≥5 cmH$_2$O

injury due to pressure effects, particularly pneumothorax)
- Restrictive fluid therapy. Avoidance of excess fluid and worsening pulmonary oedema reduces ventilator days and ICU length of stay
- Optimal PEEP and recruitment. Reduced compliance and consolidation of lung are hallmarks of ARDS. PEEP is routinely used to maintain recruitment of lung thus reducing atelectrauma (lung injury from repetitive opening and closing of alveoli) and biotrauma (systemic inflammation due to release of mediators within the lung in response to lung injury). Setting the 'correct' PEEP theoretically allows ventilation to occur on the most efficient part of the compliance curve. However, due to the characteristic heterogeneity of the lungs in ARDS, optimal PEEP for one lung region will overdistend some and fail to maintain recruitment in others. In basic terms, however, PEEP (along with FIO_2) remains one of the key influences over oxygenation as it is a determinant of the mean airway pressure. PEEP alone, will not recruit collapsed lung and after disconnections or endotracheal suction, a recruitment manoeuvre may be required. In general, recruitment techniques which can be achieved on the ventilator are superior; 'bagging the patient up', e.g. with a hand bag-valve system, inevitably involves a further disconnection after the manoeuvre, risking derecruitment. PEEP and recruitment manoeuvres are useful measures to help wean FIO_2 aggressively. Prolonged exposure to FIO_2 >0.5 is toxic to the lungs. PaO_2 >8.0 kPa or SpO_2 88–92% are accepted targets
- Permissive hypercapnia. In order to ventilate the lungs in a way that does not worsen the injury (Ventilator Induced/Associated Lung Injury – VILI or VALI), inspiratory pressures should be limited to 30 cmH$_2$O with a respiratory rate less than 30 breaths/min. This will almost inevitably lead to a rise in $PaCO_2$. Permissive hypercapnia describes the compromise to achieve these ventilation goals, accepting a respiratory acidaemia down to a pH of 7.25–7.30. If pH falls excessively, ventilation

and sedation should be optimised to minimise metabolic CO_2 production. Permissive hypercapnia should be avoided in patients with coexisting brain injury
- Neuromuscular blockade. Paralysis of intercostal and abdominal wall musculature can improve chest wall compliance thus reduce inspiratory pressure requirements. The ACURASYS study has demonstrated a mortality benefit with this strategy. In difficult cases, paralysis can also remove the excess metabolic requirements associated with ventilator dyssynchrony
- Semirecumbent positioning. A 30° head-up position is a standard of care in all ventilated patients, particularly those receiving enteral nutrition. It minimises the risk of microaspiration and improves compliance and functional residual capacity due to the postural effects on the lungs and abdominal contents
- Prone ventilation. In severe ARDS, prone positioning has been demonstrated to have a mortality benefit although only in those with a PaO_2/FIO_2 ratio <100 mmHg. There are significant risks and logistical issues with this technique, e.g. displaced lines and tubes, pressure injuries, injuries to staff in turning the patient. More studies are required to determine the optimum duration of therapy
- High-frequency oscillatory ventilation (HFOV). This therapy is well established in paediatric therapy for RDS. However, the OSCAR study, a UK multicentre trial of this therapy in adult ARDS demonstrated no 30-day mortality benefit
- Extracorporeal membrane oxygenation (ECMO). The evidence for this therapy is currently lacking and provision of the therapy extremely limited. The CESAR study demonstrated a mortality benefit in those randomised to treatment but many in that group did not actually receive ECMO, suggesting the benefit may be attributable instead to treatment in a tertiary ARDS ICU
- Corticosteroids. Numerous studies have examined this therapy as the anti-inflammatory properties would seem ideal to ameliorate the proliferative and

fibrotic phases. A study from the ARDSNet group revealed a reduction in duration of ventilation, shock and ICU stay but an overall increase in mortality, particularly if commenced later than 14 days from onset of ARDS. This therapy is therefore not currently part of the management of the condition

A selection of these interventions can be combined in a 'bundle' to optimise care of any ventilated patient irrespective of the presence of ARDS. Care bundles depend on combining a maximum of five evidence-based measures, as their success is reliant on all elements being followed.

Anaesthetic management

Preoperative

- Consider stability of respiratory status vs. urgency of surgery
    - Can surgery be safely postponed?
    - Will surgery improve respiratory status, e.g. laparotomy for abdominal compartment syndrome, source control of extrapulmonary sepsis causing ARDS?
    - Will systemic response to surgery further worsen pulmonary inflammation to unmanageable levels?
    - Can the patient safely undergo transfer around the hospital?
- Liaise with the surgical team to minimise operative time. Clear surgical goals should be set in advance and a consultant surgeon should operate in these cases

- For newly presenting patients, early liaison with the ICU team is vital. Almost any patient with mild ARDS prior to urgent/emergency surgery will worsen during and after surgery and require ICU admission

Intraoperative

- Minimise ventilator disconnections or high-flow/prolonged/frequent endotracheal suction. This avoids derecruitment of lung volume
- Consider recruitment manoeuvres following disconnection/suction
- Use PEEP in all patients and tolerate Spo_2 88–92%
- Select either pressure-control ventilation or, ideally, volume-control with pressure limitation
- Avoid airway pressures $\geq$30 cmH$_2$O
- Use frequent arterial blood gas analysis to titrate inspired oxygen and ventilation parameters
- Minimise excess fluid infusion

Postoperative

- Specific points for handover to the ICU team include ventilator pressure requirements, oxygen and PEEP settings, response to laparotomy (if applicable) and suction requirements
- Information regarding suspected aetiology is of particular relevance, particularly any therapy directed towards this which is yet to be implemented, e.g. appropriate antibiotic therapy in sepsis (and proximity to bacterial cultures)?

Further reading

Acute Respiratory Distress Syndrome (ARDS) Clinical Trials Network. Ventilation with lower tidal volumes as compared with traditional tidal volumes for acute lung injury and the acute respiratory distress syndrome. N Engl J Med 2000; 342:1301–1308.

The ARDS Definition Task Force. Acute respiratory distress syndrome: the Berlin definition. J Am Med Assoc 2012; 307:2526–2533.

Calfee CS, Matthay MA. Non-ventilatory treatments for acute lung injury and ARDS. Chest 2007; 131:913–920.

Girard TD, Bernard GR. Mechanical ventilation in ARDS: a state-of-the-art review. Chest 2007; 131:921–929.

Related topics of interest

Respiratory – asthma

Key points

- Asthma is characterised by reversible airway obstruction
- Preoperative assessment of asthma severity can predict the likelihood of perioperative problems
- The anaesthetic technique should focus on avoiding asthma precipitants
- Perioperative bronchoconstriction can be life threatening and should be treated aggressively

Asthma is a chronic disease characterised by airway obstruction and increased reactivity of the tracheobronchial tree to various stimuli (e.g. inhaled allergens, infection, exercise, anxiety, cold or drugs). It manifests as widespread airway narrowing with smooth muscle contraction, mucosal oedema and a cellular infiltrate. The pathophysiology is complex, involving inflammatory and immunological mediators (often therapeutic targets). Reversibility of airway obstruction is characteristic and distinguishes asthma from the fixed obstruction of chronic bronchitis and emphysema. The severity of airflow obstruction varies widely over short periods of time but airway resistance may be normal for long periods. The prevalence of asthma is 3–6%.

Problems

- Anxiety, anaesthetic drugs and airway manoeuvres may precipitate bronchoconstriction
- Mucous trapping
- Adrenal suppression from chronic steroid therapy

Surgery for patients with concurrent asthma

Preoperative assessment

The goal of preoperative assessment is to determine the severity of the disease and current management to allow formulation of a plan for perioperative care. Episodic wheezing, dyspnoea and cough are the most common symptoms. A detailed history should include questions regarding current symptoms and triggers, recent oral steroid use, recent or past hospital admission (particularly ICU admission and, crucially, mechanical ventilation) and current management (e.g. home nebuliser, regular inhaled steroid use). Well-controlled asthma is unlikely to cause perioperative problems. Active lung infection should trigger postponement of elective surgery.

A severe acute exacerbation may be indicated by the use of accessory muscles of respiration, pulsus paradoxus (a fall in blood pressure during inspiration, due to the effects of intrathoracic pressure on cardiac preload), cyanosis, sweating, anxiety and insufficient breath to speak. The British Thoracic Society releases evidence-based guidelines for the hospital management of acute severe asthma every few years. Disease severity is best determined by lung spirometry (FEV_1, FEV_1/FVC ratio, peak expiratory flow rate) and its response to bronchodilator therapy.

A normal PEFR in adults is ~600 mL/min. Rises in $PaCO_2$ occur only in severe cases (FEV_1 <25% normal) and may herald imminent respiratory arrest. ECG changes (sinus tachycardia, right ventricular strain, right axis deviation) are nonspecific and only present in severe cases. The chest X-ray is of little use in the diagnosis or assessment of the severity of asthma but may indicate atelectasis due to mucous trapping, pneumonia, pneumothorax, heart failure, or a foreign body in children. The commonest abnormality on chest X-ray is hyperinflation of the lungs.

Preoperative optimisation such as physiotherapy, antibiotics, oral steroids and adequate hydration can help reduce the risk of perioperative complications. Referral to a respiratory specialist may be useful in optimising current medications. Bronchodilator therapy by aerosol should be administered prior to anaesthesia and be available for nebulisation into the breathing system intraoperatively. H_2 receptor antagonists are best avoided as they may unmask H_1 receptor mediated

limit can prevent volutrauma (volume-regulated PCV)

- VCV. A constant inspiratory flow is delivered and airway pressure increases accordingly. Variations in lung compliance and resistance can lead to large increases in airway pressure as the ventilator attempts to deliver the tidal volume selected. This can cause barotrauma (see **Table 76**). Setting a peak pressure limit can reduce this risk (pressure-regulated VCV). Low inspiratory flow rates can be used to limit peak ventilatory pressure and ensure more homogeneous ventilation

Other modes and strategies

Airway pressure release ventilation (APRV)

A continuous, positive pressure is applied to the airways. Intermittent releases to a lower pressure facilitate expiration. This strategy has been used in acute respiratory distress syndrome (ARDS) patients with poorly compliant lungs. Spontaneous ventilation can occur between APRV breaths. Weaning is achieved by reducing the frequency of ventilator-delivered breaths.

Inverse ratio ventilation (IRV)

Used in neonates and, occasionally, adults with ARDS. A prolonged inspiratory phase (up to 4 times that of expiration) increases mean airway pressure and therefore oxygenation. This strategy risks barotrauma and air trapping and is contraindicated in obstructive respiratory disease.

Proning

Proning improves oxygenation but until recently no study had demonstrated a survival benefit. The PROSEVA study however, showed that in severe ARDS, early application of prolonged (16 hours) prone-positioning significantly decreased mortality.

High-frequency oscillatory ventilation (HFOV)

This is high-frequency (3–15 breaths/second), low-tidal volume (1–2 mL/kg) ventilation. The OSCILLATE and OSCAR multicentre randomised-controlled trials (RCTs) showed that in patients with severe or moderate ARDS, HFOV had no significant effect on 30-day mortality.

Extracorporeal membrane oxygenation (ECMO)

A pump-augmented, veno-venous, extracorporeal circuit oxygenates and removes carbon dioxide from the blood. Indications for use include severe hypoxaemia, uncompensated hypercapnia and excessively high end-inspiratory plateau pressures. It should be initiated early and performed in specialised centres for best outcome.

Consequences of mechanical ventilation

There are a number of physiological ramifications and specific complications associated with mechanical ventilation (**Table 77**). Similarly, there are strategies designed to mitigate these. The Department of Health published a 'High impact intervention' for ventilated patients in June 2007 with NICE guidance following in 2008. The specified care bundle is:

- Elevation of the head of the bed to 30–45°
- Sedation holding
- Deep vein thrombosis prophylaxis
- Gastric ulcer prophylaxis

Table 76 Components of ventilator-induced lung injury	
Atelectrauma	Lung injury resulting from repetitive opening and closing of collapsed alveoli
Biotrauma	Pulmonary and systemic inflammation resulting from release of inflammatory mediators from injured lung
Volutrauma	Injury resulting from overdistension, particularly stretch and rupture of capillaries leading to alveolar microhaemorrhage and oedema
Barotrauma	Inextricably linked to volutrauma and high pressures can produce the same lung injury at low volumes in the noncompliant lung

Table 77 Complications and consequences of mechanical ventilation	
Airway	Tracheal injury Accidental extubation
Pulmonary	Reduced lung compliance and FRC Ventilator associated lung injury (VALI): (see **Table 76**) Pneumothoraces Ventilator associated pneumonia (VAP)
Cardiovascular	Reduced right ventricular output (reduced venous return, cardiac output and increased pulmonary vascular resistance) Positive end expiratory pressure (PEEP) can reduced left ventricular filling and compliance
Renal	GFR may reduce by up to 40%: Reduced renal perfusion (reduced arterial pressure and increased venous pressure) Increased renin, angiotensin and vasopressin and reduced atrial natriuretic peptide
Gastrointestinal	Ileus is common; possibly caused by reduced neural activity, altered GI pressures and drug administration
Neurological	ICU delirium (due to sedative drugs and critical illness) Prolonged immobility and the use of neuromuscular blocking agents associated with critical illness polyneuromyopathy

- Appropriate humidification of inspired gas
- Appropriate tubing management
- Suctioning of respiratory secretions (including use of gloves and decontaminating hands before and after the procedure)
- Routine oral hygiene (chlorhexidine mouth wash)

Protective ventilation

The concept of protective ventilation has been established for patients with ARDS.
- Tidal volume: 6 mL/kg ideal body weight
- Peak Pressure: <30 cmH$_2$O
- Positive end-expiratory pressure (PEEP): Optimum levels of PEEP are yet to be defined.
- Early use of neuromuscular blockade
- Optimum oxygenation: Prolonged exposure to an F_{IO_2} > 0.5 is toxic. A Pa_{O_2} >8.0 kPa or Sp_{O_2} 88–92% is acceptable
- Permissive hypercapnia: With relative hypoventilation, Pa_{CO_2} will rise. A pH of 7.25–7.30 can be tolerated in most patients
- Optimum fluid balance

It is unclear whether these strategies should be extended to all patients. However, the IMPROVE study, demonstrated protective ventilation, in adult patients undergoing abdominal surgery and at risk of developing ARDS, improved clinical outcomes when ventilated according to the above guidelines.

Weaning strategies

This transition from full ventilatory support to spontaneous breathing should be started as soon as possible. Ventilatory modes which support weaning (by assisting patient efforts) are listed below. A spontaneous breathing trial should be carried out as soon as suitable (**Table 78**). If successful, the patient can usually be extubated.

Inspiratory pressure support

Weaning is achieved by progressively reducing preset airway pressure or by increasing the amount of negative pressure or flow needed to trigger a breath.

Table 78 Prerequisites for a spontaneous breathing trial	
Respiratory	Pa_{O2} > 8 kPa on F_{IO2} <40–50% and PEEP <5–8 cmH$_2$O Patient is able to initiate an inspiratory effort
Cardiovascular	No evidence of myocardial ischaemia Heart rate <140 bpm Blood Pressure normal with minimal or no vasopressor support
Cognitive	Adequate mental status; GCS>13 and rousable
Correctable comorbidity	Patient is afebrile No electrolyte abnormalities

Sickle cell disease

Key points

- Sickle cell disease should be considered in all patients originating from endemic areas
- Sickle cell trait has little impact on anaesthesia
- Maintenance of oxygenation, tissue perfusion and avoidance of the precipitants of crises are the key aims in anaesthetic management

This is a haemoglobinopathy with autosomal dominant inheritance found in African, Mediterranean and people from the Indian subcontinent. Valine replaces glutamine in position 6 on the β chain of haemoglobin A, resulting in haemoglobin S (HbS). When deoxygenated, the HbS crystallises into chains, which then deform the shape of the red cells, forming the classical crescent shape. The pathology is almost certainly more complex than this and is not simply due to the change in cell shape. Cells become 'sticky' and, combined with intravascular haemolysis, result in a significant alteration in vascular function leading to endothelial damage. This process is responsible for the more chronic effects of sickle cell disease.

The heterozygous form (sickle cell trait) has little clinical manifestation and confers some protection against Falciparum malaria. Ten per cent of people of African descent in the UK have sickle cell trait. There is a normal life expectancy, a haemoglobin greater than 110 g/L, and blood cell 'sickling' only occurs if the Sao_2 is less than 40%. There is, however, an increased risk of pulmonary infarcts.

Codominant expression of the haemoglobin gene allows normal and abnormal haemoglobin to coexist. Haemoglobin S may be produced with mutant haemoglobins such as haemoglobin C (giving SC disease), and with β thalassaemia.

Homozygous patients risk sickling cells when oxygen saturations fall below around 85% (i.e. above the saturation of venous blood). Prolonged or recurrent sickling of the red cells results in significant haemolysis and reduces cell lifespan to around 12 days. Blood haemoglobin levels are in the region of 50–80 g/L.

Red cell sickling is more likely if hypoxia, acidosis, low temperature or cellular dehydration occur. It is initially reversible, but when potassium and water are lost from the cell irreversible haemoglobin polymerisation occurs. Sickled cells lead to decreased microvascular blood flow (or occlusion) causing further local hypoxia, acidosis and thus more sickling. Local infarction causes the symptoms and signs of a sickle cell crisis. The acute chest syndrome (pleuritic pain, cough and fever), musculoskeletal complaints (bone pain, muscle tenderness, erythema), abdominal pain, splenic sequestration (acute anaemia and aplastic crisis), haematuria, priapism and cerebral vascular events transient ischaemic attacks and strokes may occur during a crisis.

Chronic haemolytic anaemia, increased infection risk and specific organ damage such as 'autosplenectomy' or renal and pulmonary damage as well as gallstones occur as the result of long-term sickling. Repeated vaso-occlusive pulmonary crises will lead to pulmonary hypertension.

Osteomyelitis and meningitis are more common and prophylactic antibiotics are often given. Homozygotes usually present in early childhood when HbF levels fall and HbS predominates. Although recent advances in care have allowed people with homozygous sickle cell disease to live beyond 70 years, average life expectancy is still in the late 40s.

Problems

- Chronic haemolytic anaemia
- Prevention of an acute sickle cell crisis
- Pre-existing organ damage
- Surgical procedure (may be sickle related)
- Infection risk, due to autosplenectomy

Anaesthetic management

Assessment and premedication

At-risk patients should have a Sickledex test, which exposes cells to sodium metabisulphite. The presence of HbS causes in vitro sickling. Sickledex does not differentiate between the homozygote and the heterozygote and, if positive, formal electrophoresis must be performed. This will quantify the types and amounts of each haemoglobin.

A haematological opinion should be sought. If homozygote and undergoing elective procedures of intermediate or high risk, exchange transfusion may be required to raise HbA concentrations to >40% with an overall target Hb of 100–120 g/L. This optimises oxygen delivery and blood viscosity and reduces the risk of perioperative sickle crises. Transfusion carries it's own complications (iron overload, transfusion-related adverse reaction, anaphylaxis and immunosuppression are increased in this patient group) and many authors now suggest transfusing less and taking a more flexible approach.

Patients are assessed for pre-existing organ damage, particularly renal and lung disease, recent admissions and sickle triggers. Other pathologies consequent upon tissue infarction (see above) should be explored. Premedicant sedatives should be avoided as they carry the risk of hypoventilation and hypoxia. Preoptimisation for elective patients includes adequate hydration, minimal fasting times and keeping warm. There should be a low threshold for deferring elective surgery in the presence of concurrent illness. The care of patients with haemoglobinopathies is often undertaken in specialised centres.

Conduct of anaesthesia

The key principle is to maintain good tissue perfusion and oxygenation, thus reducing the risk of HbS crystalisation. Normothermia, good hydration and oxygenation prevent the development of a sickle crisis. Following preoxygenation, a high F_{IO_2} is used. Controlled ventilation will prevent hypercarbia and acidosis. Cardiac output is maintained to prevent microvascular sludging and vasoconstrictors should be avoided.

Standard monitoring should be augmented with measurement of temperature and urine output to assess the state of hydration. Although alkalosis will shift the oxyhaemoglobin dissociation curve to the left (resulting in more avid binding of oxygen to haemoglobin) studies using intravenous sodium bicarbonate have not shown a reduction in complications. Similarly hyperbaric oxygen has proven ineffective. Regional anaesthesia is contentious. The benefits of vasodilation and good analgesia are attractive. However, hypotension, associated with neuraxial block can lead to poor tissue perfusion, exacerbating sickling.

Epinephrine should not be used with local anaesthetic agents, tourniquets should be avoided (they are considered safe in sickle trait) and patients should be carefully positioned to prevent venous stasis. The prone position is of particular concern, due to reduced venous return. Cell salvage is not recommended, although there are case reports of successful use. Patient warming is essential.

Postoperative care

Postoperative complications are more likely for older patients, those with sickle-lung disease or recent sickle-related complications, pregnancy and intercurrent infection. High dependency care is given to provide oxygen, multimodal analgesia and adequate hydration. NSAIDs are safe in the absence of renal disease. Opiate use can be difficult; on the one hand, there is a risk of hypoventilation with increasing doses. Conversely, patients may also be tolerant to opiates following prolonged use in previous crises. Shivering should be avoided as this increases oxygen consumption. Prophylactic antibiotics may need to be continued. If an acute crisis develops, pain control is particularly important, as the pain is characteristically very severe. Day case surgery is only appropriate for the most minor of procedures.

Further reading

Firth PG. Anaesthesia for peculiar cells – a century of sickle cell disease. Br J Anaesth 2005; 95:287–299.

Firth PG, Head A. Sickle cell disease and anaesthesia. Anesthesiology 2004; 101:766–785.

Wilson M, Forsyth P, Whiteside J. Haemoglobinopathy and sickle cell disease. Br J Anaesth: Contin Educ Anaesth Crit Care Pain Med 2010; 10:24–28.

Related topics of interest

Sleep apnoea

Key points

- Obstructive sleep apnoea (OSA) is common, affecting 4% of middle-aged men
- Patients with OSA are sensitive to opiates and at risk of postoperative respiratory depression
- Pulmonary hypertension should be excluded in patients with OSA
- The STOP-BANG index is a useful screening tool for OSA

Apnoea is defined as lack of airflow for 10 seconds. Hypopnoea is defined as a reduction in airflow with an associated drop in Spo_2 of >3% for 10 seconds. The Apnoea Hypopnoea Index (AHI) is a method used to quantify disease and is calculated as the number of events per hour during sleep (15–30 is 'moderate', >30 is considered 'severe'). OSA has a prevalence of 4% of middle-aged men, and 2% of women, increasing to approximately 40% in morbidly obese patients.

Repeated apnoeic episodes during sleep are associated with hypoxia, hypercarbia and poor sleep quality. A cycle of apnoea, arousal, hyperventilation and then return to sleep is observed throughout the night. The most frequent pathophysiology is one of exaggeration of the reduced upper airway muscle tone associated with normal sleep. This is most prevalent in rapid eye movement (REM) sleep. Other pathologies such as abnormal anatomy and derangement in central control of breathing can also be responsible.

Symptoms include snoring, poor concentration, morning headaches and daytime sleepiness. There is an increased incidence of cardiopulmonary disease due to chronic hypoxia and hypercarbia. Patients may also present having been involved in a road traffic accident after 'falling asleep at the wheel'.

OSA is of relevance to anaesthetists as sedative premedicants, anaesthetic agents and opioids reduce the effectiveness of neuronal pharyngeal dilator compensatory mechanisms and can precipitate upper airway obstruction with further impairment of ventilation.

Specific surgical treatment in adults has variable success. The most successful is probably weight reduction surgery. Uvulopalatopharyngeal surgery and operations on the tongue have questionable value and are now rarely performed. The definitive treatment for severe end-stage OSA is tracheostomy, to bypass the upper airway altogether.

In children, hypertrophy of the adenoids and tonsils can lead to chronic upper airway obstruction, which, rarely can lead to pulmonary hypertension, right ventricular hypertrophy and right heart failure. Symptoms include failure to thrive, hyperactivity, nightmares, enuresis and morning headaches. It is equally common in boys and girls, and obesity is often absent. Complete upper airway obstruction can occur with superimposed infection or sedation. Treatment with adenotonsillectomy carries a high success rate, although it can take several days for the apnoea risk to subside following surgery.

Problems

- Surgery to the upper airway
- Airway obstruction
- Right sided heart failure and pulmonary hypertension (cor pulmonale)
- Abnormal control of breathing
- Obesity

Anaesthetic management

Assessment and premedication

Whether surgery is performed to treat sleep apnoea or for an incidental indication, great care is required. The STOP BANG index (**Table 79**) is a useful screening tool for OSA and may pick up previously undiagnosed patients. OSA should be suspected in all obese adults. Other aspects of the history should focus on evidence of secondary organ damage, such as pulmonary

Table 79 The STOP BANG screening tool for obstructive sleep apnoea. Sleep Apnoea is considered likely if more than three items are present

S	Do you **S**nore loudly, enough to be heard through closed doors?
T	Do you feel **T**ired or fatigued during the daytime almost every day?
O	Has anyone **O**bserved that you stop breathing during sleep?
P	Do you have a history of high blood **P**ressure, with or without treatment?
B	**B**ody mass index (BMI) greater than 35 kg/m^2
A	**A**ge over 50 years
N	**N**eck circumference greater than 40 cm
G	Male **G**ender

Adapted from Toronto Western Hospital, University of Toronto. StopBang.ca. Obstructive sleep apnea. www.stopbang.ca

hypertension or right heart failure. Patients may be receiving long-term nocturnal nasal continuous positive airway pressure (CPAP). Haemoglobin levels may be elevated and the ECG may show right heart strain. Cardiomegaly on a chest X-ray may indicate the need for echocardiography.

Diagnostic sleep studies are the gold standard for diagnosis of OSA. Full polysomnography will measure O_2 and CO_2 airway gases, blood pressure, ECG, EEG, EMG and Spo_2. It is resource-intensive and rarely available in practice. Overnight oxygen saturation and ECG are more easily obtainable and are often used to diagnose sleep apnoea in children and adults. Such studies will provide the frequency and duration of apnoeic episodes, hypoxia and cardiovascular responses to apnoea, which will indicate the severity of the disease. Preoptimisation includes a period of noninvasive ventilation (which will take several weeks to produce benefit) and weight loss for obese patients. Sedative premedicants are avoided.

Conduct of anaesthetic

All general anaesthetic agents can precipitate upper airway obstruction. Following preoxygenation, an intravenous or gaseous induction is performed. OSA is associated with difficult and failed intubation in up to 90% of adult patients. Intermittent positive pressure ventilation is generally preferred, especially if cardiac or pulmonary involvement. Hypercarbia should be avoided, as periods of acidosis will reduce the already-blunted

respiratory drive further following extubation. Even topical local anaesthetic to the oropharynx can cause obstruction as upper airway muscle tone is reduced.

Regional anaesthesia, short acting opiates and multimodal analgesia should be used where possible as patients are sensitive to the sedative effects of opiates and benzodiazepines, risking postoperative apnoea. Deep extubation is hazardous due to the reduced respiratory drive and risk of airway obstruction. Opiate, if required, should be titrated judiciously to pain. If patients are using nasal CPAP preoperatively, the system should be available in the recovery area for immediate use.

Postoperatively

Following extubation, particular care must be taken to prevent upper airway obstruction, which can occur due to mechanical swelling related to the surgery or to tracheal intubation. Nasal CPAP may be recommended following extubation, and severe cases should be nursed in a high dependency setting.

After general anaesthesia there is a marked reduction in rapid eye movement sleep on the first postoperative night, with a rebound in REM sleep on the 3rd night. Since REM sleep is associated with decreased muscle tone, there is an increased risk of upper airway obstruction and sleep apnoea. Close monitoring may be necessary for up to 3 days, as there may problems related to rebound REM sleep. Sedative analgesics should be used sparingly and their effects closely monitored.

Further reading

Den Herder C, Schmeck J, Appelboom DJ, et al. Risks of general anaesthesia in people with obstructive sleep apnoea. Br Med J 2004; 329:955–959.

Loadsman JA, Hillman DR. Anaesthesia and sleep apnoea. Br J Anaesth 2001; 86:254–266.

Martinez G, Faber P. Obstructive sleep apnoea. Br J Anaesth: Contin Educ Anaesth Crit Care Pain Med 2011; 11:5–8.

Related topics of interest

Smoking

Key points

- One in three surgical patients smoke
- Smoking has a wide range of reversible and irreversible effects on most body systems
- Cessation should be encouraged by all health care professions; as little as 1 hour has a beneficial effect prior to anaesthesia

Approximately 30% of surgical patients are smokers. This is higher than the population average owing to increased requirement for surgery amongst smokers – coronary artery bypass grafts, tumour resections, vascular surgery to name but a few. Children presenting for surgery who live with smokers are also susceptible to perioperative complications attributable to smoke inhalation, those with current upper respiratory tract infection being at particular risk. In smoking adults, due consideration must be given to the synergistic effects of other substances of abuse as use is more frequent amongst smokers; this includes cannabis and narcotics but particularly alcohol. The perioperative morbidity associated with alcohol is dose-dependent: 6–8 units/day is associated with 1.5 times the risk of those who drink 0–4 units/day. The risk amongst those drinking in excess of 10 units/day is two–four times higher.

Problems

Chronic:
- Respiratory
  - Irritable airways (upper and lower)
  - Greater age-related rate of reduction of FRC (60 mL/year vs. 20 mL/year)
  - Reduced ciliary function
  - Reduced FEV_1
  - Increased closing capacity
  - Increased shunt fraction (independent of the other changes in pulmonary mechanics)
  - Airway and bronchogenic malignancy
  - Chronic obstructive pulmonary disease/emphysema
  - Pulmonary hypertension
- Cardiovascular
  - Ischaemic heart disease
  - Heart failure
  - Peripheral vascular disease
  - Aortic aneurysmal disease
  - Cerebrovascular disease
  - Hypertension
  - Sympathomimetic effects of nicotine
- Haematological
  - Prothrombotic (effects on platelet aggregation)
  - Hyperviscosity/polycythaemia
  - Increased carboxyhaemoglobin
- Immune
  - Immunosuppression
- Gastrointestinal
  - Gastro-oesophageal reflux
  - Peptic ulceration
  - Crohn's disease
  - Gastro-oesophageal tumours
- Genitourinary
  - Bladder tumours

Perioperative (in addition to ongoing implications of chronic effects):
- Respiratory
  - Laryngospasm
  - Bronchospasm
  - Breath holding
  - Rapid desaturation
  - Poor sputum clearance/postoperative pneumonia
- Cardiovascular
  - Ischaemia or infarction
  - Cerebrovascular events
  - Poorer outcomes following coronary artery and major vascular surgery
  - Arterial and venous thrombosis
- Immune
  - Increased postoperative infections
  - Poor wound healing (direct immunosuppression and reduced collagen synthesis)
- Gastrointestinal
  - Anastomotic breakdown

Carbon monoxide

Normal carbon monoxide levels are measured by co-oximetry as the percentage of haemoglobin circulating as carboxyhaemoglobin (normal 0–2%). In smokers this can be up to 10%. Levels of 10–30% produce symptoms, e.g. observed in house fires (fatal levels between 30% and 90%). Carbon monoxide has a range of physiological effects due to its effects on oxygen carriage and utilisation. Owing to an affinity for haemoglobin, which is up to 240 times that of oxygen, it readily saturates the blood at the expense of PaO_2. At a tissue level it causes a left-wards displacement of the oxygen–haemoglobin dissociation curve, i.e. the release to tissues of what little oxygen managed to bind is inhibited. Carbon monoxide is also histotoxic, inhibiting mitochondrial cytochrome oxidase and so the final aerobic synthesis of adenosine triphosphate (ATP) is also impaired. Finally any degree of myocardial ischaemia facilitates formation of myocardial carboxymyoglobin (carbon monoxide has 60 times oxygen's affinity for myoglobin). This causes direct myocardial depression further exacerbating poor oxygen delivery.

Fortunately carbon monoxide is one of the most rapidly reversed elements of smoking's impact on physiology. The half-life is around 6 hours in air but around 1 hour in oxygen or with exercise. It is longer in men and is up to 10 hours during sleep so patients should be encouraged to avoid the last cigarette before bed the night before surgery. Of interest, hyperbaric therapy in carbon monoxide poisoning reduces the half-life to 23 minutes at 3 atmospheres.

Investigations

Routine preoperative assessment and investigation must be augmented with a high index of suspicion for smoking related comorbidity, particular cardiopulmonary diseases; consider if echocardiography or pulmonary function tests are indicated. A low threshold should be held prior to more complex surgery for cardiology and respiratory clinic review as part of preoperative workup.

Smoking cessation

Smoking has a range of effects on the surgical patient and there is a clear benefit in stopping both in the long term and the short term (Table 80). All health care providers have a responsibility to help motivate patients to engage with stop-smoking services and in the UK, there is NICE guidance on this (Public Health Guideline 10). Studies have proven the benefits of such interventions: postoperative complications in hip and knee replacements are reduced from 52% to 18% following 6–8 weeks' cessation. Wound complications were particularly affected – 31% to 5%. Smoking reduction gained no benefits. Further studies in colorectal patients demonstrated no benefit from short-term (1–3 weeks) cessation. They also proved, however, that short-range smoking cessation interventions were not associated with increased complications as had been suggested by other less robust work.

Table 80 Timescale for benefit from smoking cessation	
Time from cessation	Benefit
1 hour	Resolution of haemodynamic effects of cigarette smoke
12–24 hours	Clearance of carbon monoxide, work capacity improved 10–20%
2–10 days	Reduced upper airways reactivity
4 weeks	Possible increase in pulmonary postoperative complications
4–6 weeks	Immune recovery with better wound healing
6–8 weeks	Reduced pulmonary complications
5–6 months	Perioperative pulmonary complications approach nonsmoker levels
Years	Reduction in ischaemic heart disease, chronic lung disease, cerebrovascular disease and malignancy

There is also compelling evidence for long-term benefits; 1-year cessation rates are up to seven times better amongst those in a preoperative stop-smoking program. Men with low nicotine dependency and a nonsmoking spouse were most likely to succeed at 1 year. Health care professionals who are smokers must make a conscious effort to remember to counsel cessation – evidence suggests they are more likely to overlook such opportunities than nonsmoking colleagues.

Further reading

Moppett I, Curran J. Smoking and the surgical patient. Br J Anaesth: Contin Educ Profess Develop Rev 2001; 1:122–124.

National Institute for Health & Care Excellence. Smoking cessation services: guidance. Public Health Guideline 10 (PH10). London: NICE, 2008.

Tønnesen H, Nielsen PR, Lauritzen JB. Smoking and alcohol intervention before surgery: evidence for best practice. Br J Anaesth 2009; 102:297–306.

Related topics of interest

- Coronary artery disease (p. 47)
- Paediatric anaesthesia – basic concepts (p. 179)
- Preoperative assessment – risk evaluation (p. 236)
- Respiratory – chronic obstructive pulmonary disease (p. 262)
- Substance abuse (p. 287)
- Vascular surgery – aortic aneurismal disease (p. 313)
- Vascular surgery – occlusive disease (p. 316)
- Venous thromboembolism – risk (p. 324)

Spinal cord injury

Key points

- Acute spinal cord injury (SCI) presents a variety of problems for the anaesthetist including management of the airway, respiratory embarrassment, neurogenic shock and any other concurrent injuries
- Patients with chronic SCI may require surgery both related and unrelated to their initial injury
- Patients with chronic SCI have specific challenges associated with management including recurrent chest infections, autonomic dysreflexia (AD), spasticity, contractures, pressure sores, chronic pain and psychological difficulties

Whilst any individual may be affected, acute SCI most commonly occurs in young males, often through road traffic collisions and falls. Around half of the injuries affect the cervical spine.

The anterior two thirds of the cord are supplied by the anterior spinal artery (formed by the fusion of branches of the vertebral arteries). Two posterior spinal arteries (from the posterior inferior cerebellar arteries) supply the posterior third of the cord. The spinal arteries are augmented by various radicular arteries along the length of the cord. Blood flow in a healthy cord is subject to autoregulation, but following injury, these mechanisms may fail, exacerbating tissue damage. Early cord oedema may temporarily raise the apparent level of injury.

After cord injury, spinal shock occurs, in which there is a temporary cessation of physiological cord function. This may last up to four weeks after which there may gradually be partial or even complete return of cord function. SCI may be complete, with total loss of function below the lesion, or incomplete, in which there is partial preservation of some aspect of neurological function at least one level below the lesion; examples include anterior cord and Brown-Sequard (hemisection) syndromes.

Problems

Airway

Until injury has been formally excluded, the spine should remain fully immobilised. When intubation is necessary, manual in-line stabilisation should be maintained. Use of bougies, fibrescopes and indirect laryngoscopes may help to limit cervical movement. Fibreoptic intubation (asleep or awake), or tracheostomy under local anaesthesia should also be considered. In the acute setting, the airway may be further at risk from other injuries and a full stomach, and a rapid sequence induction should be considered to secure the airway, bearing in mind that unstable cervical fractures are at risk of displacement from incautious application of cricoid pressure.

An upregulation of acetylcholine receptors occurs in denervated muscle following SCI, which may lead to an exaggerated potassium release following administration of succinylcholine. The time course of this upregulation is variable, and whilst succinylcholine is probably safe up to 72 hours after injury, many anaesthetists avoid its use indefinitely after this.

Breathing

Respiratory complications affect over 80% of patients with cervical SCI, with around 60% of those with lower SCI having complications at some stage during acute or rehabilitation phases of treatment. Complications include atelectasis, secretion retention, pneumonia, and ventilatory failure.

Lesions above C3 are ventilator-dependent. Lesions between C3 and C5 will maintain some voluntary diaphragmatic respiration (phrenic nerve, C3/4/5), although forced vital capacity (FVC) will be reduced by around 50% and patients may require some ventilatory support. Lesions just below C5 preserve diaphragmatic function, but intercostal activity is lost. Thoracic lesions result in a level-dependent loss of intercostal function, impairing the ability to cough and clear secretions. Patients with thoracic SCI often have additional chest trauma complicating their management.

Generally, FVC, tidal volume and expiratory reserve volume are all variably reduced depending on level. Paradoxical abdominal breathing is exacerbated in sitting positions (loss of abdominal splinting), although FVC is reduced when supine, and optimal patient position must be assessed individually.

Circulation

A (hypertensive) sympathetic storm may occur at the time of injury, followed within minutes by hypotension due to a loss of sympathetic tone causing peripheral vasodilatation (which may be exacerbated by bleeding from other injuries). Loss of cardioaccelerator fibres (T1-4) impairs chronotropic/inotropic compensatory changes in cardiac output, and there is a risk of profound bradycardia and even asystole due to unopposed vagal activity. Dysrhythmias and subendocardial ischaemia may occur, particularly with high lesions. Acutely, patients are at risk of both neurogenic and overload pulmonary oedema. Postural hypotension may occur, but often improves over time as renin activity increases. The loss of sympathetic control over vasculature impairs thermoregulation (ability to shiver, sweat and vasodilate).

Autonomic dysreflexia

Up to 90% of patients with thoracic or higher lesions suffer from AD. Stimulus below the lesion (e.g. urinary infections, bowel distension, labour, or cutaneous stimulation) triggers an autonomic discharge. Below the lesion, this (unopposed) activity results in profound vasoconstriction; above the lesion, there may be a compensatory flushing, and bradycardia, and the balance of damaged versus preserved cord function may determine the success of this compensation. AD can cause life-threatening hypertension, including cerebral bleeds. Treatment should be directed to the cause, using rapid vasodilators to control symptoms acutely.

Neurology

In the acute setting, until the spine has been formally cleared, it must be treated as unstable and manual in-line stabilisation maintained. Initially, below the lesion, there is flaccidity and areflexia (autonomic and somatic), but over the next 6 months the cord gradually becomes disinhibited and spasticity/hyperreflexia predominate and contractures may begin to form. Although there is (lesion dependent) sensory and motor deprivation below the lesion, patients may suffer from phantom limb/body pain, with more than 70% of patients with SCI suffering from some degree of chronic pain. Depression is common.

Joint consensus guidelines from the American Association of Neurosurgeons and the Congress of Neurological Surgeons in 2013 included recommendations on the use of methylprednisolone and GM-1 ganglioside in the management of acute SCI. In summary there was no evidence of clinical benefit to support the use of steroids, but clear evidence of harmful side effects and death. This represents a reversal of previous recommendations. There was also insufficient evidence to support the use of GM-1.

Other

There may be acute gastric dilation/paralytic ileus, and a risk of chronic AD from visceral stimulation. Patients are often prone to constipation and regurgitation. Patients are at risk of developing pressure ulcers, thromboembolism, osteoporosis, and latex allergy. They may develop chronic normocytic normochromic anaemia and hypoalbuminaemia.

Further reading

Denton M, McKinlay J. Cervical cord injury and critical care. Br J Anaesth: Contin Educ Anaesth Crit Care Pain 2009; 9:82–86.

Steering Committee of the Consortium for Spinal Cord Medicine. Early acute management in adults with spinal cord injury. J Spinal Cord Med 2008; 31:408–479.

Hurlbert R, Hadley M, Walters B, et al. Pharmacological therapy for acute spinal cord injury. Neurosurgery 2013; 72:93–105.

Related topics of interest

- Neuroanaesthesia – traumatic brain injury (p. 131)
- Polytrauma (p. 217)

Spinal surgery

Key points

- Generally, surgery is carried out prone, posing multiple problems for the anaesthetist, including limited access to the airway, risk of compression of vulnerable structures and the physical challenge of manoeuvring the unconscious patient into the correct position
- Deformity correction surgery may require cord function monitoring which may necessitate changes to anaesthetic technique
- Many patients suffer from significant chronic pain, and achieving satisfactory postoperative pain relief can be challenging

According to Health Episode Statistics, in 2011, over 60,000 spinal operations were carried out in the NHS in England. Disc and decompressive surgery accounted for around 40,000, spinal deformity correction 2,600, and cord surgery 3,800. Approximately 8% of procedures were carried out as emergencies and 20% as day cases. Patients may present from any age group and any ASA class. Chronic pain issues are a recurring theme and may present a significant challenge in the perioperative period.

Problems

These will be discussed in more detail but in particular include:

- Airway management – spinal instability, extubation oedema, access when prone
- Positioning issues – line displacement, patient/staff safety, pressure injuries, ventilation
- Bleeding – raw bone surfaces, vascular tumours, incessant venous bleeding
- Cardiovascular instability
- Need to facilitate neurological monitoring
- Postoperative analgesia in the chronic pain patient

Anaesthetic management

Preoperative

In addition to a standard preoperative assessment, consider:

- Pain symptoms and current analgesia
- Neurological deficits
- Joint mobility (bearing in mind the position the patient will be in for surgery)
- Patients with severe thoracic deformities may have respiratory compromise, and pulmonary function should be assessed preoperatively
- Ensure blood availability for major surgery

Intraoperative

- Airway: Cervical spine immobility may necessitate fibreoptic intubation (asleep or sometimes awake), whilst an unstable cervical spine mandates use of manual in-line stabilisation during intubation. The airway will be largely inaccessible during prone surgery, and tubes must be secured thoroughly. Cervical surgery and any procedure involving prolonged prone positioning carries a risk of airway oedema and a 'cuff-leak test' should be considered prior to extubation (a small minority of patients may require elective postoperative ventilation to allow swelling to subside). A flexi-metallic endotracheal tube is the standard choice when prone, although many anaesthetists use RAE tubes
- Breathing: There is a risk of tube migration during movement into the prone position, and inappropriate size or position of chest and pelvic supports may limit abdominal excursion, impairing ventilation. Generally, however, ventilation is unproblematic when prone. Intrathoracic pressure, especially positive end-expiratory pressure, may increase the volume of epidural veins, impairing surgical view, and a balance between surgical conditions and physiological requirements must be reached. Surgeons

occasionally require a Valsalva manoeuvre when dural leak is suspected

- Circulation: Venous return from the legs may be impaired or totally obstructed by inappropriately positioned pelvic supports. Peripheral vascular access is usually easy to obtain intraoperatively, but consideration for central access should be made before positioning. Arterial lines are used for longer cases, or for patients whose comorbidity mandates their use. Tumour resections and major, multilevel surgeries should alert the anaesthetist to the risk of substantial blood loss: consider the need for central venous access, blood availability, intraoperative cell-salvage, and point-of-care thromboelastography. In complex cases, surgeons often employ a 'haemostatic pause'. Open venous plexi, e.g. epidural veins, expose the patient to risk of venous air embolism
- Positioning: The vast majority of spinal surgery is performed prone, but some surgeons prefer alternative positions such as knee-chest. The prone position can be achieved in a variety of ways, e.g. using pillows, a Montreal Mattress, Wilson Frame or Jackson table: it is important to ensure familiarity with equipment before use, and to check that it is of an appropriate size for the patient (especially given the increasing number of obese patients presenting for spinal surgery). An unstable, or uncleared, spine mandates use of logrolling
- Neurology: Some surgeries, particularly scoliosis correction, use neurological function monitoring. Somatosensory evoked potentials (SSEP) are used to provide indirect information about the function of the motor pathways (dorsal cord), while electrically triggered electromyography (EMG) can be used to monitor individual nerve roots. In addition, motor integrity can be assessed by a 'wake up test' once the spine is straightened (ventral cord assessment). Anaesthesia lightened until the patient moves their feet to command. A benzodiazepine is given immediately and anaesthesia deepened to permit completion of the operation. Recall following the test is unusual

- Many different anaesthetic drugs (including neuromuscular blockers, volatile agents and intravenous induction agents) and physiological changes, such as reduced blood flow, have an effect on SSEP and EMG data. Thus there needs to be an open dialogue between anaesthetist and neurophysiologist to allow accurate interpretation of results. Patients presenting for spinal deformity correction often have an underlying muscular disorder. There is an association between some myopathies, such as multiminicore disease and central core disease and the development of malignant hyperthermia (MH). Although it is difficult to estimate the true risk for these patients, many anaesthetists advocate the avoidance of known MH triggers for these types of surgery
- Other: Consider urinary catheterisation for longer cases, both for monitoring and to prevent bladder over distension. Maintain normothermia, using active warming as required

Postoperative

- Remember to exclude airway oedema before extubation
- Use anaesthetic techniques which allow a rapid return to clear consciousness and which facilitate neurological assessment
- Pain control can be very challenging in these patients, particularly in those with chronic pain or who are undergoing multilevel surgery. In addition to simple oral analgesics, preoperative gabapentin or pregabalin may be of benefit. Consider the use of surgically sited epidurals, wound catheters or infiltration of muscles before closing. Postoperatively, continue regular simple analgesics with oral or intravenous opioids, e.g. patient-controlled analgesia for breakthrough pain. For patients with chronic pain, adequate control can be difficult to achieve: consider perioperative use of clonidine and ketamine. A few patients may require a postoperative infusion of ketamine
- Patients with severe comorbidity or who have undergone major surgery may require high-dependency care postoperatively

Further reading

American Society of Neurophysiological Monitoring. Intraoperative monitoring using somatosensory evoked potentials; a position statement of the American Society of Neurophysiological Monitoring, 2010. [Online] http://www.asnm.org/?page=PositionStatements [2013]

Entwistle MA, Patel D. Scoliosis surgery in children. Br J Anaesth: Contin Educ Anaesth Crit Care Pain Med 2006; 6:13–16.

Hirshey Dirksen S, Larach M, Rosenberg H, et al. Future directions in malignant hyperthermia research and patient care. Anesth Analg 2011; 113:1108–1119.

Sharma V, Verghese C, McKenna PJ. Prospective audit of the LMA-Supreme for airway management of adult patients undergoing elective orthopaedic surgery in prone position. Br J Anaesth 2010; 105:228–232.

Related topics of interest

- Malignant hyperpyrexia (p. 111)
- Pain – chronic management (p. 202)
- Positioning for surgery (p. 220)

Substance abuse

Key points

- Substance abuse commonly involves more than one agent
- Substances can cause physiological and psychotropic effects following consumption and upon withdrawal – both can be dangerous and difficult to manage
- The drug history from the patient is rarely reliable and must be considered in conjunction with objective signs

Substance abuse can be defined as consumption of any substance for purposes out with the cultural norms. This definition therefore includes deliberate self-poisoning but this will not be discussed in detail here. It may involve any substance, from misuse of prescription drugs to unconventional use of industrial solvents. The substances which carry by far and away the greatest morbidity and mortality however are legal: direct alcohol-related deaths outnumbered illicit drug-related deaths by more than 3:1 in 2012 and smoking was the cause of 18% of all deaths in 2009 in the UK according to Office of National Statistics data. The myriad effects of these particular drugs are covered elsewhere in this book.

The other face of substance abuse is when healthcare providers find themselves with a dependency. This, for example, affects around 2% of UK trainee anaesthetists (the national population average is 2.2%). The AAGBI has specific guidance on this topic which will not be covered here in any detail.

Problems

- Drug-specific features
  - The toxidrome – characteristic cluster of signs and symptoms
  - Withdrawal
- General features
  - Problems related to other substances commonly coabused (e.g. chronic obstructive pulmonary disease (COPD), from smoking, liver disease from alcohol abuse).
  - Transmission of HIV and hepatitis

- Infections due to injection
  - Local – abscess, thrombophlebitis, cellulitis, mycotic aneurysm
  - Systemic – sepsis (bacterial or fungal), infective endocarditis, septic emboli, empyema
- Difficult venous access
- Lifestyle associated issues – malnutrition, immunosuppression, poor personal care, injury/trauma
- Opportunistic infection – tuberculosis, aspergillosis

Clinical features

Broadly speaking the most common drugs of abuse can be divided into

- Sedatives: opiates, cannabis, benzodiazepines, barbiturates (less common now), GHB (gamma hydroxybutyrate)
- Stimulants: cocaine, ecstasy, amphetamine
- Hallucinogens: LSD, magic mushrooms (psilocybin), phencyclidines (PCP/angel dust, ketamine)

Key features of the toxidromes of the more common agents are given in **Table 81**. In general terms, sedatives are globally CNS depressant with varying degrees of cardiorespiratory depression and a tendency to be MAC sparing. Stimulants affect the nervous and cardiovascular systems predominantly with agitation, tremor, tachycardia, dysrhythmias and hypertension. Anaesthesia following recent consumption can lead to marked cardiovascular instability and MAC is markedly increased. Hallucinogens may also cause sympathetic activation, particularly due to anxiety and panic, and this will cause a corresponding increase in MAC. Industrial solvents abused for their hallucinogenic effects may result in hepatorenal injury.

Investigations

Those presenting for anaesthesia who are known substance abusers must be fully

Table 81 Common drugs and their features

Drug	Features	Withdrawal	Withdrawal management
Opioids	Sedative, miosis, bradypnoea, bradycardia	Sympathetic storm, seizures, dysphoria, GI upset	Benzodiazepines, clonidine, beta-blockers ± general anaesthesia
Cannabis	Sedation, hypotension (vasodilation), dysphoria in new users	N/A	N/A
Benzodiazepines	Sedation, bradypnoea, synergistic with alcohol	Anxiety, restlessness, nausea, vomiting, seizures	Long-acting benzodiazepine, e.g. chlordiazepoxide and tapered dose reduction
Cocaine	Euphoria, hallucinations, tachycardia, hypertension, myocardial ischaemia, serotonin syndrome	Paranoia, depression, anxiety, fatigue, formication (sensation of skin crawling)	Withdrawal – dexmedetomidine or clonidine: Toxicity – benzodiazepine, nitrates, calcium channel blockers (not beta-blockers)
Amphetamine inc. ecstasy	Hypertension, tachycardia, lack of appetite, tirelessness, hyperpyrexia, arrhythmias, prolonged QT	Paranoia, anxiety, derealisation, panic attacks, sleeplessness, fatigue	Withdrawal – sedatives, e.g. benzodiazepines Toxicity – cooling, dantrolene, correct hyponatraemia, neuromuscular blockade
LSD	Anxiety, hallucinations, seizures, mydriasis, hypothermia	Rarely, flashbacks	N/A
Magic mushrooms	As for LSD plus nausea and vomiting, severe renal failure and psychosis	N/A	N/A
GHB	Transient euphoria then 2–3 hours coma (date rape drug, metabolised to CO_2 and H_2O)	Autonomic instability, aggression, psychosis, seizures, hyperthermia, rhabdomyolysis	Large doses of benzodiazepine

investigated for conditions resulting from the abused substance; e.g. pulmonary function tests may be required for COPD following nicotine abuse, liver function tests for those who abuse alcohol or solvents. Have a low threshold for routine full blood count, renal function and biochemistry and clotting profile. Chest X-ray to screen for tuberculosis and echocardiography to evaluate possible endocarditic vegetations may also be appropriate in some cases. Relevant cultures should be taken where infection is suspected. In the context of acute toxicity, e.g. accidental overdose, specific management and investigation should be guided by recommendations from expert resources such as the UK National Poisons Information Service. Additional investigations in this context include paracetamol and salicylate blood assays, creatine kinase and urinary myoglobin in case of prolonged unconsciousness and rhabdomyolysis, CT head scan to exclude intracranial causes for altered consciousness and ECG to exclude arrhythmias.

Treatment

There are specific treatments for the withdrawal features of many drugs. With the exception of opiates (naloxone) however, there are very few specific antidotes. Treatment is supportive and often involves benzodiazepines to treat agitation and sympathetic overactivity. Protocolised management is often required, particularly in the management of alcohol withdraw (Clinical Institute Withdrawal of Alcohol (CIWA) score to guide benzodiazepine titration). Enlist the support of substance abuse management specialists wherever possible.

Flumazenil is a benzodiazepine antidote but should largely be reserved for the treatment of iatrogenic overdose. Substance abusers commonly use more than one agent and there is a high risk of precipitating refractory seizures by removing the inhibiting influence of the benzodiazepine on another agent.

Anaesthetic management

Preoperative assessment should include a careful drug abuse history although this will be notoriously unreliable. Clinical examination for signs of intravenous abuse, subcutaneous injection ('skin-popping') or physiological signs of withdrawal is more objective. Recent consumption is relevant in determining likely requirements for anaesthesia; e.g. recent sedative consumption will reduce anaesthetic requirements whereas less recent consumption may leave the patient in some degree of withdrawal thus increasing requirements.

Regional techniques may remove some of the uncertainty for general anaesthesia requirements but are not always possible, e.g. infection, immunosuppression, patient refusal or agitation. They also offer the benefit of ongoing postoperative analgesia which is particularly helpful in opiate addicts who otherwise have potentially massive intra- and postoperative opiate requirements.

Particularly in the case of recent stimulant abuse, invasive cardiovascular monitoring should be strongly considered. Beta-blockers should be avoided, particularly in cocaine toxicity; generalised sympathetic upregulation means these agents result in unopposed alpha stimulation. Therapeutic cardiovascular stimulants, e.g. atropine, adrenaline, salbutamol should be avoided. Anticholinergic agents should also be avoided following hallucinogen intake – sympathetic hyperactivity may also be problematic in these patients but these drugs may also exacerbate the hallucinations.

Further reading

Association of Anaesthetists of Great Britain & Ireland. Drug and alcohol abuse amongst anaesthetists; guidance on identification and management. London: AAGBI, 2011.

Jenkins BJ. Drug abusers and anaesthesia. Br J Anaesth: Contin Educ Profess Develop Rev 2002; 2:15–19.

Nicholson Roberts T, Thompson JP. Illegal substances in anaesthetic and intensive care practices. Br J Anaesth: Contin Educ Anaesth Crit Care Pain 2013; 13:42–46.

UK National Poisons Information Service. Toxbase. [Online] http://www.toxbase.org/ [2013]

Related topics of interest

Systemic inflammatory response syndrome and sepsis

Key points

- Sepsis is a common condition still associated with a high mortality rate
- The key to treatment is many simple interventions done rapidly in a coordinated manner

Infection is defined as a pathological process caused by the invasion of normally sterile tissue, fluid or body cavity by pathogenic or potentially pathogenic micro-organisms. If this is sufficient to trigger the systemic inflammatory response syndrome (SIRS) response, the resulting clinical state is termed sepsis.

SIRS is defined by two or more of the following

- White cell count <4000/mL or >12,000/mL
- Temperature <36°C or >38°C
- Respiratory rate >20 bpm
- Pulse rate >90 bpm

Severe sepsis is sepsis in the presence of end-organ hypoperfusion as denoted by signs such as lactataemia, oliguria or confusion. Severe sepsis that does not respond to fluid resuscitation is referred to as septic shock. Sepsis has an annual incidence of 3 per 1000 in Western populations.

Diffuse endothelial injury, microvascular coagulation, systemic inflammation and cellular-level dysfunction lead to multiorgan failure and death in 30–50% of patients. Many attempts have been made to arrest this chain of events but as yet there is no 'magic bullet'. The importance of basic measures done well and promptly is emphasised in the Surviving Sepsis Campaign guidelines, an expert consensus list of evidence-based recommendations. These have recently undergone their third revision since their inception in 2002. The guidelines are not without their critics and several elements have fallen from practice in the light of new evidence (see 'Controversial treatments' below).

The guidelines are now effectively divided two timed bundles:

- 3 hour bundle
  - Measure serum lactate
  - Obtain blood cultures prior to antibiotic administration
  - Administer broad spectrum antibiotics (ideally within 1 hour)
  - Administer 30 mL/kg crystalloid if hypotensive or lactate >4 mmol/L
- 6 hour bundle
  - Administer vasopressors for hypotension unresponsive to 30 mL/kg fluid aiming for mean arterial pressure (MAP) >65 mmHg
  - In event of hypotension despite fluid (septic shock) or lactate >4 mmol/L:
    - Measure central venous pressure (CVP), target of >8 mmHg
    - Measure $Scvo_2$, target of >70%
  - Remeasure serum lactate if initially elevated, target normalisation

Other bundle approaches have been suggested including the 'Sepsis 6', a group of six interventions to be achieved within the first hour from recognition of sepsis: administer 100% oxygen, intravenous fluids and broad spectrum antibiotics and take appropriate cultures, blood tests including arterial lactate and insert a urinary catheter. The recent ProCESS trial revealed early goal directed therapy (EGDT) was no better than protocolised standard care; the authors of this study suggest the key remains rapid sepsis identification and rapid instigation of these basic measures.

Other principles of intensive care unit (ICU) management of sepsis include:

- Reassess response to antibiotics and rationalise when and where possible within 12 hours
- Limit fluid when there is no further increase in perfusion with increase in cardiac filling pressures
- Select appropriate vasoactive drugs when fluid alone is insufficient to maintain perfusion
- Add low-dose intravenous hydrocortisone but only when shock

does not respond to vasoactive agents and fluid resuscitation
- Maintain haemoglobin 70–90 g/L unless signs of severe tissue hypoperfusion, active bleeding or myocardial ischaemia
- Maintain low tidal volumes, limit plateau pressures and in those with acute respiratory distress syndrome (ARDS), use positive end-expiratory pressure
- Nurse in a 30° head-up position
- Avoid routine use of pulmonary artery catheters in ARDS patients
- Wean analgesia and sedation according to a protocol once appropriate
- All patients should have deep vein thrombosis (DVT) prophylaxis and stress ulcer prophylaxis (since the 2008 revision, stronger evidence now exists for proton pump inhibitors rather than H_2 blockers)
- Maintain control of blood sugar <10.0 mmol/L
- Always be prepared to consider limitations to support when this becomes appropriate

Problems

General principles for anaesthesia

As with trauma damage control surgery, sepsis source control should be a surgical or radiological procedure with predefined and achievable goals. Advance liaison with ICU should be considered in all such patients, many of whom will require ongoing organ support as a consequence of worsening sepsis and systemic inflammation during the course of surgery. The procedure should be carried out by a senior surgeon or radiologist in a prompt manner.

In general terms, anaesthetic management of septic patients requires an attention to detail regarding simple aspects of care and an expectation that these patients will deteriorate. Care should be addressed in bundles so that simple elements, sometimes easily forgotten, e.g. DVT prophylaxis, are not overlooked. A well-integrated multiprofessional approach is the only reliable way in which to ensure all aspects of care are achieved rapidly.

Ventilatory management

- Assume the patient has ARDS (see p. 000 for full details)
- Sepsis is the leading cause of ARDS and is likely to develop either from the sepsis, the surgical stress of source control procedures or a combination of the two
- High metabolic load due to pyrexia, elevated white cell metabolism and increased catabolism will lead to high CO_2 production – this must be proactively addressed (within the limits of lung-protective ventilation) from the point of induction of anaesthesia

Haemodynamic management

- Ensure arterial pressure monitoring and central venous access to assess trends in lactate and acid–base balance, haemoglobin, electrolytes and $Scvo_2$
- Fluid should be administered with a particular goal in mind and vasoactive drugs added early to avoid overinfusion of fluid which will worsen lung injury, tissue oedema and oxygen delivery. Albumin offers no mortality benefit in this context although neither the SAFE nor ALBIOS studies demonstrate harm. Hetastarch solutions are associated with increased renal replacement therapy requirements and mortality
- Noradrenaline should be the first-line agent in adults. Adrenaline is now recommended as a second-line agent. Vasopressin can be used where these are insufficient or where reductions in noradrenaline are desirable (e.g. cardiac arrhythmia)
- Dobutamine may be a useful agent where myocardial dysfunction is evident or microvascular perfusion is inadequate despite adequate MAP and intravascular volume
- Dopamine has very limited indications and is associated with high rates of tachyarrhythmia, immunosuppression, hypothalamic–pituitary–adrenal axis dysfunction and an increased mortality risk compared to noradrenaline
- Haemodynamic end points should reflect flow/perfusion rather than arbitrary pressures

- All patients should have a urinary catheter and have hourly fluid balance calculated accurately

Early goal directed therapy is a concept derived from a moderate-sized, monocentric study however there was an impressive 60-day mortality benefit shown. Controversy remains around the components: CVP is a very poor therapeutic guide, an arbitrary MAP of 65 mmHg will not suit every patient and continuous $Scvo_2$ is rarely available. Targeting markers of end-organ perfusion with early, aggressive therapy is noncontroversial but determining the best target markers remains a topic of debate. As discussed, the ProCESS study appears to challenge the benefit of EGDT. The ARISE (Australian) and ProMISe (UK) studies may offer further evidence.

Infection management

- Prioritise microbial identification (culture screen), source control (debridement, decompression and drainage) and prompt delivery of antibiotics
- Every hour without antibiotics in septic shock decreases survival by 7.6%
- Consider methods of source control which minimise surgical stress, e.g. percutaneous drainage vs. laparotomy
- Entire team takes joint responsibility to ensure specimens reach microbiology within 2 hours of source control surgery to optimise culture yield
- Liaise with microbiology colleagues to optimise antimicrobial prescribing and subsequent rationalisation

General care

- Avoid hypothermia – coagulopathy and immune suppression result
- Permit pyrexia in sepsis
  - Physiological response, reversal of which is increasingly controversial
  - Paracetamol may worsen immune function and is relatively contraindicated in severe hepatic dysfunction
  - NSAIDs may worsen platelet and renal dysfunction commonly seen in sepsis
- Consider epidural catheters carefully
  - Pyrexia in sepsis usually occurs 90 minutes after the onset of frank bacteraemia so apyrexia is not a reliable marker of absence of bacteraemia
  - Patients are likely to have coagulopathy which may not be accurately quantified by routine coagulation tests (e.g. platelet dysfunction)
  - Patients may not benefit from the procedure if they are likely to remain sedated for 72 hours postop

Controversial treatments

- Tight glycaemic control – no longer recommended due to unacceptable rates of dangerous hypoglycaemia (NICE-SUGAR study): target 4.0–10.0 mmol/L instead
- Activated protein C – no longer recommended since publication of PROWESS-SHOCK study demonstrating no therapeutic benefit

Further reading

Dellinger RP, Levy MM, Carlet JM, et al. Surviving sepsis campaign: international guidelines for management of severe sepsis and septic shock: 2012. Intensive Care Med 2013; 39:165–228.

Rhodes A, Bennett ED. Early goal-directed therapy: an evidence-based review. Critical Care Med 2004; 32:S448–S450.

Wenzel RP, Edmond MB. Septic shock – evaluating another failed treatment. N Engl J Med 2012; 366:2122–2124.

Related topics of interest

- Respiratory – acute respiratory distress syndrome (p. 256)
- Regional anaesthesia – central neuraxial blockade (p. 242)

Thermoregulation

Key points

- Body temperature is closely regulated by the hypothalamus
- Both general and regional anaesthesia lead to a reduction in thermoregulation
- Heat is lost by radiation, convection, evaporation, respiration and conduction
- Perioperative hypothermia has multiple detrimental effects and must be avoided

Normal body temperature is 37°C +/- 0.5°C and it exhibits a circadian rhythm (lowest at 0400 hours and highest at 1700 hours). Heat is gained from metabolism, exercise and from ingestion of hot foods. It is lost by radiation (40%), convection (30%), evaporation (20%), respiration (10%) and small amounts through conduction.

The body can be considered as having two distinct temperature compartments: the core and the periphery. The core accounts for around two-third of body mass in adults, but is much greater in infants, which helps explain their susceptibility to heat loss. Although core temperature is relatively constant, the periphery varies by several degrees.

Normal thermoregulation can be considered in terms of afferent sensing, central processing and efferent responses.

The afferent thermal input is predominantly from the core (brain, hypothalamus, spinal cord, deep tissues) with around 20% of input from cutaneous temperature sensors. Cold information is transmitted via A-delta fibres and warm information via unmyelinated C-fibres (also responsible for pain sensations). This explains why intense heat sensation cannot be distinguished from pain.

The hypothalamus is responsible for controlling core temperature. Efferent responses are activated once core temperature deviates outside of strict thresholds.

Thermoregulatory responses include:
- Behavioural: moving to a warmer area, adding clothes
- Cutaneous vasoconstriction: α-adrenergic-mediated vasoconstriction of vascular beds and counter-current exchange mechanisms in the peripheries
- Shivering: heat production can be doubled but at the expense of oxygen consumption (up to 10x increase)
- Nonshivering thermogenesis: via β_3-adrenoceptor stimulation in 'brown fat' can double heat production in infants; however, it is of limited value in adults

Temperature measurement

Intraoperative body temperature may be monitored at a number of sites.
- Tympanic: infrared light emission provides an accurate measurement of brain temperature, provided there is an unobstructed path between the tympanic membrane and the sensor. Not generally suitable for continuous monitoring
- Nasopharyngeal: reflects brain temperature but is affected by respiratory gases (unless the patient is intubated). There is a risk of bleeding and dislodgment
- Oesophageal: reflects cardiac temperature, if correctly positioned
- Blood: e.g. via pulmonary artery catheter reflects core temperature
- Skin: dependent on cutaneous blood flow. The core/peripheral temperature gradient may reflect perfusion and volume status, particularly in infants
- Urinary catheter: a thermistor may be incorporated to measure core temperature
- Rectal: affected by faeces, may read slightly higher due to local bacterial metabolism. Risk of viscus perforation

Hypothermia

Perioperative hypothermia, defined as a core temperature below 36°C is increasingly recognised as cause of morbidity. It is almost inevitable in the anaesthetised patient unless measures are taken to prevent it. Particular risk groups include low BMI, critical illness, the very young (low surface area to volume ratio), the elderly and patients suffering burns.

The consequences of hypothermia are mostly due to impaired cellular function. They include an increased risk of perioperative infection due to impaired immune function, a reduced cardiac output, hypovolaemia (reduced ADH secretion), reduced tissue oxygen delivery, coagulopathy and abnormal platelet function (hypothermic patients undergoing hip replacement have increased blood transfusion requirements), prolonged drug action (e.g. muscle relaxants), slow awakening due to reduced cerebral function and shivering (increases oxygen demand, causes pain).

The consequences of severe hypothermia include coma, cardiac arrhythmias (atrial fibrillation <35°C, ventricular fibrillation <28°C), further hypovolaemia (loss of renal tubular function), and, if prolonged, gastric erosions and pancreatitis.

Effects of anaesthesia on temperature

Figure 18 indicates a typical thermoregulatory response to general anaesthesia. Heat is loss due to:

- Redistribution: peripheral vasodilatation and the internal redistribution of heat.

The core compartment expands into the peripheral compartment

- Widening of thermoregulatory interthreshold range: proportional to depth of anaesthesia, hypothalamic compensatory mechanisms are triggered at lower temperatures
- Reduced heat production (reduced metabolism and muscle activity)
- Increased heat loss: open body cavities, evaporation
- Loss of behavioural responses

Pre-existing cold peripheries will exacerbate core cooling following induction due to greater heat redistribution. This may be reduced by active warming of patients in the preoperative period. Obese patients are less affected by redistribution due to the enhanced insulating properties of adipose tissue.

The theatre environment itself increases heat loss. Surgical patients are often near naked, thus air warmed by the skin is replaced by new, cold air leading to convective heat loss. In addition, there are frequent air changes and ambient theatre temperatures are often around 20°C. Surgical cleansing fluids enhance heat loss by conduction and evaporation. Water conducts heat several thousand times more efficiently than air.

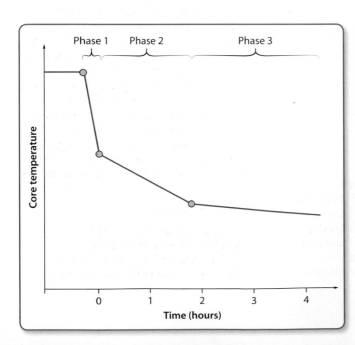

Figure 18 Pattern of perioperative heat loss following induction of general anaesthesia. Phase 1: Rapid redistribution of heat from core to peripheries. This can be minimised by pre-operative warming. Phase 2: Continued loss due to convection, conduction, radiation and evaporation. Phase 3: Plateau as heat loss is balanced by heat production. Adapted from Sessler DI. Perioperative heat balance. Anaesthesiology 2000; 92:578–596.

Regional anaesthesia also impairs temperature regulation although not to the same extent as general anaesthesia. As well as internal redistribution of heat resulting from vasodilatation, neuraxial anaesthesia appears to lower the thermoregulatory threshold. Afferent 'cold' sensory input form the lower extremities is lost, which may explain the 'warm' sensations experienced by patients. Upper body shivering fails to compensate for the loss of lower body muscle activity.

Combination of general and regional anaesthesia results in a greater risk of hypothermia than either alone.

Strategies for minimising heat loss

NICE produced guidelines for the prevention of perioperative hypothermia in 2008.

- High-risk patients should be identified in advance
- Forced-air warming or under-patient warmers, including the preoperative period
- Defer surgery if core temperature below 36°C
- Regular perioperative monitoring of core temperature (every 30 minutes)
- Increase room temperature >21°C
- Use radiant heaters, especially for neonates
- Cover the patient
- Warm all fluids used on and in the patient. Intravenous volumes of >500 mL should be warmed
- Warm and humidify gases
- Provide extra-inspired oxygen for the shivering patient
- Patient warming with appropriate blanket/ duvet in the postoperative period

Hyperthermia

Hyperthermia is defined as a core temperature >37.5°C. Severe hyperthermia is a core temperature >40°C or an increase in body temperature at a rate greater than 2°C per hour. The aetiology of hyperthermia falls into two categories; increased heat production or decreased heat loss.

Increased heat production

- Pyrogens/toxins (e.g. in sepsis, inflammatory response, following burns or blood transfusion reactions)
- Drug reactions. As a consequence of excessive dosage of the drug or as an abnormal reaction to normal doses. Potential triggers include methylene-dioxy-meth-amphetamine (MDMA, 'ecstasy'), thyroxine, monoamine oxidase inhibitors, tricyclic antidepressants, amphetamines, and cocaine. Hyperthermia following a drug reaction may manifest as the neuroleptic malignant syndrome (NMS) or serotonin syndrome
- Endocrine. Associated with hyperthyroidism or phaeochromocytoma
- Hypothalamic injury following cerebral hypoxia, oedema, or head injury/trauma
- Malignant hyperthermia (MH)

Decreased heat loss

- Excessive conservation especially in neonates and children
- Heat stroke
- Drug effects (e.g. as a predicted effect of anticholinergic administration)

Pathophysiology

Hyperthermia leads to an increased metabolic rate and oxygen consumption with associated increased cardiac output and minute ventilation to meet demand. Increased carbon dioxide production leads to respiratory acidosis, initially compensated for by tachypnoea. As the oxygen debt worsens a metabolic acidosis develops secondary to lactic acid production. Subsequent sweating and vasodilatation result in a relative hypovolaemic state and worsening of the metabolic derangement if left untreated. Neurological damage, seizures, rhabdomyolysis, acute renal failure, myocardial ischaemia and damage may all follow.

Management

- General cooling measures; decrease ambient temperature, exposure of the patient, cold air fans, application of ice packs to extremities, cooling suits/

garments. Cold fluid given intravenously or intraperitoneally, intravascular cooling devices, cardiac bypass

- Definitive treatment of underlying condition using dantrolene (e.g. in MH, NMS, MDMA poisoning) mannitol (rhabdomyolysis, acute renal failure)
- General intensive care; invasive monitoring to optimise fluid balance, sedation and ventilation if required

Neuroleptic malignant syndrome

This is an idiosyncratic complication of treatment with neuroleptic drugs such as the butyrophenones and phenothiazines. Patients are usually catatonic with extrapyramidal and autonomic effects including hyperthermia. The aetiology is unknown but appears to be related to antidopaminergic activity of the precipitating drug on dopamine receptors in the striatum and the hypothalamus suggesting a possible imbalance between noradrenaline and dopamine. There is no evidence of an association with MH. Clinical features include hyperthermia, muscle rigidity and sympathetic overactivity. Treatment comprises withdrawal of the agent and general supportive and cooling measures.

Further reading

Adnet P, Lestavel P, Krisovic-Horber R. Neuroleptic malignant syndrome. Br J Anaesth 2000; 85:129–135.
National Institute for Health and Care Excellence (NICE). Inadvertent perioperative hypothermia.

CG65. London; NICE, 2008.
Sessler DI. Perioperative heat balance. Anaesthesiology 2000; 92:578–596.

Related topics of interest

- Burns (p. 27)
- Elderly patients (p. 64)
- Endocrine disease (p. 72)
- Malignant hyperpyrexia (p. 111)
- Paediatric anaesthesia – basic practical conduct (p. 183)

Thoracic surgery

Key points

- Thoracic surgical patients are usually significantly comorbid, and a prediction of the impact of surgery on postoperative function is important prior to offering a procedure
- Some degree of hypoxia is to be expected but it should be actively managed
- Be meticulous about checking and rechecking the position of airway devices

This topic will include an overview of anaesthetic management from preassessment to postoperative care plus potential complications. Practice varies from one country to another. As an illustration, in this topic there will be a focus on the provision of thoracic anaesthesia in the UK which is based on the 2010 British Thoracic Society guidelines for lung cancer management and Royal College of Anaesthetists 2013 Service Provision guidance.

Thoracic procedures include:

- Lobar resection
- Pneumonectomy
- Mediastinoscopy
- Bronchoscopy
- Video-assisted thoracoscopic surgery: for lung resection, sympathectomy, mediastinal tumour resection and drainage and investigation of effusions
- Surgical management of air leaks, empyema
- Chest wall surgery, including minimally invasive pectus surgery and flail segment stabilisation
- Tracheal stenting

Problems

- Significant comorbidities (**Table 82**)
- Intraoperative and postoperative hypoxia
- Double-lumen tube (DLT) use and one-lung ventilation (OLV)/isolation

Investigations

Preoperative tests attempt to quantify perioperative risk and predict postoperative respiratory function. They include spirometry,

Table 82 Incidence of significant comorbidity amongst thoracic surgery patients

Comorbidity	Incidence
Smoking	27%
Cancer	11%
Chronic obstructive pulmonary disease	11%
Hypertension	10%
Ischaemic heart disease	10%
Diabetes	8%
Peripheral vascular disease	6%

carbon monoxide transfer, and quantitative CT/MRI where available. Functional tests such as shuttle walk testing (>400 m is considered good) and cardiopulmonary exercise testing to measure peak O_2 consumption (>15 mL/kg/min considered good) provide further useful information but these tests do not necessarily reflect quality of life.

Segment counting is useful to estimate postoperative lung function as part of the risk assessment for dyspnoea. The lung is divided into segments (out of a maximum of 19: 9 left, 10 right) and the following formula then predicts postoperative FEV_1 (N = number of pulmonary segments to be resected):

$$= FEV_1 \times (19\text{-}N)/19$$

Global risk scores, such as Thoracoscore, can be used to estimate risk of death. Generally patients with a predicted postop FEV_1 and TLCO <40% (lung transfer factor for carbon monoxide) have a moderate-to-high risk of postoperative breathlessness plus increased requirement for postoperative ventilatory support, and need to be informed of this as well as the potential requirement for long-term oxygen therapy.

Anaesthetic management

AAGBI minimal monitoring standards form a basic requirement plus invasive monitoring such as an arterial line and cardiac output monitoring where indicated. A decision needs to be made whether a DLT is to be used, or an alternative such as an endobronchial blocker. Consideration of analgesia and location of postoperative care also need to take place.

Double-lumen tubes

Most thoracic procedures warrant the insertion of a DLT to facilitate OLV. Various sizes and types are available but common to all is a tracheal lumen and cuff and an endobronchial lumen and cuff. The size selected depends on the manufacturer and may be influenced by height, gender and anticipated airway diameter. A left-sided tube is most commonly used as right-sided DLTs are technically more difficult to site as the operator has to correctly align an orifice with the origin of the right upper lobe bronchus. Operations where a right-sided tube should be used include a left pneumonectomy, left lobectomy, left lung transplant or abnormality of the left bronchial tree.

Initially both tracheal and bronchial cuffs should be checked and a stylet inserted into the tracheal lumen. Conventional laryngoscopy is performed with the DLT tip angled anteriorly. Once through the cords, the stylet is removed, the tube rotated 90° towards the side of choice and advanced until resistance is encountered or a predetermined depth achieved. Isolation and testing is accomplished as follows:

- Inflate tracheal cuff and ensure bilateral air entry by usual means
- Clamp tracheal lumen of Cobb connector and open tracheal port
- Confirm ventilation of operative lung and inflate bronchial cuff to ablate leak (expect to use 1–2 mL of air)
- Recap and unclamp tracheal side
- Clamp and open bronchial side
- Confirm ventilation of nonoperative lung
- Recommence bilateral ventilation
- Use fibreoptic bronchoscope to confirm position and adjust as necessary:
  - Visualise the carina via tracheal lumen to check the blue of the bronchial cuff is just visible
  - For right-side tubes verify alignment of Murphy's eye with right upper-lobe bronchus via bronchial lumen

- Recheck position after any change in position: transfer to operating table, lateral roll etc.

One-lung ventilation

There are several indications for OLV:

- Preventing cross-contamination of the other lung with pus or blood (strictly speaking this is lung isolation rather than OLV per se), i.e. during surgery to treat empyema, bronchiectasis or haemorrhage
- Controlling ventilation independently, such as for management of bronchopleural fistula
- Improving surgical access (relative indication)

The majority of cases will be undertaken in the lateral position and the upper lung allowed to collapse, whilst the dependant lung is ventilated with tidal volumes of 5–6 mL/kg. As with acute respiratory distress syndrome patients, a protective ventilation strategy should be adopted with the application of small tidal volumes and positive end-expiratory pressure (PEEP) through pressure-controlled ventilation. This is associated with a lower incidence of postoperative lung dysfunction whilst maintaining satisfactory gas exchange.

Hypoxaemia

Hypoxaemia during OLV is common and due to a number of factors. The dependant lung is susceptible to atelectasis due to compression by mediastinal and abdominal contents as well as age-related changes. Shunt occurs because some perfusion of the unventilated lung persists. It is mitigated to a degree by hypoxic pulmonary vasoconstriction (HPV), which happens in the extra-alveolar arterioles in response to low partial pressures of oxygen. This may be impaired however by excessive PEEP, vasoconstrictor use, incomplete collapse of the operative lung and the use of inhalational anaesthetic agents. When hypoxaemia occurs strategies can be undertaken to improve oxygenation once problems with gas supply and malpositioning of the DLT have been excluded (malpositioning may manifest with high airway pressures or leak and may occur on positioning). These are as follows:

- Increasing F_{IO_2}
- Increasing PEEP (effect unpredictable)
- Applying small amount of continuous positive airway pressure to operative lung
- Intermittent inflation of operative lung

Clearly good communication between anaesthetic, surgical and theatre teams is crucial. At the end of the procedure the operative lung is gently suctioned and manually reinflated under direct vision prior to returning to two-lung ventilation.

Analgesia

Optimal analgesia is of vital importance after thoracic surgery in order to facilitate physiotherapy and aid clearing of secretions. A multimodal approach is optimal with oral paracetamol, NSAIDs and tramadol if appropriate, and may include a thoracic epidural or paravertebral block, either as a single shot or infusion, +/– PCA opioid.

The UK Pneumonectomy Study was a prospective, observational cohort study including 312 patients undergoing surgery in 2005. Sixty-one per cent of patients received an epidural and 31% a paravertebral infusion. Epidural catheter use was associated with increased incidence of clinically important major complications but also reduced odds for postoperative ventilatory failure, potentially reducing the need for post-thoracotomy mechanical ventilation.

Postoperative management

These patients may need critical care support postoperatively and this should ideally be identified and arranged before the day of surgery. However, the vast majority are able to return to the thoracic surgery ward after a period of stability in recovery.

Further reading

Lim E, Baldwin D, Beckles M, et al. Guidelines on the radical management of patients with lung cancer. Thorax 2010; 65:iii1–iii27.

Ng A, Swanevelder J. Hypoxia during one-lung anaesthesia. Br J Anaesth: Contin Educ Anaesth Crit Care Pain 2010; 10:117–122.

Powell ES, Cook D, Pearce AC, et al. A prospective, multicentre, observational cohort study of analgesia and outcome after pneumonectomy. Br J Anaesth 2011; 106:364–370.

Powell ES, Pearce AC, Cook D, et al. UK pneumonectomy outcome study (UKPOS): A prospective observational study of pneumonectomy outcome. J Cardiothorac Surg 2009; 4:41.

Royal College of Anaesthetists. Guidelines for provision of cardiac and thoracic anaesthesia services. London: RCoA, 2013.

Related topics of interest

Thyroid and parathyroid surgery

Key points

- Thyroid surgery must only be undertaken in euthyroid patients
- Parathyroid surgery shares many of the potential postoperative complications of thyroid surgery
- Special consideration must be given to the airway in these patients and they should be approached as a shared airway case

Thyroid surgery is usually indicated for one or more of three main reasons; thyroid dysfunction, benign enlargement or malignancy. The majority of parathyroidectomies are undertaken for resection of secretory adenomas, but a small number are still performed for secondary and tertiary hyperparathyroidism in chronic renal failure patients who have not responded to medical management. Both procedures share some important postoperative complications but thyroid surgery, in particular, poses a number of additional considerations for the anaesthetist.

Problems

- Airway/breathing
  - Positional dyspnoea and stridor
  - Tracheomalacia
  - Airway cartilage invasion (tumour)
  - Bleeding (compressive haematomas)
  - Vocal cord palsy (pre-existing or postoperative)
  - Laryngeal oedema (postoperative)
  - Pneumothorax (especially during retrosternal resection)
- Circulation
  - Superior vena cava obstruction
  - Potential for massive bleeding (vascular tumour/gland, large vessels)
  - Risk of venous air embolism
  - Specific features of the hypo/hyperthyroid states
- Biochemistry
  - Hyperthyroidism – tachyarrhythmias especially AF, hypertension, exophthalmos, thyroid myopathy (proximal weakness), anxiety, abnormal glucose tolerance
  - Thyrotoxic crisis – pyrexia, flushing, abdominal pains, tachycardia/AF, cardiogenic shock, confusion, delirium, dehydration, ketosis, coma, death
  - Hypothyroidism – bradycardia, macroglossia, myocardial ischaemia, atherosclerosis, hypothermia and a tendency to obesity, Addison's syndrome and pernicious anaemia
  - Hypocalcaemia (intentional or inadvertent parathyroidectomy) – perioral tingling, twitching, tetany, prolonged QT interval, ventricular dysrhythmias (e.g. torsades de pointes)
- Neurological
  - Recurrent laryngeal nerve injury – partial or complete airway obstruction can result
  - Possible requirement for intraoperative nerve monitors by the surgeon (precludes use of neuromuscular blocking drugs)

Clinical features

Patients must be euthyroid on the day of surgery and clinical signs of hyper- or hypothyroidism should be sought, particularly cardiac dysrhythmias. A comprehensive airway assessment can give an indication of intubation difficulty and predict problems at induction. The latter are most likely in those who become more dyspnoeic or stridulous when supine – this indicates airway obstruction, possible tracheomalacia (more common with longstanding goitre) and also illustrates the patient will be unable to lie flat for preoxygenation and induction.

Palpation of the neck may demonstrate a thyroid mass with no inferior limit within the neck; i.e. retrosternal surgery will be required. Of particular relevance in these cases is the presence of vena cava obstruction – ask the patient to lift their arms straight up; venous engorgement of the face and neck with worsened inspiratory stridor denotes obstruction.

Investigations

A recent set of thyroid function tests should be available on the day of surgery. Electrolytes including calcium and phosphate should also be known. A full blood count, coagulation screen and group and save are required in case of haemorrhage.

Traditionally, chest X-ray and thoracic inlet radiographs were used to assess airway obstruction. This has been superseded by CT imaging either to assess the airway or the mass (with a malignancy the patient will likely have undergone staging CT to plan oncotherapy). From a clinical and medicolegal stand point, preoperative nasendoscopy is vital to assess laryngeal function. Pre-existing vocal cord palsy (prior surgery or tumour invasion of recurrent laryngeal nerves) may be asymptomatic.

Treatment

There are a number of preoperative treatments for the hyperthyroid patient:
- Propylthiouracil; blocks the iodination of tyrosine and partially blocks the peripheral conversion of thyroxine (T_4) to tri-iodothyronine (T_3)
- Carbimazole; prevents synthesis of new T_3 and T_4 by inhibiting thyroid peroxidase and the oxidation of iodide to iodine. May cause a leucopaenia and takes 6 weeks to work
- Beta-blockade (usually propranolol); reduces the sympathetic effects of thyrotoxicosis and blocks peripheral conversion of T_4 to T_3
- Iodides (such as potassium iodide); inhibits binding of iodide to tyrosine, reduces the effect of thyroid stimulating hormone and inhibits proteolysis of thyroglobulin when given at supraphysiological doses

Anaesthetic management

Parathyroid surgery for a single secreting adenoma is now usually performed as a minimally invasive procedure following localisation of the offending gland with Technetium-99 sestamibi scanning and ultrasonography. Although the majority are still performed under general anaesthesia, cervical plexus blocks or surgical infiltration allow this procedure to be performed without general anaesthesia where desirable. Similarly, thyroidectomy has been demonstrated to be safe and effective with a combination of deep and superficial plexus blocks plus sedation but this approach is very unusual, particularly in the UK.

Conventionally, intravenous induction is followed by intubation with a flexi-metallic endotracheal tube to facilitate direction of airway apparatus away from the surgical field. Gaseous induction or awake fibreoptic intubation are alternatives where airway assessment would dictate. If difficulty is envisaged, the surgeon should be prepared to offer assistance either via rigid bronchoscopy or surgical tracheostomy. Performing the latter under local anaesthesia is another option but may not be possible with a large goitre.

Remifentanil, either with vapour anaesthesia or propofol total intravenous anaesthesia (TIVA) is increasingly popular. It usually removes the requirement for neuromuscular blocking agents which facilitates neurophysiological monitoring of the recurrent laryngeal nerves (although identification and careful dissection by an experienced surgeon is the best means by which to avoid nerve injury). Remifentanil also promotes relative hypotension which minimises blood loss in the surgical field. This drug also allows a very smooth extubation without the risk of straining and subsequent bleeding into the neck. Intravenous dexamethasone to reduce oedema also helps with the extubation process which should occur with the patient sitting up to reduce venous engorgement.

Great care must be taken in securing the airway with tapes and ties as access will be limited if displacement occurs. It is also important to ensure airway devices do not infringe the surgical field. Protection of eyes is important; euthyroid patients may still have exophthalmos from recent hyperthyroidism.

Head-up positioning reduces intraoperative venous bleeding into the surgical field but this also increases the risk of air embolus. Postoperative pain is usually mild-to-moderate; simple analgesia plus surgical infiltration of local anaesthesia or superficial cervical plexus blocks should suffice. Good antiemesis is important; straining and retching risks bleeding into the neck.

Postoperative problems

Hypocalcaemia

The features of this are described above. It can occur following both parathyroid and thyroid surgery. Albumin-corrected levels above 2 mmol/L should be treated with oral supplements. Urgent treatment with intravenous calcium chloride is required below this level, or when symptomatic.

Vocal cord palsy

Semon's law describes the pattern of symptoms produced: recurrent laryngeal transection produces a cadaveric/midadducted cord with a quiet or hoarse voice whereas neuropraxia causes complete adduction. If this occurs bilaterally, airway obstruction results, requiring immediate intervention.

Tracheomalacia

This softening and collapse of the trachea is rare but would typically require immediate reintubation and tracheal stenting. The surgeon will usually assess the integrity of the trachea intraoperatively where suspected.

Thyrotoxic storm

This may occur intraoperatively or postoperatively following partial thyroidectomy but is now much less common as a result of better preoperative management of hyperthyroidism. The treatment is beta-blocker therapy, sedation, cooling, rehydration and antithyroid drugs. Esmolol and dantrolene have both been reported as specific treatments. The patient will require ongoing management in critical care.

Bleeding

Clip removers or stitch cutters must be immediately available in case of expanding haematoma in the neck which may impinge on the airway.

Further reading

Amathieu R, Smail N, Catineau J, et al. Difficult Intubation in thyroid surgery: myth or reality? Anesth Analg 2006; 103:965–968.

Farling P. Thyroid disease. Br J Anaesth 2000; 85:15–28.

Lee B, Lee J-R, Na S. Targeting smooth emergence: the effect site concentration of remifentanil for preventing cough during emergence during propofol–remifentanil anaesthesia for thyroid surgery. Br J Anaesth 2009; 102:775–778.

Malhotra S, Sodhi V. Anaesthesia for thyroid and parathyroid surgery. Br J Anaesth: Contin Educ Anaesth Crit Care Pain 2007; 7:55–58.

Related topics of interest

Total intravenous anaesthesia and target-controlled infusions

Key points

- Total intravenous anaesthesia/target-controlled infusion (TIVA/TCI) is a useful anaesthetic technique with several important potential benefits over inhalational anaesthesia
- The mathematical models used are complex extrapolations that are NOT 100% accurate representations of what is happening in vivo

TIVA is a technique for providing general anaesthesia using only drugs given via the intravenous route. TCIs are a way of delivering TIVA. They consist of devices that use specialised mathematical models to administer specific drugs at rates and doses to achieve and maintain a predicted target plasma or 'effect site' concentration (Cp or Ce respectively). Kruger-Theimer first developed the concept in 1968. The fundamental pharmacokinetic principles behind TIVA and TCIs are volumes of distribution, clearance (both of which are drug specific) and infusion kinetics.

Volume of distribution (Vd)

- Vd is the theoretical volume into which a drug must uniformly distribute to produce the concentration seen in the plasma; i.e., it relates total drug in the body to plasma concentration
- After administering an intravenous drug, some remains in the intravascular compartment and some is distributed amongst other bodily tissues
- If the drug remains in the plasma, concentration is high and Vd is low (**Figure 19a**)
- If a drug is preferentially bound to peripheral tissues, the plasma concentration will be so low as to result in a Vd greater than the patients actual volume (**Figure 19c**)
- Vd (L/kg) = Dose/C_0
  C_0 = Plasma concentration at time zero

Clearance

- Is a measure of the body's capability to remove a substance from the plasma
- It does not constitute elimination/excretion – which is the actual removal of a substance from the plasma or body
  Clearance (mL/min) = $Vd \times k_{elim}$

These two variables are linked with another group of interlinked properties:

- Half-life ($t_{1/2}$ – time for an exponential process to fall to 50%)
  - $t_{1/2} = 0.693 \times (Vd/Cl)$
- Time constant (τ – time taken for an exponential process to fall to 1/e or 37%)
  - $t = Vd/Cl$
- Rate constant (k – the marker of the rate of change of an exponential process, and the reciprocal of time constant)
  - $k = Cl/Vd$

Infusion kinetics

The movement of a drug through a volume is comprised of three basic phases: wash-in, steady-state and wash-out. TCI models tend to represent the human body as three pharmacological compartments (or volumes) (**Figure 20**):

- $V1$ = the plasma volume (drugs can only be administered to and eliminated from this compartment)
- $V2$ = the vessel rich group (brain, heart, liver, kidneys etc.)
- $V3$ = the vessel poor group (fat, cartilage etc.)
- By convention the outside world is designated $V0$

Sometimes a hypothetical compartment known as the effect site (or biophase) is included. The effect site:

- Relates the Cp over time to drug effect over time
- It is the location at which drugs exert their biological effect
- Has no effect on plasma pharmacokinetics, since the amount of drug acting at it is so small

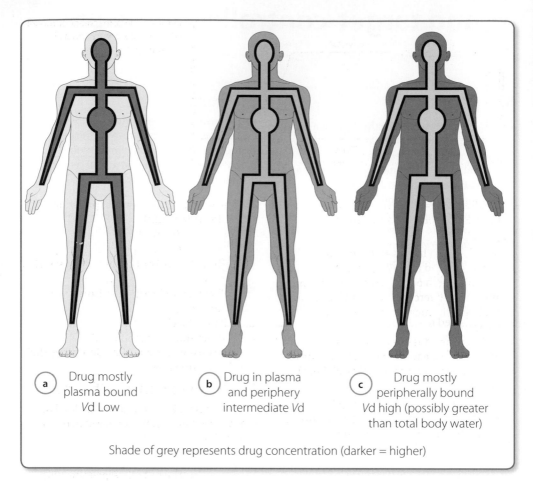

(a) Drug mostly plasma bound *Vd* Low

(b) Drug in plasma and periphery intermediate *Vd*

(c) Drug mostly peripherally bound *Vd* high (possibly greater than total body water)

Shade of grey represents drug concentration (darker = higher)

Figure 19a–c Volume of distribution of drugs according to tissue binding. Grey shading indicates drug concentration, i.e. darker grey = higher concentration.

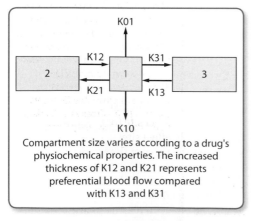

Compartment size varies according to a drug's physiochemical properties. The increased thickness of K12 and K21 represents preferential blood flow compared with K13 and K31

Figure 20 Simple three-compartment pharmacokinetic model.

- Ce is estimated because it cannot be measured (if it could be there would still be wide variations in concentration at the receptor or molecular level)

Figure 21 illustrates how concentration varies with time with a constant rate infusion.

Wash-in

- Drug is administered to $V1$ and plasma concentration rises
- Concentration rises in build-up negative exponential fashion
  - $C = 1-e^{-kt}$
- Drug is simultaneously being redistributed to V2 and V3
- Drug is also simultaneously being eliminated

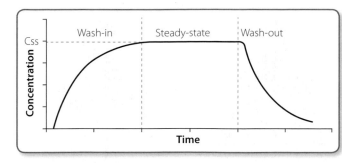

Figure 21 Pharmacokinetic model of plasma concentration with constant-rate infusion.

- Loading dose = $Vd \times Cp$ (where Cp = desired plasma concentration)

Steady-state
- After five drug half-lives steady state will be reached at which point drug administration equals drug elimination
- There is no intercompartmental movement of drug and concentration remains constant
- Maintenance dose = $C_{ss} \times$ Clearance (where C_{ss} = steady-state concentration)
- C_{ss} = Rate in (i.e. mg/min)/Cl (mL/min)

Wash-out
- After stopping an infusion, drug is redistributed from $V2$ and $V3$ back into $V1$
- Drug elimination continues and concentration falls in a triexponential fashion (**Figure 22**)
- $Ct = A.e^{-\alpha t} + B.e^{-\beta t} + C.e^{-\gamma t}$ (where Ct = Concentration at time t)
  - Phase 1 = redistribution from vessel rich group
  - Phase 2 = redistribution from vessel poor group
  - Phase 3 = elimination
- Distribution, elimination and context-sensitive half-time determine the offset of drug effect

Context-sensitive half-time

- Is the time taken for the plasma level of a drug to fall by 50% after cessation of an infusion

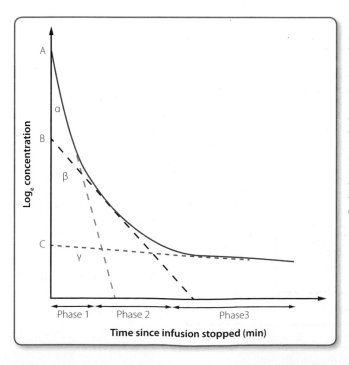

Figure 22 Tri-exponential drug elimination curve. A,B and C refer to 3 compartments with different rates of elimination and 3 different rate constants (α, β and γ). The 3 phases of elimination are governed by the compound effect of these compartments. The Concentration of the drug at any given time can be calculated as $C(t) = A.e^{-\alpha t} + B.e^{-\beta t} + C.e^{-\gamma t}$. Adapted from Physics, Pharmacology and Physiology for Anaesthetists: Key Concepts for the FRCA - Cross and Plunkett. Cambridge University Press.

- Context-insensitive drugs have a half-time that is or may become constant, e.g. remifentanil after 10 minutes or alfentanil after 4 hours (**Figure 23**)

Target-controlled infusions

- TCI models are drug specific, e.g. Marsh and Schnider (propofol) or Minto (remifentanil), and are based on various parameters, e.g. age, gender, height and weight
- Such models are developed by giving drugs as a bolus or infusion to volunteers and taking arterial and venous samples to measure concentrations and then relating dose and plasma/effect site concentration with time
- Consequently, the desired concentration is purely based on extrapolated data thus minute variations between subjects are not taken into account:
  - Pharmacodynamic variations in receptor site concentration
  - Pharmacokinetic variations in metabolism
  - Physiological variations is regional blood flow
- Furthermore, the fact that the plasma/effect site concentration cannot be easily measured can result in the potential for error
- Historically, TCI delivered drugs used a 'Bolus, Elimination, Transfer' (BET) model of administration:
  - Bolus infusion establishing a desired plasma concentration ($Vd \times Cp$)

- Elimination infusion aiming to maintain a constant plasma level (i.e. matching plasma clearance)
- Transfer infusion to account for intercompartmental transfer

The relationship between concentration and time is complex. Pharmacokinetic software combines bolus and steady infusion rates to reach the desired plasma or effect-site concentration as quickly as possible. There will always be a time-lag (and potential hysteresis) between plasma and effect site concentration.

TIVA and TCI

Advantages

- Potentially more perioperative haemodynamic stability
- Ideal for procedures in which inhalational anaesthetic delivery cannot be guaranteed, e.g. bronchoscopy, jet ventilation
- More rapid awakening than some volatiles
- Avoids problems associated with inhalational agents, e.g.
  - Postoperative nausea and vomiting
  - Increased cerebral blood flow and raised intracranial pressure
  - Need for specialised vaporisers or scavenging etc.

Disadvantages

- Plasma and/or effect site concentrations are not measured
- Most models are based on healthy volunteers
- Requires dedicated IV access which should be monitored perioperatively

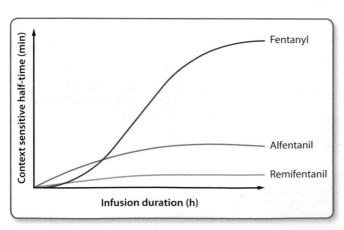

Figure 23 Context sensitive halftime for 3 commonly used opiates. Adapted from Physics, Pharmacology and Physiology for Anaesthetists: Key Concepts for the FRCA - Cross and Plunkett. Cambridge University Press.

- Requires specialist pumps – expense, potential for malfunction etc.
- Risk of accidental awareness increased due to inability to monitor effect-site concentration and cannula/infusion-related failure

Infusion pumps

- Syringe drivers with an onboard computer that is programmed with multiple syringe dimensions and a variety of infusion programmes, ranging from mL/h to more complex pharmacokinetic models (e.g. Marsh or Schnider models

for propofol or Minto model for remifentanil) (**Figure 24**)
- Models tend to use three compartments (although some experimental models used in pregnancy have up to 13 compartments to include specialised tissues, e.g. mammary, uterine and fetal)
- Important safety features including:
    - Secure locking mechanism to prevent accidental dislodging
    - Dose, weight and rate limitations
    - Alarms for occlusion, power failure, near end of infusion etc.

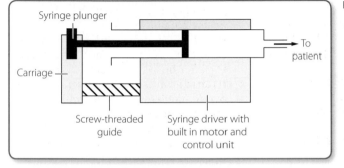

Figure 24 TCI drug infusion pump.

Further reading

Hughes MA, Glass PS, Jacobs JR. Context sensitive half-time in multicompartment pharmacokinetic models for intravenous anesthetic drugs. Anesthesiology 1992; 76:334–341.

Kruger-Thiemer E. Continuous intravenous infusion and multicompartment accumulation. Eur J Pharmacol 1968; 4:317–324.

Youngs EF, Shafer SL. Basic pharmacokinetic and pharmacodynamic principles. In: White PF (ed.), Textbook of intravenous anaesthesia. Baltimore: Williams and Wilkins, 1997:2–26.

Related topics of interest

Urology

Key points

- Urology patients are often elderly with multiple comorbidities
- Transurethral resection of the prostate (TURP) syndrome is not uncommon and can cause cardiovascular and neurological symptoms. It should be recognised and treated promptly
- Renal surgery can result in major haemorrhage due to the proximity of major vessels
- Caudal and penile blocks are suitable for paediatric urological surgery

This topic will consider the main anaesthetic considerations for urology surgery on the lower and upper renal tract. The most common urological procedures are endoscopic. Many patients with bladder tumours undergo multiple anaesthetics for repeat urological procedures over a period of years. Nephrectomy and radical prostatectomy, historically open procedures, are now often performed using the laparoscope. Robot-assisted surgery is also gaining popularity. The most common approach to prostatic surgery remains TURP.

Prostate and bladder surgery

Transurethral resection of prostate and bladder tumour present specific problems to the anaesthetist, mostly due to the risk of 'TURP syndrome' which has an incidence of 1–8%. Retropubic prostatectomy traditionally requires a laparotomy and large blood loss should be expected. General anaesthesia with epidural analgesia or abdominal plane block is usually performed.

Problems

- Elderly patients with concurrent diseases, particularly renal impairment due to chronic renal outflow obstruction
- The TURP syndrome of fluid overload and hyponatraemia
- Risk of bladder perforation
- Position – TURP is performed in lithotomy
- Blood loss

- Risk of hypothermia with TURP
- Systemic fibrinolysis due to urokinase release from raw prostate tissue

Anaesthetic management

Assessment and premedication

Particular attention should be paid to the cardiovascular history of patients presenting for prostatectomy. Prostatic hypertrophy may cause obstructive renal failure and surgery is often delayed until catheterisation has allowed renal function to normalise. Minimum investigations are a FBC, group and save, urea and electrolytes and ECG. The preoperative serum sodium should be >130 mmol/L. Other investigations may be required depending on the patient's health.

Conduct of anaesthesia

Each patient should be anaesthetised with consideration of his other pathologies. Regional anaesthesia aiming for sensory block higher than T10 is the anaesthetic of choice for TURP surgery for the reasons indicated in **Table 83** (there is little evidence of better survival outcomes, however). Supplementary O_2 and sedation, if required is often given. Blood loss should be monitored; the haemoglobin concentration in irrigation fluid can be measured in theatre. Significant hypotension should be managed with vasoconstrictors, rather than fluid loading. This may become evident at the end of the procedure when the legs are lowered from the lithotomy position.

Alternatively, general anaesthesia with or without a caudal block may be used. It may be required if patients cannot lie flat, are extremely anxious or have other contraindications to spinal anaesthesia. Antibiotics are given as standard to reduce the risk of urosepsis. If TURP syndrome is suspected perioperatively, surgery should be terminated and the urea and electrolytes measured.

TURP syndrome

Absorption of irrigating fluid occurs during prolonged endoscopic procedures (about

Table 83 Regional anaesthesia for urology surgery	
Advantages	**Disadvantages**
Reduced blood loss	Cough unsuppressed, may interfere with surgery
Assessment of cerebral function	Hypotension/high block
Bladder perforation more easily recognised (nausea, pain, abdominal distension/rigidity)	Hypoventilation
Optimum postop analgesia	Penile erection, may interfere with surgery (may be treated with glycopyrrolate)
Increased intravascular space, due to vasodilation	Psychological and patient dignity
Reduced deep vein thrombosis risk	Technical failure/usual spinal anaesthesia risks

20 mL/min), which can lead to volume overload and, crucially, hypo-osmolality. If this occurs, bradycardia, hypertension, raised central venous pressure, pulmonary oedema and later cardiovascular collapse may be seen. Hyponatraemia and hypo-osmolality can lead to cerebral oedema causing confusion, headache, 'cortical' visual disturbance, convulsions and coma. Warm glycine solution (1.5% iso-osmotic) is used as it is a poor electrical conductor but has good optical properties giving the surgeon a clear view. Glycine absorption may be minimised by limiting the height of the fluid above the patient (hydrostatic pressure) to less than 60cm and limiting irrigation time to 1 hour. In addition, an experienced surgeon is likely to take less time and may be more attentive to open blood vessels.

The treatment is fluid restriction and organ support, including respiratory support, diuretics (if pulmonary oedema), inotropic support and anticonvulsants if required. In severe cases, hypertonic saline, loop diuretics and cardiac output monitoring may be required. Raising serum sodium by >1 mmol/L/h may cause central pontine demyelination. If the sodium falls below 120 mmol/L, a mortality rate of 50% has been documented. Glycine absorption may also cause CNS problems possibly by acting as an inhibitory neurotransmitter. It is metabolised to ammonia which may contribute to the symptoms

Postoperative care

To prevent clot retention following TURP, continuous bladder irrigation is usually performed until the bleeding has stopped. Careful cardiovascular and neurological

observation must be continued as the problems of hypo-osmolar volume overload may still occur up to 24 hours after surgery. Resolution of the sympathetic blockade may decrease the intravascular space contributing to volume overload. TURP blood loss is difficult to assess and transfusion is sometimes required. Intravenous crystalloid fluids should be given sparingly and dextrose solutions avoided. Postoperative bladder spasm can be distressing and may be treated with antimuscarinic agents, such as hyoscine or oxybutynin.

Renal surgery

The commonest indications for nephrectomy are renal tumour or for removal of a nonfunctioning kidney. Preoperative assessment is as above. The anaesthetic technique may require modification in the setting of severe renal impairment.

Nephrolithotomy can be achieved by lithotripsy or by open removal of calculi. Lithotripsy can cause intense perioperative stimulation, which may be ablated by remifentanil infusion. Patient may be positioned in the prone position for this procedure.

Whether laparoscopic or open, nephrectomy surgery requires large bore intravenous access, intubation and IPPV, warmed fluids and, depending on patient and surgical factors, cardiac output monitoring and arterial access. Care should be taken to avoid limbs with arteriovenous fistulae. The anaesthetist should remain vigilant for sudden unexpected haemorrhage due to the vascular nature of the kidney and its proximity to other vascular structures, in particular the inferior vena cava.

Patient positioning is usually lateral, with the table 'broken' to improve surgical access to the flank. Patients should be carefully padded to prevent pressure areas and cardiac output should be closely monitored due to the possibility of caval compression.

In addition to haemorrhage, pleural and diaphragmatic breaches are possible complications. Although usually noted and repaired during surgery, this may lead to tension pneumothorax. Regional anaesthesia, either epidural or abdominal plane blocks/subcostal catheters allow for good postoperative chest physiotherapy following open surgery. Epidural anaesthesia carries the risk of hypotension, which may be detrimental to the remaining kidney.

Paediatric urology

- Most paediatric surgery in district hospitals is performed as day case procedures, e.g. circumcision, orchidopexy. More complex surgery often involves congenital malformations, with associated comorbidities and is usually undertaken in tertiary centres.

Considerations for preoperative assessment and perioperative conduct are the same as other paediatric surgeries and are covered elsewhere except for regional anaesthesia, which has a particular place in urological surgery. Caudal anaesthesia is safe and effective and provides around 6 hours of analgesia when plain local anaesthesia is used. Adjuncts to prolong the block have questionable safety and should be avoided. NAP3 data found 0/100,000 cases of permanent harm following caudal anaesthesia use in paediatric surgery. Ilioinguinal/iliohypogastric block is performed when a groin incision is to be made; e.g. for orchidopexy, but carries around 20% failure rate. Penile block is particularly useful for circumcision and prepucal surgery.

Further reading

Gandhi M, Vashisht R. Anaesthesia for paediatric urology. Br J Anaesth: Contin Educ Anaesth Crit Care Pain Med 2010; 10:152–157.

Hart EM. Week 19: Anaesthesia for renal surgery. World anaesthesia tutorial for the week. London; Anaesthesia UK, 2006.

O'Donnell AM, Foo ITH. Anaesthesia for transurethral resection of the prostate. Br J Anaesth: Contin Educ Anaesth Crit Care Pain Med 2009; 9:92–96.

Related topics of interest

Vascular access

Key points

- Ultrasound can reduce the complications associated with central access
- Catheter-related infection is least likely with subclavian venous access and most likely with femoral access
- The intraosseous (IO) route is the preferred method of gaining emergency vascular access. Mechanical insertion devices allow for reliable access to be rapidly secured

Vascular access is one of the most commonly performed practical procedures by anaesthetists. All patients undergoing general anaesthesia should have vascular access secured as soon as is practically possible. Vascular access is often not considered necessary for many regional anaesthesia techniques (e.g. for ophthalmic surgery). Vascular access plays a significant role in hospital-acquired infection. An aseptic technique should be used whenever vascular access is obtained.

Peripheral

Commonly used sites include the veins on the dorsum of the hand, the brachial or cephalic veins in the antecubital fossa and the long saphenous vein. Cannulae should be inserted using an 'aseptic non-touch technique'. Gloves and 2% chlorhexidine/70% alcohol skin preparation are mandatory. A Cochrane review in 2013 concluded that there is no benefit in routinely replacing cannulae every 72–96 hours. Cannulae should be inspected daily, however, and removed if there is suspicion of infection. Safety cannulae should be used where possible.

Central

Common sites for central venous access include internal jugular, subclavian and femoral veins. Central access also may be obtained via a peripheral insertion point, e.g. antecubital veins. Central access can provide monitoring of central venous and pulmonary arterial pressures allow administration of irritant drugs and parenteral nutrition, measurement of core temperature, haemofiltration/dialysis and transvenous cardiac pacing.

In 2002, NICE published guidelines supporting the use of ultrasound for the insertion of internal jugular central lines. Although controversial at the time, there is now substantial evidence of improved safety when it is used. Ultrasound is increasingly used to facilitate vascular access in other sites. It is particularly useful in patients with poor vascular access and the obese.

A Cochrane review of antimicrobial-impregnated central catheters in 2013 revealed a reduced rate of catheter colonisation and catheter-related bloodstream infection, particularly in the ICU setting, but found little evidence of reduced sepsis or mortality.

Complications of central access

Early

- Pneumothorax/haemothorax
- Haemorrhage
- Haematoma
- Thoracic duct injury (for left sided jugular/subclavian approaches)
- Air embolism
- Guide wire embolism
- Arterial puncture/inadvertent cannulation
- Arrhythmia
- Cardiac tamponade
- Brachial plexus injury

Late

- Infection – local or bloodstream, including endocarditis
- Erosion – particularly pericardial
- Thrombosis
- Pulmonary embolism
- Venous stricture and stenosis

Complications may be minimised by:
- Use of ultrasound
- Vein selection: subclavian access carries the lowest infection rate, and the femoral route carries the highest

- Strict aseptic technique, antimicrobial-impregnated lines and tunnelling of lines
- Head-down positioning of the patient during insertion to prevent air embolism
- Removal of lines at the earliest opportunity

Emergency access

Surgical venous cutdown has largely been superseded by IO access, especially with the development of mechanical access devices such as the EZ-IO. Use in recent military conflicts has proven the benefits of such devices in securing fast and reliable access.

IO access sites in adults include the proximal tibia, humeral head, sternum, femoral trochanter and iliac crest. The medial aspect of the proximal tibia is the favoured paediatric site. Local anaesthetic infiltration prior to insertion allows for use in the awake patient.

Access is confirmed by aspiration of bone marrow and absence of local extravasation when used. Bone marrow is extremely vascular and drug onset time is equivalent to the intravenous route. Blood may be sampled, including cross-match, provided the laboratory is informed, as it requires alternative processing. Fluid boluses must be administered under pressure as free-flow is slow. All intravenous medications, including induction agents may be administered via the IO route. Rapid sequence induction can be performed safely and effectively via IO access.

Complications of IO access include failure, dislodgement, extravasation, osteomyelitis (rare), compartment syndrome, and, in children, growth plate disruption and fracture. Contraindications include insertion into a bone with proximal fracture, previous recent IO access at the same site and local infection.

Further reading

Lai NM, Chaiyakunapruk N, Lai NA, et al. Catheter impregnation, coating or bonding for reducing central venous catheter-related infections in adults. Cochrane Database Syst Rev 2013; 6;6:CD007878.

Pratt RJ, Pellowe CM, Loveday HP, at al. epic2: National evidence-based guidelines for preventing healthcare-associated infections in NHS hospitals in England. J Hosp Infect 2007; 65S:S1–64.

Resuscitation Council (UK). Use of intraosseous (IO) access during cardiac arrest. 2011 http://www.resus.org.uk/pages/IOaccess.pdf

Related topics of interest

- Emergency anaesthesia (p. 70)
- Polytrauma (p. 217)

Vascular surgery – aortic aneurysmal disease

Key points

- Aneurysm repair is a high-risk procedure and the patients are typically high-risk candidates
- Repair was traditionally open but endovascular techniques offer shorter hospital stay and lower 30-day mortality
- Open repair remains the typical method for an acute rupture

Aneurysms may form in any artery in the circulation with potentially fatal consequences. This topic will focus on abdominal aortic aneurysms (AAA). Cerebral aneurysms are covered *Neuroanaesthesia – subarachnoid haemorrhage.*

Dilation to >30 mm diameter of any section of the aorta defines an aneurysm. There is a 5:1 preponderance in men; however, once >55 mm, the annual rupture rate is 50% higher in women (18% vs. 12%) with an increased mortality compared with men. Predisposing factors include smoking, hypertension and diabetes. Consequently, as with all vascular surgery patients, it must be remembered that other vessels, particularly the coronary and cerebral vessels, will also be pathological. Furthermore, related renal and pulmonary comorbidities are similarly ubiquitous; these are high-risk procedures performed on high-risk patients.

Endovascular aortic repair (EVAR) was first successfully performed in 1990. This offers repair without the inherent risks of a laparotomy or general anaesthesia. Several large, multicentre studies in the last 10 years have demonstrated that EVAR offers better 30-day mortality compared with open repair with up to 60% reduction in blood loss, reduced transfusion requirements and a halving of hospital and Critical Care length of stay. Unfortunately by around 2 years the mortality benefit seems to disappear. EVAR is also associated with up to 25% reintervention rates and is significantly more expensive. Experience and technology continue to improve but the technique has yet to fully replace open repair. Some aneurysms remain anatomically unsuitable for the procedure and the use of EVAR in the context of acute rupture is still relatively undeveloped.

Problems

- Patient comorbidity particularly pulmonary and cardiac/cerebral vascular disease
- Postoperative complications: pulmonary embolism, pneumonia, myocardial infarction (MI), dysrhythmias, confusion, acute kidney injury, spinal ischaemia/paraplegia, graft/wound infections, lower limb and gastrointestinal ischaemia
- Open repair
    - Bleeding and coagulopathy
    - Pain
    - Stress response to laparotomy
    - Ileus
- EVAR
    - Possibility of remote-site anaesthesia in radiology suite
    - Contrast load to kidneys
    - Requirement to suspend breathing during stent deployment
    - Potential for conversion to open surgery:
        - Mid-procedure rupture
        - Failure of device in controlling aneurysm

Clinical features

AAA is typically an incidental finding during investigation for some other cause of intra-abdominal pain or pathology. Men over 65 years are screened in the UK.

The diagnosis of rupture must be made carefully but expeditiously. Abdominal pain radiating to the back, profound hypotension and shock with absent femoral pulses strongly suggest the diagnosis in the context of a patient with appropriate risk factors who presents with an expansile, pulsatile mass. Due care must be given to exclude pancreatitis, MI or acute gastrointestinal perforation with peritonitis. Aortic dissection is another important differential; it is two to three times more common than rupture and more common amongst those with aneurysmal disease.

Investigations

Ultrasound and CT angiography are the investigations of choice. Aortography, once the gold standard, is rarely performed. Preanaesthetic investigations should be identical for open repair or EVAR: their requirement is dictated by the comorbidity of the patient and the fact that an EVAR carries the risk of progressing to an open procedure. Full-blood count, electrolytes, coagulation screen, serum group and save and ECG are a minimum. Consider echocardiography and pulmonary function tests. Elective surgery may well be best deferred until after coronary angioplasty or bypass surgery if required.

Treatment

Elective patients should have had diligent hypertension management in the community. There is some evidence that statins reduce the rate of annual aneurysm expansion. Aneurysms of less than 55mm diameter are associated with <1% annual rupture risk and so repair is not offered before this point.

For aneurysms >55 mm radiologists and surgeons liaise to determine feasibility of EVAR. If not suitable, open repair or ongoing surveillance is offered (considering surgical/anaesthetic risk and risk of rupture).

Anaesthetic management
EVAR

Arterial and large-bore venous access are the minimum standard regardless of anaesthetic technique. There should be consideration of a strategy in case of conversion to an open procedure. Arterial and vascular access are best inserted in the right arm as the left axillary artery may occasionally be required for anterograde access to assist

with deployment of the proximal end of the stent. There is evidence demonstrating that spinal or local anaesthesia infiltration techniques significantly reduce postoperative pulmonary complications and hospital length of stay compared with GA (although with no mortality benefit). These benefits have not been observed with epidurals however. Periods of breath holding may be required at the moment of stent deployment; this requires either a paralysed anaesthetised patient or a cooperative awake patient. Perioperative heparin is administered once the femoral arteries are exposed. The procedure usually takes around 2 hours and blood loss is around 600 mL. Postoperative blood-pressure monitoring and close assessment of fluid status may necessitate Critical Care admission.

Open repair

These cases are significantly more complex for the anaesthetist. In addition to preparations made for EVAR, postinduction central venous access is typically obtained; multiple vasoactive infusions may be required and the central venous pressure can be used for crude assessment of volume status. Some attempt to monitor cardiac performance is helpful although oesophageal Doppler is unreliable after cross-clamping (pulse contour analysis techniques are an alternative although reliability data are lacking). The induction must aim to avoid swings in blood pressure; these strain the heart and increase aneurysm wall-stress. Epidural anaesthesia is commonly used in conjunction with GA but, owing to the haemodynamic effects, it should generally not be used until surgery is nearing completion.

Cross-clamping of the aorta will be preceded by a requirement for heparin IV bolus. The clamping itself causes significant cardiovascular disturbance with a marked rise in mean arterial pressure and systemic vascular resistance (SVR). This increases myocardial work and risks ischaemia. Deepening of anaesthesia or vasodilator infusions (e.g. glyceryl trinitrate, sodium nitroprusside or hydralazine) may be helpful.

Whilst the aorta is clamped, the patient should be fluid loaded in preparation for clamp release. Fluid loading prior to cross-clamping should be avoided; it exacerbates the myocardial strain associated with this part of the procedure. Upon release of the clamp, blood pressure drops significantly for a variety of reasons (**Table 84**). The surgeon should give due warning to allow time for fluid loading and preparation of inotropic and vasopressor drugs as required.

In general, perioperative measurement and proactive treatment of temperature, coagulation status and arterial blood gases are required. Haemoglobin should be maintained at 90–100 g/L and cell salvage can be used to limit transfusion requirements. Active warming will maintain acid–base status and coagulation function but avoid warming regions distal to the cross-clamp.

In the context of an acute rupture (surgical mortality ~35%), a haemodynamically stable induction is crucial and agents such as ketamine should be considered. Induction should be performed in theatre with the patient fully prepped and the surgeon ready to open the abdomen. Relaxant-only intubation in the apparently moribund patient has been associated with a 43% incidence of awareness amongst survivors. These cases require a larger anaesthetic team – keeping up with the transfusion requirements and liaison with Critical Care and haematology can distract from the central task of delivering a safe anaesthetic and communicating with the surgeon.

Table 84 Reasons for post-clamp removal hypotension
Increased run-off, i.e. large SVR drop
Vasodilatory effects of acidosis in reperfused tissues
Myocardial depression of
Cold, acidotic blood rejoining circulation
Reduced coronary flow secondary to fall in diastolic pressure
Inadequate fluid loading
Anastomotic leak/failure

Postoperative

EVAR patients should ideally receive ongoing invasive pressure monitoring for several hours and optimal hydration and renal monitoring in the context of radio-contrast loading is important. In the absence of significant pre-existing renal disease, there is little evidence for pretreatment with mannitol, N-acetyl cysteine or sodium bicarbonate; good hydration at all phases is adequate.

Open repair patients should all return to a Critical Care environment. They are at significantly greater risk of postoperative complications due to the invasiveness of surgery and their nursing requirements are greater. Timing of extubation is guided as always by consideration of whether temperature, acid–base balance, coagulopathy and bleeding and gas exchange are adequately addressed.

Further reading

Al-HashimiM, Thompson J. Anaesthesia for elective open abdominal aortic aneurysm repair. Br J Anaesth: Contin Educ Anaesth Crit Care Pain, 2013; doi:10.1093/bjaceaccp/mkt015

De Bruin JL, Baas AF, Buth J, et al. Long-term outcome of open or endovascular repair of abdominal aortic aneurysm. N Engl J Med 2010; 362:1881–1889.

Edwards MS, Andrews JS, Edwards AF, et al. Results of endovascular aortic aneurysm repair with general, regional, and local/monitored anesthesia care in the American College of Surgeons National Surgical Quality Improvement Program database. J Vasc Surg 2011; 54:1273–1282.

Related topics of interest

Vascular surgery – occlusive disease

Key points

- Patients undergoing limb revascularisation surgery are at the advanced stage of their disease
- As with all vascular patients, carotid and peripheral vascular patients have significant comorbidity
- Perioperative myocardial and cerebrovascular events leading to death are common

Occlusive vascular disease includes both peripheral vascular disease (PVD) and central disease. Of most common importance under the latter headings are lower-limb ischaemic disease and carotid occlusion and these will be the focus of this topic. Both offer particular challenges to the anaesthetist. The precipitating lifestyle factors and comorbidities such as smoking, alcohol, diabetes, hypertension and hyperlipidaemia must be considered. Only 8% of PVD patients have normal coronary arteries and >60% have severely diseased vessels – this increases to over 90% in those requiring amputation for their PVD.

In modern practice, most of those presenting for surgical revascularisation in PVD have previously failed angioplasty and so, by definition, have more advanced and complex disease. Similarly, with carotid disease, it is comparatively unusual for the contralateral carotid to be completely free of disease thus perioperative stroke is a significant risk, particularly with urgent procedures following a recent cerebral event. This is of notable relevance where guidelines exist, as in the UK from NICE, specifying surgery within 2 weeks of neurological symptoms and, where possible, within 48 hours to maximise the secondary preventative benefit.

Problems

Common to most vascular patients:
- Comorbidity
  - Chronic obstructive pulmonary disease (COPD) (3x risk of pulmonary postoperative complications)
  - Coronary disease or vascular disease
  - Renovascular disease and chronic kidney disease
  - Hypertension (risk of cardiomyopathy, diastolic dysfunction, altered organ autoregulation)
  - Diabetes – requires careful perioperative control to maintain blood sugar <10 mmol/L
- Exercise tolerance becomes nonspecific and nonsensitive: many factors may limit exercise before symptoms of cardiac, respiratory or vascular insufficiency become apparent
- Often elderly – comorbid and frail, multiple medications, possibly unable to lie still or flat long enough to undergo procedures under local/regional anaesthesia (LA/RA)
- May still be actively smoking

Specific to lower-limb PVD patients:
- Ischaemia, gangrene and ulcers may result in chronic low-grade infection
- Therapeutic heparinisation for acute ischaemia may preclude RA
- Duration of surgery may unexpectedly outlast regional techniques, e.g. if distal perfusion remains inadequate and a secondary bypass is required
- Five to eight per cent 30-day mortality for elective cases, >25% for emergency cases

Specific to carotid surgery:
- Perioperative stroke, MI or death (target combined risk <5% at 30 days)
- Bleeding
- Cardiovascular and cerebral autoregulatory instability for 2 weeks poststroke
- Complications of shunt insertion:
  - Gas/clot embolisation
  - Carotid dissection
  - Displacement
  - Kinking
  - Haemorrhage
  - Failure to recognise need for shunt with subsequent cerebral ischaemia

- Failed or nontolerated RA – requirement for GA/intubation with open surgical field
- Postoperative complications:
  - Haematoma/bleeding
  - Cerebral hyperperfusion syndrome – hypertension, encephalopathy, seizures with potential for cerebral oedema and cerebral haemorrhage (latter has 70% mortality in this context)
  - Postoperative stroke/MI/death

Clinical features

Cerebrovascular insufficiency presents as a transient ischaemic attack (by definition resolving fully within 24 hours) or stroke. Symptoms vary from sensory-motor deficits in the limbs to visual disturbances, vertigo, headache, speech difficulties or facial weakness. Carotid bruits may be heard but a careful neurological examination and duplex scanning of the carotid and vertebral vessels is more useful.

PVD of the lower limbs may present as varying degrees of resting leg pain, claudication and skin ulceration. The classical presentation of acute, limb-threatening ischaemia is the '6 P's' – painful, perishingly cold, pale, pulseless, paralysed with paraesthesia. Whilst PVD is the commonest cause of such a presentation, a similar limb-threatening state may be produced by trauma involving the arterial supply to a limb or iatrogenic injury, e.g. femoral dissection following interventional radiological procedures.

Investigations

The extent of comorbidity largely dictates that in the elective setting, these patients are investigated extensively. Full blood count, electrolytes and renal biochemistry, coagulation screen and a group and save are required. Blood gas analysis and spirometry or comprehensive pulmonary function tests should be considered in those with COPD. ECG and, where time allows, echocardiography and stress-echocardiography or myocardial perfusion scanning are useful. The American College of Cardiology and American Heart Association guidance on perioperative management of cardiac patients for noncardiac surgery delineates which patients should be referred to cardiology for preoperative assessment and intervention. This includes all patients suffering an MI within 30 days, severe angina, decompensated heart failure, severe left-sided valvular stenoses or significant arrhythmias (AF >100, heart blocks, ventricular tachycardias or bradycardias).

In the setting of acute limb ischaemia a pragmatic approach should be taken. Surgery should occur within 6 hours; thus, only those investigations which can both be performed and acted upon in this time should be considered.

Treatment

Many of these patients will present on multiple cardiovascular medications. These should be continued perhaps with the exception of ACE inhibitors and angiotensin-II blockers (omitted on the day of surgery). Omission of statin therapy is associated with up to a 7.5x increase in perioperative MI and death in vascular surgery. Similarly, beta-blockers should not be omitted. Commencement of these agents perioperatively is not recommended – evidence is lacking as yet for statins and there is evidence of harm for beta-blockers.

First-line treatment for PVD is commonly now angioplasty and stenting. Embolectomy under LA may be tried for acute limb ischaemia. If these fail, surgical bypass and/ or endarterectomy is the salvage therapy. Endarterectomy is the principal therapy for carotid disease currently.

Anaesthetic management

There are specific considerations for PVD and carotid surgery but, in the main, they share a common aim – to provide maximal cardiovascular stability and optimal intra – and postoperative analgesia. Both serve to limit stress on the heart. Invasive arterial monitoring is typical in most cases. 5-lead ECG monitoring with ST analysis is useful in detecting myocardial ischaemia. Under GA, some form of cardiac output monitoring is also beneficial. Careful control of fluid-state/perfusion, blood glucose, acid–base balance and temperature are vital in these patients.

Carotid surgery

Since the landmark GALA study (2008) and subsequent Cochrane review it seems the choice of LA/RA versus GA for this surgery is a matter of preference on the part of the surgeon and patient. RA was associated with lower rates of postoperative bleeding but major outcomes were similar; the importance of the surgeon and anaesthetist being familiar with the selected technique is paramount.

RA offers the distinct benefit of optimal monitoring of cerebral perfusion (both intra- and postoperatively) and is associated with less frequent shunt requirement. It is most commonly achieved by superficial cervical plexus block. Surgical infiltration of LA in addition usually negates the requirement for deep cervical block with its inherent risks. GA protects the airway from the start, optimises CO_2 tension and is helpful in the patient who cannot tolerate the procedure awake (inability to lie flat, claustrophobia, distended bladder). Cerebral monitoring however defaults to complex and less-sensitive means, e.g. processed EEG, transcranial Doppler or near-infrared spectroscopy. GA is also associated with intraoperative hypotension and postoperative hypertension (the inverse of the optimal state often produced by RA; mild hypertension intraoperatively and normotension postoperatively). Cerebral autoregulation is also disturbed above 1 MAC of inhalational agents and with total intravenous anaesthesia. A ceiling systolic blood pressure of 170 mmHg or within 20% of the patient's baseline systolic is the consensus target.

PVD surgery

This may involve femoral endarterectomy, distal embolectomy or any variety of bypass procedures. The latter usually involve synthetic graft with the inherent risk of infection. These patients typically have reduced wound healing thus wound problems are common.

Most procedures for the lower-limb lend themselves to RA although this must be weighed up against the risk of infection, duration of procedure, heparin/warfarin therapy, the ability of the patient to lie flat and any degree of aortic stenosis. RA has the benefits of avoiding GA in a high-risk population as well as minimising cardiac stress from pain and mitigating the stress response to surgery. If necessary it may be supplemented with sedation or indeed balanced GA. Pain, hypothermia and hypoxia are amongst the most detrimental factors to arise in the postoperative phase and these must be carefully avoided.

Gross metabolic disturbance following revascularisation of tissue should be anticipated and treated aggressively with fluid and vasoactive drugs. Active management of hyperkalaemia may also be required. These aspects are particularly important during surgery for acute limb ischaemia but are also relevant during the reperfusion stage of elective bypass surgery.

Where amputation is indicated, phantom limb pain and chronic postsurgical pain are common. Numerous strategies have been investigated (pre-emptive RA, intraoperative ketamine, postoperative gabapentin amongst others), but conclusive evidence of benefit is lacking and this remains a difficult phenomenon to treat.

Further reading

Fleisher LA, Beckman JA, Brown KA, et al. ACC/AHA 2007 Guidelines on perioperative cardiovascular evaluation and care for non-cardiac surgery. Circulation 2007; 116:e418–e500.

Ladak N, Thompson JP. General or local anaesthesia for carotid endarterectomy? Br J Anaesth: Contin Educ Anaesth Crit Care Pain 2012; 12:92–96.

National Institute for Health and Care Excellence. CG68. Stroke: Diagnosis and initial management of acute stroke and transient ischaemic attack. London: NICE, 2008.

National Institute for Health and Care Excellence. CG147. Lower limb peripheral arterial disease: diagnosis and management. London: NICE, 2008.

Rerkasem K, Rothwell PM. Local versus general anaesthesia for carotid endarterectomy. Cochrane Database Syst Rev 2008;CD000126.

Tovey G, Thompson JP. Anaesthesia for lower limb revascularization. Br J Anaesth: Contin Educ Anaesth Crit Care Pain 2005; 5:89–92.

Related topics of interest

Venous thromboembolism – prevention and treatment

Key points

- Prevention of thromboembolic disease should be considered for every surgical procedure
- There are now multiple antithrombotic agents available. Their mechanisms of action vary and care should be taken regarding their half-lives, side effects and reversibility
- Bleeding risk should be assessed prior to prescription of pharmacological prophylaxis
- Pulmonary embolism (PE) is a significant cause of perioperative mortality. CT pulmonary angiography is the gold-standard investigation and anticoagulaton is the most common treatment

Prevention

The prevention of venous thromboembolism (VTE) will be considered in the preoperative, perioperative and postoperative periods.

Preoperative

Oestrogen-containing contraceptives should be stopped the cycle before major surgery. Hormone replacement therapy should be stopped 6 weeks before. Obese patients should be encouraged to lose weight before surgery. Patients presenting for emergency should be adequately fluid resuscitated prior to surgery.

Peri- and postoperative

Mechanical

Graduated compression stockings: reduce the volume of blood pooling in the lower limbs and increase flow velocity. There is evidence of a 50% reduction in deep vein thrombosis (DVT), particularly in orthopaedic surgery; however, the benefit has not been demonstrated so clearly in general medical patients. There is a risk of limb loss and compartment syndrome in patients with pre-existing vascular compromise. Correct fitting

is essential if they are to be effective and safe. They are contraindicated in pulmonary or peripheral oedema, peripheral vascular disease, peripheral neuropathy and local skin damage.

Intermittent pneumatic compression devices: either foot pumps of calf pumps; Supporting evidence indicates that they should be worn for at least 16 hours to be effective.

Efficacy of stockings and pneumatic devices seem comparable, although use of stockings and compression devices together may be less effective than either one alone.

Pharmacological

The most common pharmacological therapy used in the perioperative period is indicated in **Table 85**. Pharmacological prophylaxis should be used with caution in the presence of bleeding risk factors (**Table 86**). Rates of DVT can be reduced by around 50–60% in general and orthopaedic surgery through the use of heparin/low molecular weight heparin (LMWH). Pharmacological prophylaxis should be continued for up to 35 days following hip surgery and 14 days following knee surgery.

Other methods employed to reduce perioperative VTE include:

- Caval filters: used in patients with particularly high risk, pre-existing proximal DVT or patients in whom pharmacological methods are contraindicated. Filters are deployed percutaneously through the femoral vessels and are often removable postoperatively. They are rarely offered and evidence of effectiveness is limited
- Regional anaesthesia: There is good evidence from a number of studies that neuraxial anaesthesia is associated with a lower incidence of VTE compared with general anaesthesia
- Early mobilisation and physiotherapy: Although there is little robust evidence, it is generally accepted that immobility

Table 85 Pharmacological therapy for thromboprophylaxis

Low molecular weight heparin (LMWH)	Factor Xa inhibitor E.g. Dalteparin, enoxaparin often given the night before or after surgery No requirement for monitoring and low incidence of thrombocytopaenia More effective than unfractionated heparin Care in renal failure (enoxaparin is better tolerated)
Unfractionated heparin	Factor Xa and thrombin inhibitor Easily reversed 2–3% risk of thrombocytopaenia
Oral direct factor Xa inhibitors	E.g. Rivaroxaban, apixaban Usually started the day after surgery Difficult to reverse and some concern regarding postoperative haematoma Licensed for hip and knee replacement therapy
Warfarin	Inhibits hepatic recycling of vitamin K which is required as a cofactor in coagulation factor synthesis Requires close monitoring and takes some days to reach therapeutic effect Has a paradoxical procoagulant effect early in therapy due to inhibition of protein C (anticoagulant) prior to full inhibition of coagulation factor synthesis Risk of drug interactions
Aspirin	Inhibits thromboxane A2 synthesis in platelets Limited bleeding risk compared with others, but performs less well in trials when compared with LMWH for prevention of venous thromboembolism (VTE). Better than no therapy at all
Fondaparinux	Factor Xa inhibitor Difficult to reverse if bleeding, doesn't require monitoring Given parenterally, it may be more effective than LMWH
Direct thrombin inhibitors	E.g. Dabigatran, hirudin, lepirudin No risk of thrombocytopaenia, some are given as infusion Used if patients have heparin-induced thrombocytopaenia

Table 86 Risk factors for bleeding

Significant active bleeding
Untreated thrombophilia- congenital or acquired (e.g. severe liver disease, thrombocytopaenia)
Recent anticoagulant therapy
Neuraxial block in the last 4 hours, or expected in the next 12 hours
Uncontrolled hypertension (>230/120mmHg) – cerebrovascular event
Adapted from National Institute for Health and Care Excellence (NICE). Venous thromboembolism: reducing the risk. London; NICE, 2010.

increases the risk of VTE through venous stasis, particularly in the lower limbs. It thus follows that early mobilisation will reduce the risk, although this has not been quantified

Diagnosis

In addition to clinical suspicion, the gold standard for DVT diagnosis is venography.

Doppler ultrasound is a less invasive technique, but is less sensitive. Measurement of D-dimers in the postoperative period is not helpful due to elevation in response to surgery itself.

DVT has a reported incidence of 40–60% on venogram following hip replacement. However, many of these are asymptomatic and are of questionable relevance if they never embolise or become clinically evident.

Therapeutic treatment of VTE

The mainstay of treatment is unfractionated heparin, LMWH and warfarin. Newer agents for extended treatment of thromboembolism after initial treatment phase include rivaroxaban, apixaban and dabigatran. Aspirin may be used after the initial treatment phase, but is less effective, reducing the risk of further DVT by a third.

Pulmonary embolism

Pulmonary emboli due to thromboembolic disease almost always originate from thromboses of the lower limbs, deep pelvic veins, or inferior vena cava (IVC).

Clinical presentation

PE may present with one of three clinical syndromes:

- Pulmonary infarction/haemorrhage (60% of cases of PE)
- Isolated shortness of breath (25% of cases of PE)
- Sudden circulatory collapse (10% of cases of PE). One third of these patients die within a few hours of presentation

The three most common symptoms are dyspnoea, tachypnoea and pleuritic chest pain. There may be little in the way of positive clinical signs. Those that are present are usually nonspecific and at best support the diagnosis. They include signs of right heart strain, pulmonary hypertension and DVT. The ECG may show sinus tachycardia, new-onset atrial fibrillation, nonspecific ST segment changes, axis changes, or occasionally, in the case of a large PE, an S wave in lead I and a Q wave and T wave inversion in lead III ('S1, Q3, T3'). The chest X-ray often shows a parenchymal abnormality (e.g. atelectasis). There may also be an elevated hemidiaphragm. The patient may have a mild pyrexia and elevated white cell count. The finding of a low PaO_2 also supports the diagnosis.

Diagnosis

Clinical diagnosis of a DVT is often incorrect. Both false positives and false negatives occur.

CT pulmonary angiography

Now the most frequently used method and is the gold standard for diagnosis of PE. It has 97% sensitivity for lobar/main vessels. As with any angiography, it should be used with caution in patients with renal impairment.

V/Q scanning

V/Q scanning has been superseded by CT angiography. Although a normal scan is useful in ruling out PE, over 50% of scans give equivocal results, requiring further investigation. An intermediate scan result is usually followed up by CT angiography or repeated leg ultrasound scans to detect DVT.

D-dimer

Plasma D-dimer (formed when plasmin digests cross-linked fibrin) may be useful as a low D-dimer level is strong evidence against the diagnosis of a PE.

Management

- Anticoagulation. Evidence suggests equal efficacy with LMWH, unfractionated heparin and fondaparinux during the initial treatment stage. Warfarin is usually commenced during the first few days to establish an international normalised ratio (INR) of 2.0–3.0. Oral factor Xa inhibitors (e.g. rivaroxaban) are being increasingly used for the treatment of PE. In the absence of ongoing risk factors, treatment is usually continued for 3 months
- IVC filters, as discussed above, reserved for patients with proximal venous thrombosis and contraindications to pharmacological therapy
- Thrombolytic therapy, such as tissue plasminogen activator. Lysis of PE occurs more rapidly when thrombolytics are given than with anticoagulation alone; however, there is little evidence of survival or outcome benefit. Furthermore, there is a recognised increase in major bleeding and haemorrhagic stroke
- Pulmonary embolectomy. Patients who have suffered a massive PE, and are shocked despite resuscitative measures and thrombolysis, may benefit from open embolectomy. Mortality remains high, even in patients offered surgery

- Direct thrombolysis. Either by catheter-based fragmenting of clot or by direct injection of thrombolytic agents into the clot. Due to dependence on local expertise, there is little evidence of benefit, mostly due to small trial numbers

Further reading

Barker RC, Marval P. venous thromboembolism: risks and prevention. Br J Anaesth: Contin Educ Anaesth Crit Care Pain 2011; 11:18–23.

Lapner ST, Learon C. Diagnosis and management of pulmonary embolism. Br Med J 2013; 346:28–32.

National Institute for Health and Care Excellence (NICE). Venous thromboembolism: reducing the risk. CG92. London; NICE, 2010.

Related topics of interest

Venous thromboembolism – risk

Key points

- Thromboembolism may be attributed to Virchow's **triad**: stasis of blood, damage to vessel walls or abnormal coagulation
- Preoperative assessment of thromboembolism risk allows for the correct perioperative preventative measures to be taken

In 2005, it was estimated that around 25,000 people died from preventable hospital-acquired venous thromboembolism (VTE) each year. There has been an increased emphasis on the prevention of perioperative thromboembolic disease in recent years. For example, in 2010 in the UK the National Institute for Health and Care Excellence (NICE) published guidance on prevention of VTE in hospital patients: all patients with identified risk factors should have VTE prevention measures in place. Deep vein thrombosis (DVT) prevention is included in the WHO surgical safety checklist.

Historically, thromboembolic disease has been attributed to any of three factors which comprise Virchow's triad:
- Stasis of blood flow
  - Abnormalities in rheology and turbulence around stenoses
- Damage to blood vessels
  - Endothelial dysfunction, inflammation and atherosclerosis
- Abnormal coagulation
  - Platelet, coagulation and fibrinolysis dysfunction, including metabolic and hormonal influence

Venous thrombus tends to be fibrin and red-cell rich (sometimes referred to as 'red clot') as opposed to arterial thrombus, which has a higher platelet concentration ('white clot'). This explains the tendency to use antiplatelet drugs to treat or prevent arterial thrombosis.

The 2010 NICE guidance consider surgical and trauma patients at increased risk of VTE if the following features are present:
- Total surgical and anaesthetic time >90 minutes (pelvic/lower limb surgery >60 minutes)

- Significant reduced mobility
- Acute inflammatory or intra-abdominal condition
- One or more specific risk factors:
  - >60 years of age
  - cancer
  - admission to critical care
  - dehydration
  - thrombophilic condition
  - body mass index >30
  - 'significant medical comorbidities', e.g. cardiovascular/respiratory disease, metabolic/endocrine disorders, severe acute infection
  - family history or previous VTE
  - hormone replacement therapy/oral contraceptives containing oestrogen
  - varicose veins with phlebitis

Relevant inherited thrombophilias include protein C deficiency (protein C is responsible for inactivating cofactors Va and VIIIa), protein S deficiency, factor V Leiden (protein C resistant), antithrombin deficiency and dysfibrinogenaemias. There are also acquired thrombophilias such as Lupus disease, antiphospholipid syndrome, nephrotic syndrome and pregnancy (including the 6-week postpartum period).

Surgeries that carry particularly high risk include orthopaedic (over 50% DVT incidence reported when no prophylaxis used for elective hip surgery), abdominal and pelvic surgery. The 'million women' study indicated that the risk of VTE continues up to 12 weeks into the postoperative period, particularly for orthopaedic and cancer surgery.

Anaesthetic factors

In addition to the above patient and surgical factors, the anaesthetic conduct itself can influence the development of VTE. Regional anaesthesia carries a reduced incidence of VTE compared with general anaestheia, probably due to venodilation in the lower limbs and reduced surgical stress response. Prolonged hypotensive anaesthesia and patient positioning (lithotomy, inadvertent compression of major vessels) may increase the incidence of VTE. In-dwelling intravenous devices, such as tunnelled or longer-term central lines, are susceptible to venous thrombosis.

Further reading

Barker RC, Marval P. Venous thromboembolism: risks and prevention. Br J Anaesth: Contin Educ Anaesth Crit Care Pain 2011; 11:18–23.

National Institute for Health and Care Excellence (NICE). Venous thromboembolism: reducing the risk. CG92. London, NICE, 2010.

Sweetland S, Green J, Liu B, et al. Duration and magnitude of the post-operative risk of venous thromboembolism in middle aged women: prospective cohort study. Br Med J 2009; 339:b4583.

Related topics of interest

- Blood physiology (p. 19)
- Positioning for surgery (p. 220)
- Venous thromboembolism – prevention and treatment (p. 320)

Index

Note: Page numbers in **bold** or *italic* refer to tables or figures, respectively.